AF614789

Oncofertility Communication

Teresa K. Woodruff • Marla L. Clayman
Kate E. Waimey
Editors

Oncofertility Communication

Sharing Information and Building Relationships across Disciplines

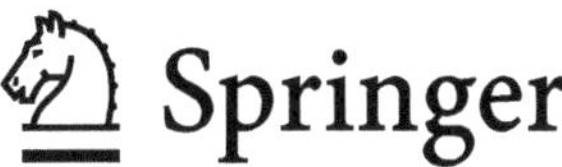

Editors
Teresa K. Woodruff, Ph.D.
Feinberg School of Medicine
Department of Obstetrics and Gynecology
Northwestern University
Chicago, IL, USA

Kate E. Waimey, Ph.D.
Feinberg School of Medicine
Department of Obstetrics and Gynecology
Oncofertility Consortium
Northwestern University
Chicago, IL, USA

Marla L. Clayman, Ph.D., M.P.H.
Feinberg School of Medicine
Division of General Internal Medicine
Robert H. Lurie Comprehensive Cancer Center
Northwestern University
Chicago, IL, USA

ISBN 978-1-4614-8234-5 ISBN 978-1-4614-8235-2 (eBook)
DOI 10.1007/978-1-4614-8235-2
Springer New York Heidelberg Dordrecht London

Library of Congress Control Number: 2013947800

Printed on acid-free paper

Springer is part of Springer Science+Business Media (www.springer.com)

Foreword

As a 17-year young adult survivor of brain cancer whose life plan and career path were eviscerated by the disease, I speak from experience as someone who recognizes the overwhelming mandate to disrupt and rethink our deeply flawed healthcare system. Now more than ever, the next generation of patient/caregiver stands the most to lose without the imperative of improved—and thusly more meaningful—communication with their providers.

Young adults are not special but they are different, with unique and underserved issues that present significant barriers to improved patient outcomes. This new, young, and empowered citizen is a different breed of consumer who demands the latest in sophisticated Web tools and mobile tech, access to trusted patient networks like StupidCancer.org, age-appropriate aggregated support resources, and a medical team who "gets it" that cancer is a chronic disease and this is not 1995.

I applaud the few and proud innovators in medicine; the academic leadership who dedicate their sleepless lives trying to discover and implement best practices in OC communication. And while it's easy to say "there's still much work to be done," that work is actually getting done. We have become the change we wished to see, and resultantly, the young adult cancer movement no longer has legs… it has wings.

New York, NY — Matthew Zachary

Foreword

When someone first learns that he or she has cancer, the primary question that comes to mind is "will I survive?" Yet, at the time of diagnosis, it is critical that people also focus on their personal hopes and dreams for life after cancer, especially when the cancer treatments being considered or planned could dramatically alter one's future. Such is the case with fertility. A number of the curative therapies for adolescents and young adults diagnosed with cancer have the potential to compromise sexual and reproductive function. Therefore, while these are difficult conversations to have, discussions about cancer treatments' effects on reproductive capacity must occur alongside those about treatment itself, before exposure to any therapy; patients and families cannot wait until treatment ends to discuss whether to have children after cancer.

So how do you broach this deeply personal topic, for many still very much a taboo, at a time of such emotional turmoil? In this much-anticipated volume, over two dozen scientists and clinicians—pioneers in the evolving, young field of oncofertility research and practice—offer clear and thoughtful guidance about how to conduct these sensitive conversations. This guidance includes consideration of personal preferences, patient age, cultural values, health literacy, spouse and partner perspectives, physician attitudes, implications of genetic testing for decision-making, ethical/legal concerns, and the specific communication skills necessary for approaching and having productive conversations touching upon these complex topics. The growing array of tools (print, online, DVD, digital applications, phone, media) now available to inform both patients and providers about state-of-the-art techniques for fertility preservation is also highlighted. Importantly, the editors included chapters on two of the key barriers to successful communication about oncofertility: insurance challenges and lack of public awareness.

This volume is a natural outgrowth of the Oncofertility Consortium project, a unique collaboration funded by the National Institutes of Health as one of its Roadmap initiatives, and directed under the outstanding leadership of Dr. Teresa Woodruff. This new text complements and builds upon another highly acclaimed product of the project, the rich Website resource http://MyOncofertility.org.

It is unlikely that the founders of the National Coalition for Cancer Survivorship were thinking specifically about the oncofertility concerns of the growing population of cancer survivors when they redefined what it meant to be a "cancer survivor" in 1986. Indeed, across the US at that time, we hardly spoke about cancer, much less anything to do with sexuality or intimacy. At that historic coalition meeting in Albuquerque, New Mexico, this intrepid group of individuals, which comprised survivors, clinicians, service delivery leaders, and advocates, argued that we should no longer adhere to the medical definition of what it meant to be a survivor, which held that an individual had to remain disease-free for 5 years after treatment to be called a survivor. They advocated that an individual should be considered a survivor from the moment of diagnosis and through the balance of life, regardless of the cause of death. With this definition change, they wanted to accomplish two goals: to send a clear message of hope to those newly diagnosed that there could be life after cancer; and second, most critically, they wanted to change the philosophy of cancer care. Specifically, they wanted to be sure that patients and oncology clinicians took the time at the outset of care to talk about the potential impact of cancer and its treatment on each individual's life and the options available for simultaneously ensuring the best chances for survival and a rich and valued future life.

This new volume is a testament to the revolution we have seen in the care of our growing population of survivors. While geared more for the research and clinical community, the topics covered are likely to be of great interest to diverse audiences. Indeed, it is my hope that, armed with the information contained in this work, cancer survivors, their healthcare providers, partners and loved ones, diverse advocates, and the broader public will feel equipped with the knowledge and skills they need to openly discuss and act on concerns related to the sexual and fertility consequences of having cancer. Given that well over a million individuals each year are diagnosed with cancer as children or during their childbearing years, the human and deeply life-affirming impact of this work has the potential to be quite profound.

Bethesda, MD Julia H. Rowland

Preface: Communicating Reproductive Science

This is the fourth book in a series that has examined the development of a new field: "Oncofertility." Our purpose in creating this new term was to communicate a simple concept: that fertility preservation for cancer patients is imperative to oncology doctors *and* to fertility doctors. The intention of a new word, without hyphenation, was to illustrate that solidarity. Oncofertility has entered the lexicon, but whether it surpasses the term that is otherwise used—"fertility preservation"—will be borne out by time.

Oncofertility arose from our recognition of the needs of young cancer patients and the development of technologies to mitigate the inevitable loss of reproductive function in some treatment settings [1]. Approximately 140,000 Americans under the age of 40 are diagnosed with cancer each year [2]. While many patients have a good prognosis, depending on the diagnosis and treatment regime, the impact on fertility can be significant. At the outset of our work in 2007, fewer than 50 % of cancer patients were receiving adequate fertility information before starting treatment [3–5]. In centers where strong fertility preservation programs exist, that number is now upwards of 80 %. We know that physicians want to provide every option for a healthy recovery for all of their patients. Helping physicians and patients stay abreast of the latest services and breakthroughs in fertility preservation will require authoritative, cutting-edge, and mobile resources.

The first book in this series (Oncofertility, Ed. Woodruff, Snyder, 2007) was written at a time when most patients were not receiving formalized information at the time of diagnosis about the fertility threats posed by the life-preserving cancer treatments they would soon be receiving. The book outlined the basic science activities that would "span the gap of knowledge" about fertility concerns in cancer and described some of the new basic science work that would ultimately provide additional options for patients [6]. The second book examined issues in Oncofertility associated with the law, economics, religious concerns, ethics, and education (Oncofertility, Ethical, Legal, Social and Medical Perspectives, Ed. Woodruff, Zoloth, Campo-Engelstein, Rodriguez, 2010) [7]. This compendium of "the humanities" represented important thinking about the concerns of the *public* regarding the use of new fertility interventions and the needs of patients and their families for real-time data. The third book in the series was an important summary of the latest thinking on the medical practices necessary to provide fertility preservation options to cancer patients (Oncofertility Medical Practice, Ed. Gracia, Woodruff, 2012) [8]. When that volume was released in 2012, the medical community not only embraced the concept but also actively asked for more information—with none of the reluctance we faced from the medical community in 2007. This final book, on communicating fertility preservation topics, is the last that we will write as a team. The contents represent some of the best thinking from a group of transdisciplinary investigators who unified their efforts under a pioneering research consortium grant from the NIH that asked the scientific community to tackle "the most intractable biomedical problems of our day using teams" [9]. Oncofertility was an intractable problem at the time this book series started; because of tremendous advances in basic science, our tenacity in addressing critical issues of ethics and law, our investments in medical practice descriptions that help busy clinicians provide Oncofertility care, and our commitment to making sure every voice was heard through unique communication platforms, we did "not lose time or momentum" in achieving our goals. We have done what we set out to do and at the end, I believe that patients' needs are now being addressed and the outcome that we measure is their ability to retain reproductive capacity and have a family one day.

As the reader will see, one of our main goals was to develop a suite of tools necessary to communicate information across disciplines rapidly. At the outset of our work, we set out several principles of technology development that were meant to guide our thinking. The first principle is that technology implementation and delivery is a collaboration between people, ideas, message needs, and infrastructure and that the methods and tactics should match the need. We also agreed that creating a robust interdisciplinary intellectual environment depends on a common language—a set of terms, ideas, and methods of work that everyone can understand. We also posited that the needs and expectations of the medical enterprise (patients and providers), research enterprise, and community vary but can be integrated into a seamless product. In following these principles, our hypothesis was that technology (anthropomorphically) participates in the work, and in doing so can increase the pace and quality of the communication activity. We believe that this hypothesis has been proven and a few products and tangible outcomes of our work are described in the chapters that follow.

Some of the products that I am most proud of include our Oncofertility Website (oncofertility.northwestern.edu), which was developed as an authoritative resource for professionals and was partnered with our "patient, parent, and partner" Website, myoncofertility.org. The Website offers information protocols for basic scientists, patient data sheets for providers, law reviews and ethics discussions, and videos that tell the Oncofertility story over time, and it also acts as our social medial hub (Facebook, blog, Twitter feed, etc.). We are neither an advocacy group nor a for-profit enterprise. Our purpose is to ensure that we are good stewards of the knowledge that we develop in the academy and that we communicate this knowledge in a way that can be understood by patients, providers, and researchers alike. Our materials are provided in English and Spanish (at minimum) and more translations are taking place every day. Our materials were built with mobile compatibility (responsive design). We also built a standalone app and microsite for our iSaveFertility pocket guides for physicians and fact sheets for patients (savemyfertility.org). These guides can be used in the consultation room and help provide the continuity of information necessary for patients to make the urgent decisions that are necessary in the context of cancer diagnosis and treatment. We link these materials to the general public through CME activities at our annual international Oncofertility Conference, which includes presentations from thought leaders, patients, and the next generation of research and clinical trainees. Our poster session has been equally innovative, using 54″ monitors to display movies, surgical procedures, and animations in a way that lets attendees learn and grasp complex information—in many cases outside of their field of expertise—quickly and memorably. We've also used communication technology to link research labs such that our work can be shared in real time with other expert labs. No single lab will ever make all of the discoveries entirely on its own—certainly not at the pace that I believe we need to move—and these technologies have permitted us to conduct team research on a truly global scale. Thus, we have moved beyond the ordinary process of discovery and publication to embrace multi-platform communication as an integral part of our work leading up to publication. This is a completely new way of thinking about basic science!

Finally, we recognize that the terms that we use are sometimes inaccessible because they are frankly unfamiliar or because people are "nervous" about reproductive terminology and think they should "know" concepts like "luteal phase" or "capaciation" and are afraid to ask. To address this issue, we created a communication tool called repropedia.org, a wiki that provides definitions of words within the context of any blog or Website. The API for repropedia can be linked to any Website, thus making those terms accessible and improving the knowledge of reproductive science for all of us.

You will be introduced to these and many more tools in the pages of this book. As this is the last book of its kind, I want to thank my co-editors Kate Waimey Timmerman and Marla Clayman for their vision and inventiveness in the development of our communication strategy and for ensuring that our blogs are filled with the latest information presented in ways that our community can best use it. I also want to thank the co-editors from the other three volumes, Karrie Snyder, Lisa Campo-Engelstein, Sarah Rodriguez, Laurie Zoloth, and Clarisa Gracia. Each of them has been an extraordinary partner during the 6 years of this grant process. I also thank the coPIs of the original roadmap grant—Lonnie Shea, Richard Stouffer, Mary Zelinski, Jeff Chang, Kerry Snyder, Clarisa Gracia, Marla Clayman, Kathleen Galvin, Kemi Jona, Gwen Quinn, and Christos Coutifaris. They have been passionate in the pursuit of better fertility options for cancer patients and patient with a big, multidisciplinary grant that took much more effort than an individual R01. I also want to thank my former student, friend, and scientific editor extraordinaire, Stacey Tobin. She has helped me communicate my ideas without grammatical error in a tireless way. She is a great communicator.

Finally, this book and all that it represents is dedicated to the patients we serve who have ever had to worry about fertility in the face of cancer. While the true mortality associated with cancer has been somewhat mitigated by the advances in cancer treatment, the existential crisis associated with that devastating diagnosis still exists, especially in a young person with all the expectancy of a future life and family. My hope is that in some small way, we have contributed to the lives of these patients by enabling a field that relies on interdisciplinary teams to solve problems and then work together to get these concepts into practice. I don't know of another example where translation of ideas became tangible so quickly. One would be hard-pressed to find an oncologist today, in 2013, who is not aware that a young person facing a cancer diagnosis wants to not only beat the disease but also return to the life that they once had—with the fullness of life and family. Oncofertility is a word, a field, and a hope for us all.

Chicago, IL, USA Teresa K. Woodruff

References

1. Redig AJ, Brannigan R, Stryker SJ, Woodruff TK, Jeruss JS. Incorporating fertility preservation into the care of young oncology patients. Cancer. 2011;117:4–10.
2. Surveillance Epidemiology and End Results (SEER). Program populations (1969–2009) National Cancer Institute, DCCPS, Surveillance Research Program, Cancer Statistics Branch. www.seer.cancer.gov/popdata. Accessed Jan 2011.
3. Kohler TS, Kondapalli LA, Shah A, Chan S, Woodruff TK, Brannigan RE. Results from the survey for preservation of adolescent reproduction (SPARE) study: gender disparity in delivery of fertility preservation message to adolescents with cancer. J Assist Reprod Genet. 2011;28:269–77.
4. Quinn GP, Vadaparampil ST, Malo T, Reinecke J, Bower B, Albrecht T, et al. Oncologists' use of patient educational materials about cancer and fertility preservation. Psychooncology. 2011 Jul 14. doi: 10.1002/pon.2022. [Epub ahead of print].
5. Quinn GP, Vadaparampil ST, Gwede CK, Miree C, King LM, Clayton HB, et al. Discussion of fertility preservation with newly diagnosed patients: oncologists' views. J Cancer Surviv. 2007;1:146–55.
6. Woodruff TK, Snyder KA, editors. Oncofertility: fertility preservation for cancer survivors. New York, NY: Springer Science+Buisness Media, LLC; 2007.
7. Woodruff TK, Zoloth L, Campo-Engelstein L, Rodriguez S, editors. Oncofertility: ethical, legal, social, and medical perspectives. New York, NY: Springer Science+Business Media, LLC; 2010.
8. Gracia C, Woodruff TK, editors. Oncofertility medical practice: clinical issues and implementation. New York, NY: Springer Science+Business Media, LLC; 2012.
9. Woodruff TK. The Oncofertility Consortium—addressing fertility in young people with cancer. Nat Rev Clin Oncol. 2010;7:466–75.

Preface: Oncofertility Communication as a Model for Multidisciplinary and Patient- and Family-Centered Care

Communication is central to the human experience. With every technological advance, from telegraphs and telephones to mobile devices and webcams, people are able to communicate with others in ways that previous generations had not. Just as interpersonal communication has changed, mediated communication has undergone a radical transformation in the last two decades.

For patients, their families, and the healthcare system, these changes have accelerated patients' ability to be involved in their healthcare. With the advent of the Internet and widespread adoption of devices on which to access it, individuals have greater access to health information as well as their social and familial networks than ever before. These may interact in a myriad of ways. Although there is still some concern about the "digital divide," in many cases, the issue is not simply about access to information. Patients need provision of information that is reputable, comprehensible, relevant, and timely. In some ways, technology has made this task more difficult. Information may be available, but it is of uncertain value and voluminous. Simultaneously, reputable information can be found relatively easily (if one knows where to look) and passed along speedily.

Patient-centered communication in cancer care has been expressed as a goal for both compassionate and quality healthcare in general and cancer care specifically [1–4]. Yet achieving patient-centered care through communication is still an elusive goal. This book comprises the many types of communication necessary for optimal cancer and oncofertility care. First are the chapters about clinical and interpersonal communication: communication to and from patients, family members, and clinicians. Included in this part are tools designed for patients and their families to enhance their ability to participate in their care and guide in their decision-making. One of the things that makes this volume unique is that it is not focused solely on the communication needs of the adult cancer patient. In addition to explicitly addressing the needs of partners, other family-oriented chapters focus on the needs of pediatric cancer patients and their parents.

The second part of the volume begins with a framework for interprofessional and interdisciplinary communication. This is essential, as cancer care is often complicated and involves several different clinical specialties. Physicians routinely include surgeons, medical oncologists, radiation oncologists, and primary care physicians. In addition, patients may interact with cancer-specific clinicians in addition to the treating oncologists, including nurse practitioners, nurse educators, dieticians, and psychotherapists. When incorporating oncofertility, reproductive endocrinologists are added to the care team. Parallel to the presentation of patient- and family-focused resources, this part includes healthcare-provider tools. Broadening the scope beyond the patient–clinician or clinician–clinician relationship, the latter chapters address the need to further educate and/or collaborate with various stakeholder groups, including patient advocacy organizations, insurers, policy makers, and the general public.

Oncofertility is not the only clinical arena in which communication among many parties is necessary for optimal care, but rarely are the stakes higher. The prospect of thinking about family-building in the face of a cancer diagnosis is highly emotional and personal. In addition, decisions must often be made quickly, and patients cannot be expected to be familiar with the topics at hand. As more patients require specialized care with multiple clinicians, communication fostering exemplary oncofertility care can serve as a model for exemplary care for many chronic or life-threatening illnesses. Technology and treatments may change, but patients and their families will continue to want, need, and deserve the best in communication so that they may benefit from the best in care.

Chicago, IL, USA Marla L. Clayman

References

1. Arora NK, et al. Facilitating patient-centered cancer communication: a road map. Patient Educ Couns. 2009;77(3):319–21.
2. Epstein R, Street RJ. Patient-centered communication in cancer care: promoting healing and reducing suffering. Bethesda, MD: National Cancer Institute; 2007.
3. Ethical Force Program. An ethical force program consensus report: improving communication—improving care. How health care organizations can ensure effective, patient-centered communication with people from diverse populations. Chicago, IL: American Medical Association; 2006.
4. Institute of Medicine. Crossing the quality chasm: a new health system for the 21st century. Washington, DC: National Academies Press; 2001.

Contents

Contributors

Hoda Badr, PhD Department of Oncological Sciences, Mount Sinai School of Medicine, New York, NY, USA

Anna R. Brandon, PhD, MSCS Department of Psychiatry, University of North Carolina, Chapel Hill, NC, USA

Robert E. Brannigan, MD Department of Urology, Feinberg School of Medicine, Northwestern University, Chicago, IL, USA

Marla L. Clayman, PhD, MPH Division of General Internal Medicine, Robert H. Lurie Comprehensive Cancer Center, Northwestern University, Chicago, IL, USA

Alice Crisci, BS Fertile Action, Manhattan Beach, CA, USA

Gregory Dolin, MD Center for Medicine and Law, University of Baltimore School of Law, The Johns Hopkins University School of Medicine, Baltimore, MD, USA

Amanda B. Fuchs, BA Feinberg School of Medicine, Northwestern University, Chicago, IL, USA

Sara Barnato Giordano, MD Division of Hematology and Oncology, Medical University of South Carolina, Charleston, SC, USA

Allison Goetsch, BS, MS Center for Genetic Medicine, Northwestern University, Chicago, IL, USA

Clarisa R. Gracia, MD, MSCE Department of Reproductive Endocrinology and Infertility, University of Pennsylvania, Philadelphia, PA, USA

Lisa B. Hurwitz, BA Department of Communication Studies, Northwestern University, Evanston, IL, USA

Jacqueline S. Jeruss, MD, PhD Department of Surgery, Northwestern University, Chicago, IL, USA

Lauren N.C. Johnson, MD Department of Reproductive Endocrinology and Infertility, University of Pennsylvania, Philadelphia, PA, USA

Laxmi A. Kondapalli, MD, MSCE Division of Reproductive Endocrinology and Infertility, Department of Obstetrics and Gynecology, University of Colorado Denver Anschutz, Medical Aurora, CO, USA

Stefani Foster LaBrecque, BS Northwestern University Advanced Media Production Studio, Evanston, IL, USA

Alexis R. Lauricella, PhD, MPP Department of Communication Studies, Northwestern University, Evanston, IL, USA

France Légaré, MD, PhD Centre Hospitalier Universite de Quebec Research Centre, Hôpital St-François D'Assise, Quebec, QC, Canada

Department of Family Medicine and Emergency Medicine, Laval University, Quebec, QC, Canada

Donna Rosene Leff, PhD Medill School of Journalism, Media, Integrated Marketing Communications, Northwestern University, Chicago, IL, USA

Kathleen Lin, MD, MSCE Reproductive Endocrinology and Infertility, Seattle, WA, USA

Natalia C. Llarena, BA Department of Surgery, Northwestern University, Chicago, IL, USA

Jennifer E. Mersereau, MD, MSCI Department of Obstetrics and Gynecology, University of North Carolina, Chapel Hill, Chapel Hill, NC, USA

William Pearse, MS Chicago Medical School, Rosalind Franklin University, Chicago, IL, USA

Gwendolyn P. Quinn, PhD Department of Health Outcomes and Behavior, Moffitt Cancer Center, Tampa, FL, USA

Ivana Sehovic, MPH Department of Health Outcomes and Behavior, Moffitt Cancer Center, Tampa, FL, USA

Megan Johnson Shen, PhD Department of Psychiatry and Behavioral Sciences, Memorial Sloan-Kettering Cancer Center, New York, NY, USA

Karrie Ann Snyder, BA, MA, PhD Department of Sociology, Northwestern University, Evanston, IL, USA

Dawn Stacey, RN, PhD Faculty of Health Sciences,, School of Nursing, University of Ottawa, Ottawa, ON, Canada

Clinical Epidemiology Program, Ottawa Hospital Research Institute, Ottawa, ON, Canada

H. Irene Su, MD, MSCE Division of Reproductive Endocrinology and Infertility, Department of Reproductive Medicine, University of California, San Diego, La Jolla, CA, USA

Alexandra Tate, MD Department of Sociology, University of California, Los Angeles, Los Angeles, CA, USA

Susan T. Vadaparampil, PhD Department of Health Outcomes and Behavior, Moffitt Cancer Center, Tampa, FL, USA

Amber Volk, MS Department of Medical Genetics, Mayo Clinic, Rochester, MN, USA

Kate E. Waimey, PhD Department of Obstetrics and Gynecology, Feinberg School of Medicine, Northwestern University, Chicago, IL, USA

Harlan Wallach, BFA, MFA NUIT—Northwestern University Information Technologies, Chicago, IL, USA

Ellen Wartella, PhD School of Communication, Northwestern University, Evanston, IL, USA

Teresa K. Woodruff, PhD Department of Obstetrics and Gynecology, Feinberg School of Medicine, Northwestern University, Chicago, IL, USA

Part I
Communicating with Patients and Their Families

Chapter 1
How Do Cancer Patients Learn About Fertility Preservation? Five Trajectories of Experience

Karrie Ann Snyder and William Pearse

Introduction

Cancer-related infertility has become an increasingly discussed topic in both the medical and cancer advocacy communities due to the growing awareness that some cancer treatments (e.g., radiation and chemotherapy) can impair future fertility—including treatments for nonreproductive cancers. Continuing advances in assisted reproductive technologies that may be applied to preserve the fertility potential of those afflicted with cancer have also helped to highlight the issue [1, 2]. Organizations including the American Society of Clinical Oncology (ASCO) [3] and the American Society for Reproductive Medicine (ASRM) [4] have developed guidelines to help oncologists and cancer centers integrate discussions of fertility impairment and fertility preservation treatment options early into the diagnosis and treatment process. Most experts agree that the most effective fertility preservation options (e.g., embryo freezing and sperm banking) are those that are made available to cancer patients *before* treatment begins. ASCO [3] suggests "Patients who are interested in fertility preservation should consider their options as soon as possible to maximize the likelihood of success." (p. 2922). In the *New England Journal of Medicine* article by Jeruss and Woodruff [2], the authors contend that, "A discussion about the threat treatment poses to fertility is a critical part of the care of young patients with cancer, in order to allay concerns or offer options for preserving fertility." (p. 905). ASRM [4] also affirms that, "Unless patients are informed or properly referred before treatment, options for later reproduction may be lost." (p. 1623).

K.A. Snyder, B.A., M.A., Ph.D (✉)
Department of Sociology, Northwestern University, 1810 Chicago Avenue, Evanston, IL 60208, USA
e-mail: karrie-snyder@northwestern.edu

W. Pearse, M.S.
Chicago Medical School, Rosalind Franklin University, Chicago, IL, USA

T.K. Woodruff et al. (eds.), *Oncofertility Communication: Sharing Information and Building Relationships across Disciplines*, DOI 10.1007/978-1-4614-8235-2_1,

Yet despite these calls-to-action within the medical and advocacy communities, survey research has shown that many cancer patients, both pediatric and adult, do not recall having any discussion with a physician regarding potential fertility impairment or preservation options prior to treatment [1, 5–7]. In developing the ASCO guidelines [3], Lee et al. found that "recent surveys of male and female cancer survivors of reproductive age concur that at least half have no memory of a discussion of fertility at the time of their treatment disposition." (p. 2926). Moreover, they concluded that, "Even when patients do recall infertility discussions, many are dissatisfied with the quality and amount of information provided." (p. 2926). Surveys with physicians (most often oncologists) have similarly found that doctors do not always inform patients of fertility-preserving treatment options, even those that are fairly routine and effective, such as sperm banking [8]. Moreover, research conducted since 2006 has found that, "the majority of physicians are not following [the ASCO] guidelines." (p. 338) [9].

While the information gap regarding fertility preservation is well recognized, we lack a nuanced understanding of what information is exchanged during patient–physician discussions, how these discussions evolve, and how patients experience this information exchange. We wanted to examine how discussions about treatment unfold between women of reproductive age with cancer and their oncologists, with the goals of improving best practice fertility preservation guidelines and shaping future research. We conducted interviews with women who had been diagnosed with breast cancer during their reproductive years. Although most research in this area has focused on whether or not a discussion regarding infertility has taken place, we found that the issue is more complicated than a "yes" or "no" answer. We identified five trajectories of experience among our respondents that describe not only if the topic of infertility was raised, but also the depth to which it was discussed. By looking at clinical discussions of fertility preservation from the perspective of women who have experienced a breast cancer diagnosis, we also identified key factors that facilitated or inhibited such discussions.

Study Design

We gathered data from interviews with 67 women who were diagnosed with breast cancer prior to 40 years of age (with 88.1 % being most recently diagnosed within the past 3 years and all diagnosed within the past 5 years; Table 1.1). Data collection took place between March 2008 and October 2009. The sample was recruited through advertisements placed in breast cancer advocacy organization newsletters (print and e-newsletters), email lists, and message boards aimed at cancer patients. We were initially concerned that the resulting sample would be much more politicized than the general population of younger women with breast cancer. To explore this possibility, we specifically asked women about their level of participation in breast cancer advocacy organizations and support groups. We found that only a few women

Table 1.1 Sample characteristics ($n=67$)

Race/ethnicity	
% Caucasian, non-Hispanic	62.7 %
% African-American	29.8 %
% Caucasian, Hispanic	4.5 %
% Asian	3.0 %
Educational attainment	
% with Bachelor's degree or higher	86.6 %
Family status	
% Married/Partnered[a]	59.7 %
% Engaged to be married	9.0 %
% with Children[b]	40.3 %
Mean age at time of interview (years)	35.0
Mean age at time of first diagnosis (years)	32.8
Age range at time of first diagnosis (years)	23–40
Less than 3 years since most recent diagnosis	88.1 %
4–5 years since most recent diagnosis	11.9 %
% with Health Insurance	98.5 %

[a]Partnered includes those women who are not legally married but consider themselves to be in permanent partnerships
[b]This category indicates women who identify themselves as a parent. Although the overwhelming majority of women have biological children, this category also includes nonbiological children including foster and stepchildren

in our sample could be classified as highly involved in such networks or groups. Since being involved in the cyber community (such as joining an email list from an advocacy group or occasionally checking a message board) involves minimal, if any, commitment, we do not think the sample over represents those who are very immersed in the breast cancer advocacy community. In some cases, the respondent had no involvement in any advocacy organization, and a friend or family member forwarded the recruitment advertisement onto them. The sample was characterized by high educational attainment and health insurance coverage, and included both married and single respondents as well as parents and nonparents (Table 1.1).

Interview Procedure

We conducted semi-structured phone interviews averaging 60 min in length; all respondents were read an IRB-approved statement of informed consent before agreeing to participate in the study. Interviewers were well versed on the topic of breast cancer as well as fertility preservation and all had completed IRB training. Interview topics included family background, diagnosis experiences, treatment concerns and decisions, and future family plans.

Data Analysis

We examined—from the patient's perspective—the interactions between a patient and her oncologist regarding discussions of infertility and fertility preservation. While cancer patients can learn about treatments and make treatment decisions based on interactions with a wide range of healthcare workers and interested parties, including family members, our focus was on the relationship between a patient and her oncologist. Most of our respondents identified their oncologist as their main information source and most survey work and fertility-preservation guidelines have identified this clinical exchange as vital for patients to learn about fertility impairment and potential treatment options.

Information about cancer and fertility runs the gamut, from how soon after adjuvant treatment can one start trying to conceive to whether or not a future pregnancy will lead to a reoccurrence of breast cancer. Our analysis, however, focused on two distinct issues:

1. The potential of breast cancer treatment to impair fertility.
2. The availability of fertility preservation treatment options (both standard treatments such as embryo banking and investigational treatments such as ovarian cryopreservation).

We limit our focus to these two topics because it is the exchange of this information that is considered *necessary* for those facing cancer to make effective choices to safeguard their fertility prior to beginning cancer treatment.

Coding and Development of Five Trajectories

We took an inductive approach to data analysis—meaning that we did not start with set hypotheses of how these discussions evolve. Rather, our respondents' narratives led to the identification of the five trajectories of experience we identified. The trajectories schema emerged through a three-stage coding process as described below (Fig. 1.1).

Stage 1: Was fertility impairment discussed?

We first determined if a conversation regarding potential fertility impairment took place prior to the patient starting potentially damaging cancer treatment. Respondents were asked if they discussed cancer-related infertility with their oncologist, and if so, when this discussion took place. "Fertility Discussed" indicates a discussion took place prior to treatment and "Fertility Not Discussed" indicates that no discussion took place prior to treatment. The latter group was categorized as Trajectory 1.

Stage 2: Who initiated the discussion?

During the coding for Stage 1, we found that, among those who had discussed cancer-related fertility issues, *who* brought up the topic differed. For some, the patient initiated the topic and, for others, their oncologist had. Since this point of comparison seemed to be a primary difference in the experience of discussing or

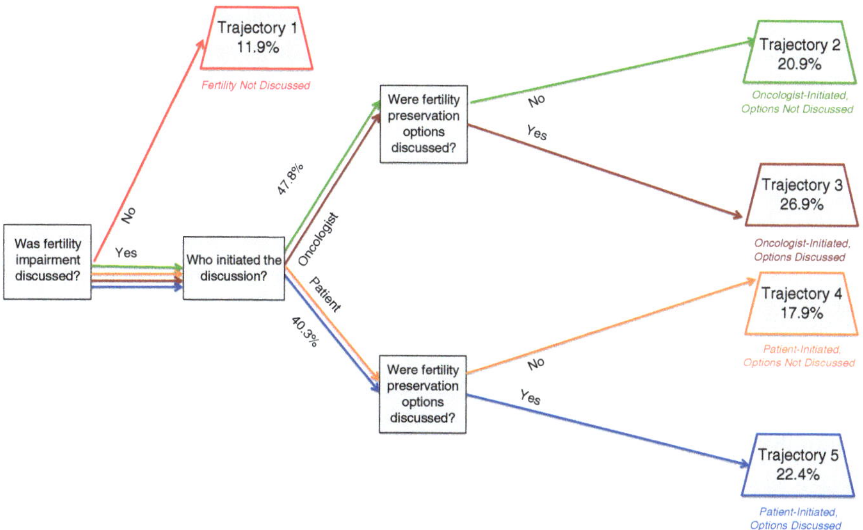

Fig. 1.1 Five trajectories of experience

learning about fertility preservation, we coded interviews as either "Oncologist-Initiated" or "Patient-Initiated." During their interviews, respondents who had discussed fertility preservation with their oncologist were asked who brought up the topic. Respondents were also asked if they discussed the issue with any other healthcare workers, such as nurses, before starting cancer treatment. The vast majority did not. In a couple cases, the issue was brought up by another healthcare worker (e.g., a breast surgeon), which then prompted the patient to approach her oncologist. Respondents who initiated the conversation were categorized in Trajectories 4 or 5; those who indicated that their oncologist started the conversation were categorized in Trajectories 2 or 3.

Stage 3: Were fertility preservation options discussed?

Throughout the coding of Stages 1 and 2, it was evident that fertility preservation options were not routinely discussed even if fertility impairment was. Therefore, we further coded interviews where fertility was discussed into two categories—"Options Discussed" and "Options Not Discussed." We defined fertility preservation treatment options as procedures performed prior to radiation and chemotherapy, where the goal is to preserve fertility functioning; procedures included standard options (e.g., oocyte/embryo freezing) as well as investigational options (e.g., ovarian cryopreservation; see [2] for further discussion.) "Options Discussed" included situations where respondents recalled their oncologist discussing *some* range of fertility-preserving options and/or referred the respondent to a fertility specialist prior to treatment to explore available procedures. "Options Not Discussed" included experiences where a respondent did not remember being told about any fertility-preserving options, was not sent to a fertility specialist prior to the start of her treatment, and/or was told not to worry about the issue until after her treatment was completed. Consistent with the description by Jeruss and Woodruff [2], even when respondents discussed options with their oncologist, rarely were they given the complete range of existing and investigational fertility preservation options and alternatives to biological parenthood such as adoption. Nonetheless, this distinction was meant to determine if respondents were told that cancer-related infertility was a potential roadblock to future family goals *or* that it was a situation that they could be proactive about prior to treatment.

Patient Trajectories

All of the respondents were assigned one of five distinct trajectories of experience (Fig. 1.1). While a small number of respondents (Trajectory 1–11.9 %) did not discuss the topic at all with their oncologists, most patients did (88.1 %). However, we found that for women who did discuss the topic with their oncologist, there was a range of experience in both the depth of information received and whether or not respondents felt that their concerns were adequately addressed. In 47.8 % of cases, oncologists brought up the subject and over half of this group did go on to discuss a range of potential options (Trajectory 3; 26.9 % of overall sample). Yet, even if an oncologist did bring up the topic of potential fertility impairment, a discussion of options was not guaranteed, with 20.9 % of the overall sample falling into Trajectory 2. Though most guidelines have focused on the importance of oncologists to broach the topic of fertility, our respondents frequently initiated this discussion (40.3 %). As with oncologist-initiated discussions, there was a range of ways in which the topic was discussed, from in-depth conversations regarding the options available (Trajectory 5–22.4 % of overall sample) to instances where an oncologist told a patient that she should not worry about fertility until after she was cancer free as in Trajectory 4 (17.9 % of overall sample).

Inhibiting and Facilitating Factors

We also examined patterns and common characteristics of how these conversations evolved or abruptly ended. Figure 1.2 identifies inhibiting and facilitating factors related to the patients, their oncologists, and their relationship that shaped the experiences of our respondents.

Oncologist Interest and Knowledge

Although this was a study of patients' experiences, a fundamental question is whether or not oncologists feel responsible for raising the topic of fertility and have

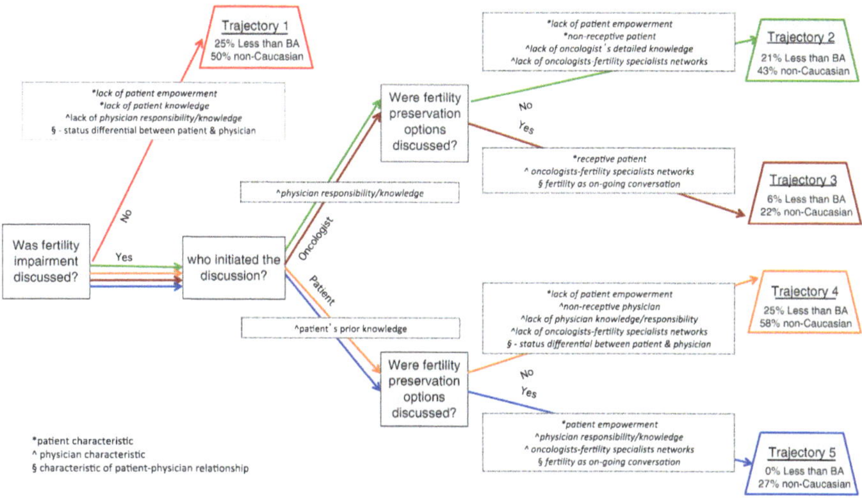

Fig. 1.2 Inhibiting and facilitating factors

detailed knowledge about fertility preservation options. There were several cases in which respondents described very proactive oncologists who either took the lead in the conversation or were very open to discussing the matter further. But there were as many instances in which patients described that their physicians were not interested in the topic; in these cases, the oncologists made it clear that their main goal was battling the patient's cancer first and foremost, or they offered information that was inaccurate/vague, or they simply responded that they did not know what would happen to fertility or where the patient could go for help.

Oncologists' Networks with Fertility Specialists

One factor that influenced whether or not a fertility impairment discussion progressed to a discussion of fertility preservation treatment options was the presence of a network connecting oncologists with fertility specialists. This relationship was a primary way in which patients were able to learn about their fertility preservation options. In some cases, respondents felt their oncologists passed them off to a fertility specialist, while others reported a close collaboration between their physician and fertility specialists. These experiences stand in stark contrast to those who specifically asked their oncologists directly for a referral, but were told that their oncologist did not know any fertility specialists; unfortunately, this was a common occurrence among our respondents. For example, JoAnne (Trajectory 2), a 37-year-old married mother of one, was shocked when her oncologist informed her that chemotherapy could impact her fertility. She then recalled a discussion about the odds of her resuming menstruation after chemotherapy and a very cursory mention from her doctor that women sometimes freeze eggs. So while she was informed of the threat of potential fertility impairment, JoAnne felt there was no discussion of options beyond the vague comments from her doctor, and she did not receive guidance on where to go for further information:

> It was very brief and really he said, 'I've known there are women who have gotten eggs harvested. If you want to look into that, you need to go do it now.' That was about the extent of the entire conversation about that. And then I really felt kind of on my own. I said, 'Great, do you know any?' And his answer was really no. I mean that kind of—we felt kind of left off on our own of how to figure that out.

When the fertility specialist/oncologist link was lacking, patients had to be proactive to find a fertility specialist to consult. Several respondents were successful and received the desired information; however, JoAnne's Internet research led her to believe that the only option was oocyte harvesting and that it would delay her treatment. Without much guidance, she and her husband decided just to "deal with the cards we were dealt" and hope her fertility would be unharmed. Those who recalled oncologists giving them referrals had a much easier time finding out desired information and were able to weigh their options more effectively. In fact, an important point of departure among those whose oncologist brought up the topic (Trajectories 2 and 3) and whether or not they discussed options was this existing link or relationship between their oncologist and a fertility specialist. Clearly, if an oncologist brought up fertility, they had at least some rudimentary knowledge of the issue and at least some sense of responsibility to discuss the issue (through self-initiative or in order to follow guidelines at their healthcare institution). Divergence in the progression of the discussion often came from whether or not the oncologist was able to offer a referral to a fertility specialist.

Patient Receptiveness

How receptive a patient is to fertility-related information is also an important factor that influences the progression of discussions with their oncologist. Women in this study varied in what their future family plans were and whether or not they wanted to have biological children. Of those patients whose doctors raised the subject of fertility but no options were relayed (Trajectory 2), several women said they were not interested in having future children or becoming first-time parents. These respondents were comfortable with their decision not to pursue the topic further, but they thought that it was information that women facing cancer should hear.

Patient Knowledge and Empowerment

A patient having some sense that infertility matters can change the discussion of fertility preservation, particularly if her oncologist does not bring up the topic. In our study, sometimes this knowledge was obtained through the patient's occupation (such as being a physician themselves), occasionally it came from knowing someone else who had breast cancer, and sometimes it was just a gut instinct at the time of diagnosis. How much someone knows prior to being diagnosed with cancer matters as well. Respondents who were physicians and those in other health-related occupations knew (or heavily suspected) not only that their fertility may be at risk but also what follow-up questions to ask.

What is puzzling is why some women who had a feeling that fertility might have been an issue did not pursue the topic or did not push the topic further if they had unanswered questions. The level of self-efficacy that respondents described in their relationship with their oncologist shaped how empowered they felt to push the topic of infertility further. For example, Janet (Trajectory 4), a 32-year-old community college student and married mother of one child, had asked her oncologist about fertility issues prior to beginning treatment but described her concerns as being "dismissed" by her oncologist and that she was not offered any fertility preservation options. When asked about her role in her overall treatment, Janet presented herself as having a passive role, saying "I really had no choice." Though she described not being happy with her oncologist overall, when we asked why she did not change doctors she replied, "He seemed to know what he was doing so I just stayed."

Janet's experience represents those of many respondents in Trajectories 1, 2, and 4. The women in these categories more often described themselves as following doctor's orders in all aspects of their cancer care, even if they were not getting the information or treatment they desired. Other respondents, particularly those in Trajectory 5, described themselves as being proactive to the point of being pushy, at times even fighting what they perceived to be the ambivalence of their physicians and advocating in general to ensure they received the best treatment available. When Fiona (Trajectory 5), a 31-year-old single grant writer with no children, was diagnosed, she quickly suspected that radiation and chemotherapy could harm her future fertility. Fiona's energies quickly turned to her fertility, "then almost my primary focus was fertility. Without a doubt. I was willing to forgo chemotherapy if it meant that I couldn't have kids." Fiona broached the topic of fertility and she felt her oncologist was less than enthusiastic about discussing the issue further:

> Then, after doing a bit of research on the Internet, and I asked my oncologist directly about it. I had to bring it up ... [My oncologist] reacted as if—I got the feeling that she didn't want me thinking about that. I got the feeling that her focus was to keep me alive. And I got the feeling like maybe if I hadn't brought it up, I'm not sure she would have mentioned it to me. But honestly knowing her, I think she would have told me because just to cover herself. But it wasn't one of the first things—she wasn't as concerned about it as I was, of course.

Despite this initial resistance, Fiona took charge by continuing to ask questions and she was able to set up consultations between her oncologist and a fertility specialist she found online. Fiona's outcome was largely shaped by her own self-described pushiness and self-efficacy. Our point here is not to blame respondents for not learning about fertility impairment or options, but to point out that patients' quality of knowledge concerning potential fertility impairment prior to diagnosis and the level of self-efficacy, or empowerment, they feel when interacting with their oncologist were key factors in the outcomes for our respondents.

Status Differences Between Patient and Physicians

So what shapes empowerment? One potential answer suggested by our data is the nature of the relationship between patient and doctor in terms of status similarity/ difference. There are varying perspectives on what empowerment entails, see [10]. We use the definition of Linhorst et al. [11]: "having decision-making power, a range of options from which to choose and access to information." (p. 427). Respondents who felt less empowered to pursue the topic of infertility were also those respondents for whom there was potentially the greatest social status difference between patient and physician in terms of occupation/education level and race/ethnicity. The empowered group that included Fiona (Trajectory 5) also included two physicians, a physician's assistant, and a professor, whereas groups that described far less self-efficacy (Trajectories 1, 2, and 4) had occupations outside of healthcare as well as lower educational attainment. In Trajectories 3 and 5, where respondents described far higher levels of self-efficacy, fewer than 6 % of women did not have at least a Bachelor's degree compared to over 21–25 % of respondents in Trajectories 1, 2, and 4. Occupation and education not only determine what a patient knows about the potential for fertility impairment, but also shape the relationship between patient and physician and influence the patient's level of comfort with bringing up topics or even challenging their physician. Some research supports the idea that the likelihood of an oncologist discussing fertility preservation may be related to perceived status similarities between themselves and their patient. Rieker et al. [12] suggest that oncologists may be more likely to discuss the issue of sperm banking with patients who they believe to have a similar status (e.g., highly educated patients). Situations where there is a greater perceived social distance between patient and oncologist may impede fertility-related conversations.

Moreover, cultural background differences could exacerbate feelings of status differences. As shown in Fig. 1.2, Trajectories 1, 2, and 4 included most of the women in this study who were non-Caucasian and most of these women described their oncologists as being Caucasian. Differences in race and ethnicity could further inhibit self-efficacy on part of the patient or serve as barrier to the oncologist broaching the topic. This latter assertion is supported by Quinn et al. [9], who found that oncologists felt cultural and language differences with patients were barriers to the discussion of fertility preservation.

Research of oncologists' behavior found that some are reluctant to bring up fertility preservation because of concerns about a patient's ability to afford these procedures [8, 9]. While concerns over costs may not indicate issues related to social status differences, it does raise the possibility that how oncologists perceive patients and their class or socioeconomic position may influence whether or not the topic of fertility preservation gets discussed.

What Doesn't Matter?

Within our sample, age of the patient did not seem to influence who was told what. We had thought that younger women would be given more options, either because they had no children yet or because of a general assessment that their fertility may be better to begin with. However, many younger patients were told to "just wait and see" what happens to their fertility posttreatment. Similarly, patients did not feel that oncologists withheld (or offered) information based on their partnership or parental status.

Also, the quality of the relationship between patient and physician from the patient's perspective did not matter. Many who did not discuss fertility-related issues/options still described their overall relationship with their physician as good, even if they felt they would have made different choices had they been given more information. Conversely, oncologists who were described by their patients as motivated on the topic of infertility did not predict a good relationship overall.

Shaping Future Research and Guidelines

Our sample was disproportionately insured and highly educated, with many having professional occupations. Addressing a more diverse sample could reveal a greater number of trajectories of experience, including family-initiated discussions for groups where having children is seen as a community responsibility. Also, by focusing on a relatively privileged range of respondents, our findings may actually underestimate the lack of information received by the general population of younger women facing breast cancer. Among women who would seem to have the most access to personalized care, information, and financial resources for elective fertility-preservation procedures (which are not routinely covered by health insurance), many were not told that their fertility could be compromised nor were they given treatment options. It is likely that those lacking economic resources would have even less access to fertility-related information and options. Our study also focuses on women exclusively. Since men and women (as well as different cancer types) have different fertility risks, treatment options, and success rates for fertility preservation, a more in-depth look at the barriers and facilitators specific to men's discussions of fertility with their oncologists as well as studies that include women with other types of cancer are needed. Nevertheless, the preliminary findings we describe here and the suggestions below will help guide future research regarding patient–oncologist communication on the topic of fertility preservation.

Moreover, our aim is not to conclude what percentage of female cancer patients experience a particular outcome versus another, but to understand what matters in how these discussions evolve, at what points the exchange of information breaks down, and where interventions could help facilitate more comprehensive conversations between patient and physician. Based on our respondents' experiences, we suggest the following future research directions and considerations for the development of clinical guidelines:

Understanding the oncologist's Role in Fertility Preservation

It is important that we further investigate what oncologists know about fertility issues, as well as available fertility preservation options. Several respondents were not confident about their oncologist's knowledge regarding fertility impairment. Some even reported being given responses that were unclear at best and simply wrong and misleading at worst. Although relying on patients' perspectives, there does seem to be the assumption in many discussions of fertility preservation that oncologists are well versed on the issue. However, Schover et al. [8] in a survey of 718 oncologists found that with regard to sperm banking, oncologists' knowledge is largely "not up to date" (p. 1895). While the authors failed to find a significant correlation between knowledge and "how often they mentioned sperm banking to eligible patients" (p. 1892) [8], in a study of 16 oncologists, Quinn et al. [13] found that oncologists are not always well informed about fertility preservation and this influenced whether or not they felt comfortable with the topic and ultimately discussed the issue with patients (also see [9]). Quinn et al. [13] also reported that the physicians in their sample "were unaware of any guidelines, either for their specialty or for the institution regarding [fertility preservation]" (p. 152) and most had not received formal training on the issue (p. 152).

Moreover, studies of oncologists have found that patient characteristics such as the gender or marital status of a patient [8, 13], a patient's prognosis [8, 9, 13], and other considerations such as the time available to meet with patients [8, 13], influenced the degree to which oncologists addressed fertility, if at all. Future research should also focus on oncologists and cancer centers who do integrate informed fertility preservation discussions into their care routines, to understand how they learn about and stay current on the topic, and how they implement best-practice guidelines and develop effective strategies for counseling patients on fertility preservation.

Examining the Role of Fertility Specialists

Access to fertility specialists was clearly an influential factor in how fertility discussions progressed for our responders. Several guidelines, including from ASRM and ASCO, discuss the importance of networks between oncologists and fertility specialists and how to encourage discussions across these specialties. However, Quinn et al. [14]

found that less than half of physicians routinely refer patients of childbearing age to reproductive endocrinologists. Moreover, Schover et al. [8] found that the most cited barrier among the oncologists they surveyed for not referring men to sperm banking was "a hard time finding convenient banking facilities" (p. 1895). Our research also identified the relationship between fertility specialists and oncologists as critical for patients to receive desired information. It is imperative that future research explores when and how these networks emerge and when are they the most effective for patients. Moreover, future research should look to fertility specialists as subjects of interest. What do they know regarding cancer-related infertility? Are fertility specialists aware of investigational procedures such as ovarian cryopreservation?

What Factors Allow Patients to Raise Concerns?

Our respondents' feelings of self-efficacy were often the determining factor in whether they obtained information on fertility. Future research should investigate factors within the patient–physician relationship that allow patients to share their concerns. Is it when patients feel more "comfortable" with their physician? Is it when the conversation of fertility is not touched upon in a laundry list of potential side effects? How does the presentation of fertility-related information (e.g., educational brochures versus physician talking points) influence whether or not a patient feels they can ask follow-up questions?

Empowerment Through Information

Women who did not discuss fertility or fertility preservation options with their oncologist often used the word "dismissed" to describe their experiences and concerns. It is impossible from our data to know how physicians assessed their individual cases and what potential options would have been available (if any). However, it is clear that all but one respondent who did not discuss the topic at all eventually learned about fertility impairment and treatment options after the fact, with most becoming upset that they were not more fully informed before starting treatment. Clinical guidelines could be explicit in that if standard fertility preservation options are not advised for a particular patient, physicians should offer some amount of explanation as to why. If women find out after the fact, their reactions to this unsettling information could affect their quality of life post-cancer. Having information—even if the answer is that standard options are not advised—is more empowering to patients than simply being kept in the dark. This conversation could also open the discussion to include other parenting options (e.g., surrogacy, adoption) as outlined by Jeruss and Woodruff [2].

Understanding Social Inequality and Barriers to Information

The most distressing part of our study was that some groups were less likely to receive fertility-related information, even when they directly asked about infertility. Fertility-preservation options prior to treatment (e.g., IVF) and posttreatment (e.g., adoption) can be costly, and economic and social resources will play a key role in determining which groups are able to become parents post-cancer. Here, we reveal that this potential inequality can be traced back to the initial patient–physician interaction, where inequality in access to vital information was tied to educational attainment, occupation, and even racial/ethnic background for many of our respondents. In their survey, Schover et al. [8] found that oncologists reported that they would be less likely to refer men for sperm banking who were HIV+ or openly homosexual (pp. 1894–5). Best-practice guidelines and researchers must address more openly how specific subsets of patients have been overlooked or may require more specialized educational techniques. For example, some racial/ethnic groups may be less likely to pursue a topic not initiated by their physician because of cultural and community differences in how to interact with experts and institutional agents such as physicians.

In this study, there was a clear distinction between those able to make a decision, even if that decision was to not pursue fertility preservation, and those who felt they were not allowed to make a choice. Clinical guidelines should not recommend that all patients have a biological child, but must ensure that cancer patients are informed about infertility as a potential side effect of cancer treatment and that patients are able to have an open dialogue with their healthcare team about possible fertility preservation options. Receiving information, feeling involved in medical decision making, and communicating openly with their physician shapes patient empowerment. A great deal of research has shown that patient empowerment can lead to "improvements in health status, increased satisfaction, and self-efficacy" ([10], p. 25) as well as better health and emotional outcomes, even for patients with potentially life-threatening illnesses like breast cancer [15, 16]. If a patient is unable or chooses not to take steps to preserve their future fertility, the feeling of being fully informed and capable of weighing options, and that their concerns are addressed would benefit cancer patients.

Acknowledgement This work was supported by the Oncofertility Consortium NIH 5UL1DE019587 and RL1HD058296.

References

1. Snyder KA, Pearse W. Discussing fertility preservation options with patients with cancer. JAMA. 2011;306:202–3.
2. Jeruss JS, Woodruff TK. Preservation of fertility in patients with cancer. N Engl J Med. 2009;360:902–11.

3. Lee SJ, Schover LR, Partridge AH, Patrizio P, Wallace WH, Hagerty K, Beck LN, Brennan LV, Oktay K. American society of clinical oncology recommendations on fertility preservation in cancer patients. J Clin Oncol. 2006;24:2917–31.
4. Ethics Committee of the American Society for Reproductive Medicine. Fertility preservation and reproduction in cancer patients. Fertil Steril. 2005;83:1622–8.
5. Duffy CM, Allen SM, Clark MA. Discussions regarding reproductive health for young women with breast cancer undergoing chemotherapy. J Clin Oncol. 2005;23:766–73.
6. Partridge AH, Gelber S, Peppercorn J, Sampson E, Knudsen K, Laufer M, Rosenberg R, Przypyszny M, Rein A, Winer EP. Web-based survey of fertility issues in young women with breast cancer. J Clin Oncol. 2004;22:4174–83.
7. Thewes B, Meiser B, Taylor A, Phillips KA, Pendlebury S, Capp A, Dalley D, Goldstein D, Baber R, Friedlander ML. Fertility- and menopause-related information needs of younger women with a diagnosis of early breast cancer. J Clin Oncol. 2005;23:5155–65.
8. Schover LR, Brey K, Lichtin A, Lipshultz LI, Jeha S. Knowledge and experience regarding cancer, infertility, and sperm banking in younger male survivors. J Clin Oncol. 2002;20: 1880–9.
9. Quinn GP, Vadaparampil ST, King L, Miree CA, Wilson C, Raj O, Watson J, Lopez A, Albrecht TL. Impact of physicians' personal discomfort and patient prognosis on discussion of fertility preservation with young cancer patients. Patient Educ Couns. 2009;77:338–43.
10. Bridges JFP, Loukanova S, Carrera P. Patient empowerment in health care. In: Heggenhougen K, Quah S, editors. International encyclopedia of public health, vol. 5. San Diego, CA: Academic; 2008. p. 17–28.
11. Linhorst DM, Hamilton G, Young E, Eckert A. Opportunities and barriers to empowering people with severe mental illness through participation in treatment planning. Soc Work. 2002;47:425–34.
12. Rieker PP, Fitzgerald EM, Kalish LA. Adaptive behavioral responses to potential infertility among survivors of testis cancer. J Clin Oncol. 1990;8:347–55.
13. Quinn GP, Vadaparampil ST, Gwede CK, Miree C, King LM, Clayton HB, Wilson C, Munster P. Discussion of fertility preservation with newly diagnosed patients: oncologists' views. J Cancer Surviv. 2007;1:146–55.
14. Quinn GP, Vadaparampil ST, Lee JH, Jacobsen PB, Bepler G, Lancaster J, Keefe DL, Albrecht TL. Physician referral for fertility preservation in oncology patients: a national study of practice behaviors. J Clin Oncol. 2009;27:5952–7.
15. Deadman JM, Leinster SJ, Owens RG, Dewey ME, Slade PD. Taking responsibility for cancer treatment. Soc Sci Med. 2001;53:669–77.
16. Lantz PM, Janz NK, Fagerlin A, Schwartz K, Liu L, Lakhani I, Salem B, Katz SJ. Satisfaction with surgery outcomes and the decision process in a population-based sample of women with breast cancer. Health Serv Res. 2005;40:745–67.

Chapter 2
Communicating Across Diverse and Differently Literate Audiences

Jennifer E. Mersereau and Anna R. Brandon

Barriers to Communication: The Scope of the Problem

The majority of health information is delivered in English [1]. Yet, according to the US Census Bureau, about 20.3 % of the population speaks a language other than English in the home, a number that increased by 140 % between 1980 and 2007 [2, 3]. More than 400 languages are spoken in the United States [2]; more than 50 million people residing in the United States (16 %) are of Hispanic or Latino origin alone, an increase of 15.2 million just in the last decade, and growing at 4 times (43 %) the growth of the total population (10 %). Practically illustrating the disparities, one cross-sectional study revealed that while whites received 57 % of all eligible health services, only 35 % of Hispanics with limited English proficiency received the health services for which they were eligible [4]. Although inequities in health care result from multiple factors, research suggests that those minorities with limited English proficiency are among the groups treated most unfairly [1].

Communication, however, is more than speaking the same "language." Attitudes, beliefs, and values passed down through generations in families and societies have a significant impact on both the clinician and the patient regarding expectations for care and outcomes. A sample of 74 Russian-speaking cancer patients in San Francisco, California highlighted that cultural taboos about the word "cancer" and other dynamics of care benefit from interpreters trained to understand the interaction of language and culture [5]. Cultural "mismatches," occurring when provider and

J.E. Mersereau, M.D., M.S.C.I. (✉)
Department of Obstetrics and Gynecology, University of North Carolina, Chapel Hill, 4001 Old Clinic Building, Chapel Hill, NC 27599, USA
e-mail: jmerse@med.unc.edu

A.R. Brandon, Ph.D., M.S.C.S.
Department of Psychiatry, University of North Carolina, Chapel Hill, NC, USA
e-mail: anna_brandon@med.unc.edu

T.K. Woodruff et al. (eds.), *Oncofertility Communication: Sharing Information and Building Relationships across Disciplines*, DOI 10.1007/978-1-4614-8235-2_2,

patient have disparate attitudes, beliefs, and values about disease and treatment, have been found to negatively impact not just patient satisfaction but the actual quality and effectiveness of health care [6].

Low Health Literacy: A National and International Epidemic

In the United States, approximately half of the adult population has been found to have low health literacy, or the ability to successfully obtain, process, and appropriately act on health information [7]. Census reports indicate that 15 % of adults have not completed high school education, and estimates are that approximately 43 % of American adults had "basic" or "below basic" prose literary skill (the lowest of four levels) [3, 8, 9]. Particularly concerning in the health arena, 20 % of adult Americans read at a fifth grade level or lower, and the resulting low health literacy has been associated with increased cancer disparities [7, 10]. Further support for this association is found in a study of men in the US Veteran's Administration system suggesting that, compared to men with better reading abilities, men with a reading level below the sixth grade had a were 69 % more likely to be diagnosed with late-stage prostate cancer, despite equal access to screening tools [11].

Discussion cancer, reproductive function, and technology utilized for fertility preservation (FP) require the use of language often unfamiliar even to individuals with high school and above educational levels, further disadvantaging those with limited proficiency in English and those in lower socioeconomic groups.

Internet-Based Information

In the United States in 2012, over 81 % of adults reported routinely accessing the Internet, and 80 % of these individuals endorsed gathering health-related information on the web [12]. The US National Cancer Institute's "Health Information Trends Survey" (HINTS) found that 28 % of Americans specifically searched for cancer information on the Internet in 2005, and that a significant majority went to the Internet first, before seeking care with a health professional [13]. Potential explanations for this trend have not been fully studied, but may include limited accessibility to their healthcare provider, hesitancy to ask providers sensitive issues about reproduction, or limited ability for the healthcare professionals to answer questions outside their area of expertise.

The term "e-health" has been coined to describe the use of the Internet (or related technologies) to gather health information and locate services. Such technology affords user flexibility for access, and provider tailoring of content and language to unique user needs. Online tools can be adjusted based on user's culture or language, using interactive tools to enhance learning. E-health programs potentially could provide substantial opportunities in low-health literate populations by providing pictures, and consistency in navigation [14]. In addition, E-health strategies have other potential benefits, such as broad reach, 24-h availability, anonymity or a social interaction (whichever is preferred), multimedia options, and the potential to tailor to the needs of groups or individuals [15].

However, despite these advantages, e-health has not been demonstrated to be universally beneficial in providing information in a way that improves health outcomes. There are several potential reasons why internet-based information may fail to provide adequate information to high-literacy or low-literacy populations. For example, the overall readability for many cancer-focused websites is at a high-school level or beyond [16]. In a study of a sample of Spanish-language health-related websites, 86 % were written at a college-level readability [17]. Other HINTS research has shown that people who have lower subjective health literacy are more likely find online material frustrating and "took a lot of effort" to understand [18].

The Unequal Burden of Cancer

Current advances in the field of oncology have great potential to improve survival and quality of life after cancer treatments. However, the above-discussed barriers to communication and low health literacy mean vulnerable populations of patients often have limited access and comprehension of new options and strategies to prevent and treat cancer. More than a decade ago, the US Institute of Medicine document "The Unequal Burden of Cancer," described and prioritized addressing the disparities of cancer incidence and mortality among the US populations [19]. Unfortunately, in certain minority groups, cancer continues to be often poorly understood, with significant misperception about screening techniques. For example, in a 2005 cross-sectional US study, more than 25 % of Hispanics and about 18 % of African Americans, compared to 14 % of whites, believed that there was nothing they could do to reduce their risk of cancer [20]. In another study, 75 % of Vietnamese-American women, a group with high rates of cervical cancer, did not know the purpose of Pap smears [21]. Finally, nonwhite cancer survivors report a higher number of information needs, including more health promotion, interpersonal and emotional, side effects and symptoms, and insurance needs [22].

Unmet Needs About Information Regarding Fertility and Cancer

Research in young adults with cancer consistently supports that these patients have an interest in their fertility and that they believe they should have, at the very least, the opportunity to understand that the treatment they undergo for cancer may end fertility potential. In the area of breast cancer, 57 % of women reported substantial concern at diagnosis about losing fertility, and 29 %

admitted that those concerns influenced treatment decisions [23]. However, while young survivors express an interest in fertility, many women felt that they had inadequate exposure to information about fertility before and after cancer treatments [24]. Unfortunately, a recent study suggested that only 28 % of patients reporting fertility concerns actually reported meeting with a fertility specialist [25]. On the other hand, healthcare providers are challenged by the lack of consensus about what characteristics identify patients as "appropriate" to refer for a fertility preservation consultation (FPC).

Recent evidence suggests that there are racial, social, and demographic disparities that distinguish which young women with cancer receive FP information and treatment vs. those who do not [26]. For example, nonwhite racial groups have greater unmet information needs regarding fertility and cancer, compared to Caucasians [27]. In a retrospective chart review of 199 medical records of women with a new cancer diagnosis, Caucasian women were referred twice as often for fertility preservation consultation (FPC) than women of other ethnicities, and patients with insurance coverage were 40 % more likely to be referred for FPC [28]. According to the study, only 22 % (9/51) of eligible African American women received FPC, and no Hispanic women (0/19) received FPC. A survey study from the California Cancer Registry found that Latina women were 80 % less likely to pursue FP treatments than Caucasians [26]. They also reported that of 31 African American women, none pursued FP strategies. Beyond racial and ethnic factors, the level of education also predicts a woman's access to information about FP. In a survey-based study of 918 young women receiving cancer treatment, women were significantly more likely to have fertility addressed by their oncologist if they were educated at the Bachelor's level or beyond (Adjusted OR [95 % CI] 1.4 [1.0–2.1], $p=0.005$) [26]. Only one study to date has addressed sexual orientation and FP access; the investigators reported that, compared to 32/813 heterosexual women, none of the 29 women who self-identified as non-heterosexual pursued FP treatment [26]. Potential explanations for these differences have not been adequately explored but are likely to include language barriers, health literacy, and cultural beliefs about the issues of cancer and reproduction [26, 29, 30].

What Are Unique Communication Challenges with Fertility Preservation?

Fertility Preservation Topics Are Complex

In all young men and women with a new cancer diagnosis, discussion about fertility and cancer treatments can be challenging. Advances in assisted reproductive technology provide ways to preserve fertility in young women, with four clear options: (1) oocyte cryopreservation, (2) embryo cryopreservation, (3) ovarian suppression by administration of a GnRH agonist, a medication that puts the ovaries "at rest" during cancer treatment, or (4) ovarian tissue cryopreservation.

A final option is to elect to "wait and see" if fertility is compromised after treatment. Each of these FP options carries unique risk factors as well as varying probabilities for later pregnancy. It is difficult to discuss these risk factors with patients because outcomes are dependent upon the dose and duration of cancer treatment, the age of the patient, and the patient's baseline ovarian reserve when treatment begins, all alongside other risk factors for infertility that women face independent of cancer or cancer treatment [31]. Perhaps in part because of this complexity, less than half of the female cancer patients of reproductive age receive sufficient information about these options or an appropriate referral for FPC before cancer treatment begins [26, 31–34].

Because the FPC covers such complex topics, women who have a higher level of education are at an advantage to understand and integrate the concepts quickly enough to pursue intervention. In addition, women with a higher education background may be more assertive and proactive with their providers, bringing up the topic of FP themselves, important since many oncologists are NOT routinely discussing FP unless their patients bring it up [35]. The complexity of FP options has led to research elucidating what patients know, need to know, and what they retain after receiving an FP consultation. Using objective measures of FP knowledge, investigators consistently find poor FP knowledge in patients prior to the FPC [36, 37]. After the FPC, findings suggest that the objective measures of overall FP knowledge remain poor, with an average score on a validated FP knowledge scale of about 50 % correct [38]. Specifically focusing on those questionnaire items addressing patient comprehension about the risks associated with FP (e.g., cancer recurrence risk, birth defects in future children), approximately half of the sample responded with inaccurate assessments of these risks. Such misperceptions of risk may prevent women from making informed decisions not just about immediate FP, but also about any future pursuit of biological reproduction. On the other hand, those women in the sample who demonstrated higher pre-visit and post-visit knowledge also had higher levels of education or had actively sought out information prior to a FPC. These data suggest that significant numbers of young women need basic preparation for the information they will receive at the FPC and the decision-making processes involved in choosing an option (or not choosing FP at all).

Time Limitations Exist to Absorb Complex FP Information

Understandably, most oncology providers themselves do not have the time or expertise to take responsibility for the essential communications about FP [39, 40]. Even more than other medical fields, the language used during an FPC is highly specialized, filled with interrelated medical, embryological, and statistical concepts about processes and probabilities for achieving later pregnancy. When FP is discussed with patients, methods vary from simply providing printed information from organizations such as Fertile Hope or LiveSTRONG, to counseling by the oncology provider and to formal consultation with a fertility specialist. Surveys of breast cancer survivors identify limitations to these methods, suggesting that at least 25–50 % do not receive adequate or appropriate education, counseling, or resources about reproductive decisions prior to their cancer treatments [25, 41]. Unlike an infertile woman who may have been attempting pregnancy for years and is already familiar with basic concepts of assisted reproduction, young women newly diagnosed with cancer have to assimilate unfamiliar information regarding their FP alternatives simultaneously with the details of cancer treatment.

Beyond the time and expertise required for conveying this complex set of alternatives to patients are the serious concerns oncologists may have about delaying cancer treatment long enough for FP to occur [42, 43]. One cycle of ovarian hyperstimulation may take several weeks; physician and patient alike may believe that this delay could have adverse survival consequences that outweigh the benefits of consideration of fertility options. However, at least one qualitative investigation suggests that women benefit from at least being informed that there are ways for preserving fertility even if the oncologist believes the risks of FP are too great [24, 32].

Appropriately Translated FP Material Does Not Exist

Language has been considered the "lowest common denominator of cultural sensitivity," and language barriers are an obvious problem in populations who may have difficulties maneuvering through health information. In the United States in 2007, 20 % of the population over the age of five spoke a language other than English at home [44]. However, it is estimated that only 2 % of websites use a language other than English [15]. Literal translation alone does not always allow for effective communication of complex health topics and regional and cultural nuances may add extra challenges. Ideally, complex medical topics, such as FP, would be linguistically and culturally adapted, rather than literally translated, to meet the needs of the intended audience. However, this type of adaptation can be expensive and resource-intensive.

Cultural Sensitivities

Cultural variation adds an extra level of difficulty beyond language and literacy in the effective communication of complex medical topics such as FP. Intangible concepts such as values, risk perceptions, and family/community/religious relationships may affect the comprehension of and satisfaction with communication about fertility and cancer. Healthcare providers, with their own medical culture, may not be fully aware of their own communication skill level, assumptions about cultural values, or personal biases [6]. Cultural beliefs and norms affect views about screening and early detection, compliance with treatment, and even the disease of cancer [45]. To demonstrate this complexity, one team identified at least seven domains impacting the view of aging Chinese women toward cancer screening and treatment: fatalism, the use of herbs, self-care, hot-cold balance, lifestyle, medical examination, and Western medicine [46]. Although at least one group has piloted a counseling intervention for female breast cancer survivors at risk for reproductive health problems, outside of documenting ethnic and social predictors of care little is known about the cultural beliefs and values of specific populations of women surrounding cancer and FP [47].

Because both the diagnosis of cancer and of the possibility of future motherhood are emotionally charged topics, discussion by health professionals necessitates sensitivity to the cultural standards influencing patient expression of emotion. Unfortunately, behavioral science research suggesting how clinicians might better accommodate and regulate emotion specifically during FP conversations is lacking [40]. Social psychologists, on the other hand, have published extensive research on communication processes. The so-called difficult conversations generally have three core elements: Establishing what has/is happened/happening, exploring feelings, and establishing what the impact is upon an individual's self image [48]. There are cultural and individual variations of how these three features are negotiated between speakers, but they are always in play. Most clinicians have little difficulty establishing a diagnosis or a recommended treatment plan, but often exploring a patient's feelings may be more of a challenge. Yet most research suggests that patient-centered care requires a working alliance, that is, a physician–patient relationship that moves beyond fact sharing and treatment planning to discussions that include psychosocial and experiential issues the patient may be facing [49]. Unexpressed feelings make it hard for patient and clinician to hear each other, and could be one reason why women may hear an oncologist mention a referral for an FPC, but not attend to the details regarding the options or probabilities for later conception success. The simple question, "What are your feelings about having a child at some later point in your life?" not only opens the conversation but assures the patient that these feelings are normal, valid, and important to the clinician as treatment recommendations are being formed. Following that question up with "How important is it to you to have your own biological child?" moves the conversation then toward how important natural conception is to the identity of the patient to a mental health professional. If a patient appears to be at risk for depression or anxiety, an appropriate referral can be made, normalizing the distress by pointing out many women seek out additional support when considering important decisions like this one.

Strategies to Improve Communication: Addressing the Challenges

There are potential strategies that exist to improve communication about complex topics such as FP and cancer in all populations, especially vulnerable populations who may have racial, educational, and language barriers. For example, prior research has shown that cancer survivors of lower socioeconomic status may need assistance and training in how to gain access to information and may benefit the most from training [50].

Table 2.1 Strategies to improve communication in clinical care

Pay close attention to patient cues
Repeat your message
Slow down your speech
Avoid colloquial expressions
Present information in more than one way (diagrams, pictures, notes)
Verify the patient's response
Provide hand-outs in simple English for the patient to bring home
Use a formal translator when possible, rather than a family member or friend

Practical Advice for Clinical Care

Strategies for enhancing communication with patients are not specific to FP or cancer. However, these topics are emotionally and technically difficult for patients. The following section includes some evidence-based recommendations. First, paying close attention to patient cues is imperative for assessing comprehension and understanding [51, 52]. Patients that do little more than nod and smile, demonstrate self-conscious mannerisms, or use vague responses may be revealing a lack of understanding. If a clinician suspects that a patient does not fully comprehend the discussion or understand the terms, he or she should find a graceful way to repeat the message. Slowing down one's own speech in a relaxed manner and speaking clearly and without colloquial expressions, jargon, or slang will minimize confusion and reduce stress for a listener. This is useful when discussing topics that are difficult emotionally, technically complicated for a layperson, or when the patient is processing a nonnative language. Also, ensuring that the patient is given enough time to complete his or her own thoughts will increase comprehension and encourage him or her to ask for clarity when needed.

Second, clinicians should be as complete and explicit as possible, presenting information in more than one way (i.e., diagrams, pictures, notes). The clinician should verify the patient's response, taking a moment to restate concretely what he or she heard and concluded, perhaps saying, "As I understand, you are concerned about…Is that correct?" Clinicians need to be aware that certain words and phrases have multiple meanings in English—beyond making sure that the patient understands you, clinician's need to make sure they understand what their patient is trying to say (Table 2.1).

Although there are definite cultural norms, clinicians need to beware of stereotyping patients. They should ask questions, make observations, and gather history, setting assumptions aside until they have a better assessment of what their patients may need or desire in the consultation. Inaccurate physician assumptions, may act to reduce the number of referrals for consultation [53].

Table 2.2 Recommendations for study personnel approaching minority and disadvantaged women for research participation [55, 56]

Be alert, clear spoken, and a good listener
Be positive and assertive, but not aggressive
Be responsive to the patient's reasons for reluctance
Be respectful and culturally sensitive
Be confident, sincere, and spontaneous in introducing self and the study
Be credible, by knowing the objectives of the proposed study and what is involved in participation
May be helpful for a senior doctor to initiate the invitation to participate
Utilization of staff representing the population being recruited
Tailor consent forms to the population
Consider audio consent aids where language fluency is low
Engage community leaders to publicize research benefits
Highlight the role of Ethics Committees or Institutional Review Boards (IRB) in safeguarding patients

Often reading a nonnative language (passive fluency) is less difficult than using the language in real time (active fluency). If translated materials are unavailable, writing down (or providing brochures) in simple English allows the patient to take the information home, read in a less stressful environment, and offers the opportunity to consult English-speaking family or friends to help. If the clinician cannot understand the patient, it is sometimes helpful to ask the patient if he or she could write out his or her questions for improved communication.

The Conduct of Research

Mirroring the disparities in treatment and survivorship are the disparities in minority representation in clinical research. Racial and ethnic diversity have been documented in the access to FP (referral and treatment), but no similar investigations have been conducted surrounding access to research trials [26, 28, 54]. Potential explanations for our lack of empirical research in this area likely go beyond socioeconomic status to include overarching recruitment challenges such as mistrust of the medical system, lack of understanding about the benefits and risks of research participation, and communication barriers. For example, investigators involved with stroke-prevention in African-Americans described a "recruitment triangle" that predicted a patient's probability of participation in a clinical trial. The patient, key family members or others in the patient's support system, and medical personnel form this triangular relationship, and each must be considered in establishing strategies to recruit and retain minority research participants. Other work has provided recommendations for study personnel approaching African American and Latina women for research participation (Table 2.2) [55, 56].

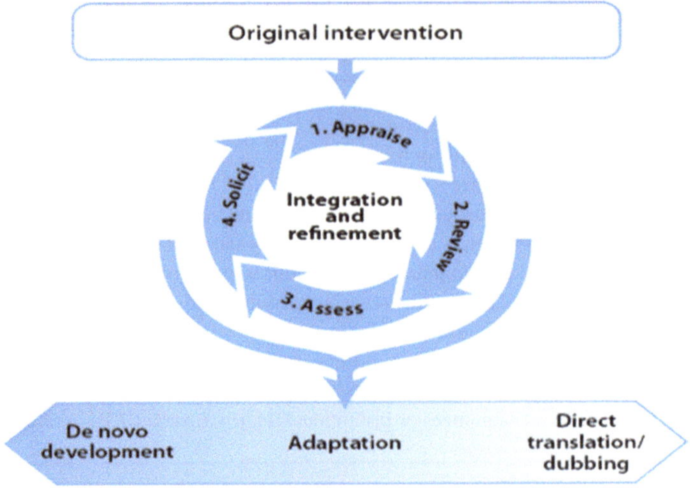

Fig. 2.1 Cultural adaptation of educational materials [57]

Developing Culturally Relevant Patient Literature and Decision Aids

Specific techniques have been developed to facilitate the cultural and linguistic adaptation of existing educational materials. For example, to modify educational and/or decision aid materials for Spanish speakers, researchers have conceptualized the adaptation process as one of locating an optimal point along a spectrum between complete de novo development of an intervention at one extreme, and simple, literal translation of the existing English decision aid (or the simple addition of dubbing or subtitles, in the case of a video) at the other extreme [57, 58]. Utilizing a cyclical framework and an iterative process, culturally relevant decision aids for FP can be developed through the following process:

1. Appraising the current FP educational material to identify essential concepts and information that must be retained in the new version.
2. Reviewing previously identified recurring themes in published literature relevant to FP and the patient population (e.g., cultural norms regarding family size) to enable development of appropriate materials [59–61].
3. Assessing the regional context of the population and engaging the patient stakeholders.
4. Soliciting direct input through interview and focus group processes regarding stakeholder perspectives on fertility potential post-cancer treatment, collecting specific suggestions for making the adapted version both linguistically and culturally relevant.
5. Integrating the feedback and refining the educational materials, such as worksheets or decision aids (Fig. 2.1) [57].

The aim is thus to neither abandon the useful and applicable knowledge already gained from development and refining the original English language version nor merely translate the text of the existing decision aid, but to consider the broader cultural considerations critical to making decision aids and patient literature relevant, appealing, and accessible to the target population.

Improving Online Communication

Several studies and guidelines provide strategies to improve the quality of online educational material. In a study designed to guide the development of E-health tools, focus group members identified several critiques of the use of current E-health resources [62]. For example, one theme that emerged was the distrust of websites with and ".edu" or ".gov" address, with concerns that .edu websites would not be constructed with layman's terms and .gov websites could not be trusted to provide unbiased information. Another theme that was exposed involved websites being too simple, with videos that moved too slowly or animations that were too basic. Take-home messages from this study include considering "layering content" to allow users at various literacy levels to utilize the site in methods and a pace that is appropriate for them, as well as the suggestion to develop simple E-health content that is intended for families (parents and young children) to explore together [62].

Several institutions provide guidance about how to make one's website content more accessible to a low literacy population. For example, the US National Cancer Institute and the Department of Health and Human Services furnish general information and instruction about developing accessible online content at www.usability.gov and a PDF handbook called the "Research-based Web Design and Usability Guidelines" at www.usability.gov/guide-lines/guidelines_book.pdf. They provide a step-by-step guide to produce a "user-centered" website that will allow for appropriate content and easy navigation (Fig. 2.2) [63].

Conclusion

As we become more successful in treating cancer, the numbers of survivors will only continue to increase. We echo the call to close the divide in regard to the stark inequalities and disparities that exist in the access to treatment and the subsequent survival rates of nonwhite patients [64]. For female survivors, this can only begin with the dissemination of FP information that reflects an understanding of the culturally influenced beliefs and boundaries that motivate women's responses to cancer, treatment, and survivorship.

Acknowledgments This work was supported by the Oncofertility Consortium NIH 5UL1DE019587.

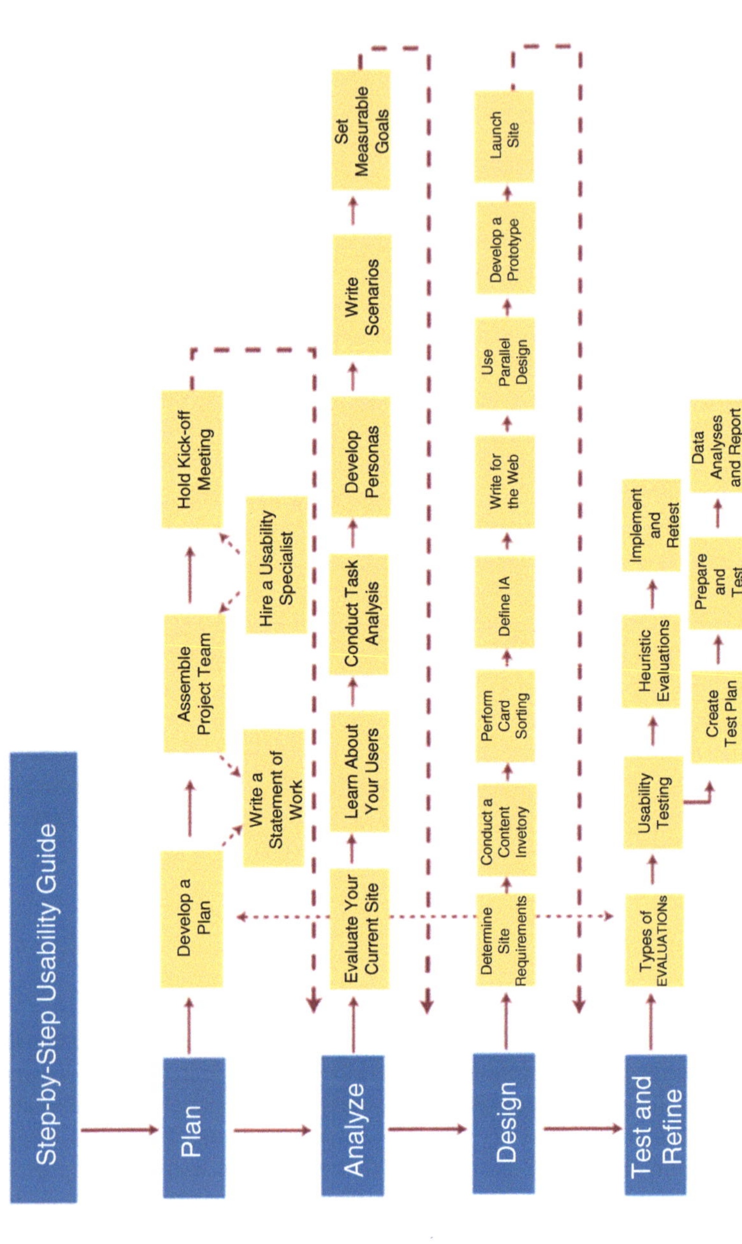

Fig. 2.2 U.S. Department of Health and Human Services. The research-based Web design and usability guidelines, enlarged/expanded edition. Washington: U.S. Government Printing Office, 2006

References

1. Saha S, Fernandez A, Perez-Stable E. Reducing language barriers and racial/ethnic disparities in health care: an investment in our future. J Gen Intern Med. 2007;22 Suppl 2:371–2.
2. Shin HB, Kominski RA. Language use in the united states: 2007: U.S. Department of Commerce, U.S. Census Bureau; April 2010.
3. United States Census Bureau. U.S. Census Bureau: state and County QuickFacts. 2012. http://quickfacts.census.gov/qfd/states/00000.html
4. Cheng EM, Chen A, Cunningham W. Primary language and receipt of recommended health care among Hispanics in the United States. J Gen Intern Med. 2007;22 Suppl 2:283–8.
5. Dohan D, Levintova M. Barriers beyond words: cancer, culture, and translation in a community of russian speakers. J Gen Intern Med. 2007;22:300–5.
6. Quinn GP, Jimenez J, Meade CD, et al. Enhancing oncology health care provider's sensitivity to cultural communication to reduce cancer disparities: a pilot study. J Cancer Educ. 2011;26(2):322–5.
7. Nielsen-Bohlman LPA, Kindig D. Health literacy: a prescription to end confusion. Washington, DC: National Academy of Science; 2004.
8. OECD and Statistics Canada. Literacy in the information age: final report of the International Adult Literacy Survey. Paris and Ottowa; 2000.
9. Kutner M, Greenberg E, Baer J, National Assessment of Adult LIteracy (NAAL). A first look at the literacy of America's adults in the 21st century. Washington, DC: US Department of Education, Institute of Education Sciences; 2005.
10. Doak LG, Doak CC, Meade CD. Strategies to improve cancer education materials. Oncol Nurs Forum. 1996;23(8):1305–12.
11. Bennett CL, Ferreira MR, Davis TC, et al. Relation between literacy, race, and stage of presentation among low-income patients with prostate cancer. J Clin Oncol. 1998;16(9):3101–4.
12. http://www.pewinternet.org/Static-Pages/Data-Tools/Get-the-Latest-Statistics.aspx. Accessed Dec 2012.
13. Hesse BW, Nelson DE, Kreps GL, et al. Trust and sources of health information: the impact of the internet and its implications for health care providers: findings from the first health information national trends survey. Arch Intern Med. 2005;165(22):2618–24.
14. Campbell MK, Honess-Morreale L, Farrell D, Carbone E, Brasure M. A tailored multimedia nutrition education pilot program for low-income women receiving food assistance. Health Educ Res. 1999;14(2):257–67.
15. Neuhauser L, Kreps GL. Online cancer communication: meeting the literacy, cultural and linguistic needs of diverse audiences. Patient Educ Couns. 2008;71(3):365–77.
16. Wilson FL, Baker LM, Brown-Syed C, Gollop C. An analysis of the readability and cultural sensitivity of information on the national cancer Institute's Web site: CancerNet. Oncol Nurs Forum. 2000;27(9):1403–9.
17. Berland GK, Elliott MN, Morales LS, et al. Health information on the Internet: accessibility, quality, and readability in English and Spanish. JAMA. 2001;285(20):2612–21.
18. Manganello JA, Clayman ML. The association of understanding of medical statistics with health information seeking and health provider interaction in a national sample of young adults. J Health Commun. 2011;16 Suppl 3:163–76.
19. Institute of Medicine. The unequal burden of cancer: an assessment of NIH research and programs for the ethnic minorities and the medically underserved. Washington, DC: National Academies Press; 1999.
20. Rutten LF, Beckjord EB, Hess BW, Croyle RT. Cancer communication: Health Information National Trends Survey. Washington, DC: National Cancer Institute. NIH Pub. No. 07-6214.
21. Schulmeister L, Lifsey DS. Cervical cancer screening knowledge, behaviors, and beliefs of Vietnamese women. Oncol Nurs Forum. 1999;26(5):879–87.
22. Kent EE, Arora NK, Rowland JH, et al. Health information needs and health-related quality of life in a diverse population of long-term cancer survivors. Patient Educ Couns. 2012; 89(2):345–52.

23. Partridge AH, Gelber S, Peppercorn J, et al. Web-based survey of fertility issues in young women with breast cancer. J Clin Oncol. 2004;22(20):4174–83.
24. Gorman JR, Bailey S, Pierce JP, Su HI. How do you feel about fertility and parenthood? The voices of young female cancer survivors. J Cancer Surviv. 2012;6(2):200–9.
25. Thewes B, Meiser B, Taylor A, et al. Fertility- and menopause-related information needs of younger women with a diagnosis of early breast cancer. J Clin Oncol. 2005;23(22): 5155–65.
26. Letourneau JM, Smith JF, Ebbel EE, et al. Racial, socioeconomic, and demographic disparities in access to fertility preservation in young women diagnosed with cancer. Cancer. 2012;118(18):4579–88.
27. Hammond CT, Beckjord EB, Arora NK, Bellizzi KM, Jeffery DD, Aziz NM. Non-Hodgkin's lymphoma survivors' fertility and sexual function-related information needs. Fertil Steril. 2008;90(4):1256–8.
28. Goodman LR, Balthazar U, Kim J, Mersereau JE. Trends of socioeconomic disparities in referral patterns for fertility preservation consultation. Hum Reprod. 2012;27(7):2076–81.
29. Richardson LD, Norris M. Access to health and health care: how race and ethnicity matter. Mt Sinai J Med. 2010;77(2):166–77.
30. Fedewa SA, Lerro C, Chase D, Ward EM. Insurance status and racial differences in uterine cancer survival: a study of patients in the National Cancer Database. Gynecol Oncol. 2011;122(1):63–8.
31. Matthews ML, Hurst BS, Marshburn PB, Usadi RS, Papadakis MA, Sarantou T. Cancer, fertility preservation, and future pregnancy: a comprehensive review. Obstet Gynecol Int. 2012;2012:953937.
32. Niemasik EE, Letourneau J, Dohan D, et al. Patient perceptions of reproductive health counseling at the time of cancer diagnosis: a qualitative study of female California cancer survivors. J Cancer Surviv. 2012;6(3):324–32.
33. Schover LR, Rybicki LA, Martin BA, Bringelsen KA. Having children after cancer. A pilot survey of survivors' attitudes and experiences. Cancer. 1999;86(4):697–709.
34. Forman EJ, Anders CK, Behera MA. A nationwide survey of oncologists regarding treatment-related infertility and fertility preservation in female cancer patients. Fertil Steril. 2010; 94(5):1652–6.
35. Duffy CM, Allen SM, Clark MA. Discussions regarding reproductive health for young women with breast cancer undergoing chemotherapy. J Clin Oncol. 2005;23(4):766–73.
36. Balthazar U, Fritz MA, Mersereau JE. Fertility preservation: a pilot study to assess previsit patient knowledge quantitatively. Fertil Steril. 2011;95(6):1913–6.
37. Peate M, Meiser B, Friedlander M, et al. It's now or never: fertility-related knowledge, decision-making preferences, and treatment intentions in young women with breast cancer—an Australian fertility decision aid collaborative group study. J Clin Oncol. 2011;29(13):1670–7.
38. Balthazar U, Deal AM, Fritz MA, Kondapalli LA, Kim JY, Mersereau JE. The current fertility preservation consultation model: are we adequately informing cancer patients of their options? Hum Reprod. 2012;27(8):2413–9.
39. Lee SJ, Schover LR, Partridge AH, et al. American society of clinical oncology recommendations on fertility preservation in cancer patients. J Clin Oncol. 2006;24:2917–31.
40. Quinn GP, Vadaparampil ST, Bell-Ellison BA, Gwede CK, Albrecht TL. Patient-physician communication barriers regarding fertility preservation among newly diagnosed cancer patients. Soc Sci Med. 2008;66(3):784–9.
41. Meneses K, McNees P, Azuero A, Jukkala A. Development of the fertility and cancer project: an internet approach to help young cancer survivors. Oncol Nurs Forum. 2010;37(2):191–7.
42. Peddie VL, van Teijlingen E, Bhattacharya S. A qualitative study of women's decision-making at the end of IVF treatment. Hum Reprod. 2005;20(7):1944–51.
43. Peddie V, Porter M, Barbour R, et al. Factors affecting decision making about fertility preservation after cancer diagnosis: a qualitative study. BJOG. 2012;119(9):1049–57.
44. https://www.census.gov/hhes/socdemo/language/data/acs/index.html. Accessed Dec 2012.

45. Navon L. Cultural views of cancer around the world. Cancer Nurs. 1999;22(1):39–45.
46. Wenchi L, Wang JH, Chen MY, et al. Developing and validating a measure of chinese cultural views of health and cancer. Health Educ Behav. 2008;35(3):361–75.
47. Schover LR, Rhodes MM, Baum G, et al. Sisters Peer Counseling in Reproductive Issues After Treatment (SPIRIT): a peer counseling program to improve reproductive health among African American breast cancer survivors. Cancer. 2011;117(21):4983–92.
48. Stone D, Patton B, Heen S. Difficult conversations. New York, NY: Penguin; 1999.
49. Meystre C, Bourquin C, Despland JN, Stiefel F, de Roten Y. Working alliance in communication skills training for oncology clinicians: a controlled trial. Patient Educ Couns. 2013;90(2):233–8.
50. McInnes DK, Cleary PD, Stein KD, Ding L, Mehta CC, Ayanian JZ. Perceptions of cancer-related information among cancer survivors: a report from the American cancer Society's studies of cancer survivors. Cancer. 2008;113(6):1471–9.
51. Mast MS. On the importance of nonverbal communication in the physician-patient interaction. Patient Educ Couns. 2007;67(3):315–8.
52. Schouten BC, Meeuwesen L. Cultural differences in medical communication: a review of the literature. Patient Educ Couns. 2006;64(1–3):21–34.
53. Quinn GP, Vadaparampil ST, King L, et al. Impact of physicians' personal discomfort and patient prognosis on discussion of fertility preservation with young cancer patients. Patient Educ Couns. 2009;77(3):338–43.
54. Lee S, Heytens E, Moy F, Ozkavukcu S, Oktay K. Determinants of access to fertility preservation in women with breast cancer. Fertil Steril. 2011;95(6):1932–6.
55. Symonds RP, Lord K, Mitchell AJ, Raghavan D. Recruitment of ethnic minorities into cancer clinical trials: experience from the front lines. Br J Cancer. 2012;107(7):1017–21.
56. El-Khorazaty MN, Johnson AA, Kiely M, et al. Recruitment and retention of low-income minority women in a behavioral intervention to reduce smoking, depression, and intimate partner violence during pregnancy. BMC Public Health. 2007;7:233.
57. Ko L, Reuland D, Jolles M, Clay R, Pignone M. Cultural and linguistic adaptation of a multimedia colorectal cancer screening decision aid for Spanish speaking latinos. J Health Commun. (in press).
58. Reuland DS, Ko LK, Fernandez A, Braswell LC, Pignone M. Testing a Spanish-language colorectal cancer screening decision aid in Latinos with limited English proficiency: results from a pre-post trial and four month follow-up survey. BMC Med Inform Decis Mak. 2012; 12:53.
59. Quinn GP, Hauser K, Bell-Ellison BA, Rodriguez NY, Frias JL. Promoting pre-conceptional use of folic acid to Hispanic women: a social marketing approach. Matern Child Health J. 2006;10(5):403–12.
60. Sawyer L, Regev H, Proctor S, et al. Matching versus cultural competence in research: methodological considerations. Res Nurs Health. 1995;18(6):557–67.
61. Simmons VN, Cruz LM, Brandon TH, Quinn GP. Translation and adaptation of smoking relapse-prevention materials for pregnant and postpartum Hispanic women. J Health Commun. 2011;16(1):90–107.
62. Mackert M, Kahlor L, Tyler D, Gustafson J. Designing e-health interventions for low-health-literate culturally diverse parents: addressing the obesity epidemic. Telemed J E Health. 2009;15(7):672–7.
63. http://usability.gov/about/index.html. Accessed March 2013.
64. Guidry JJ, Torrence W, Herbelin S. Closing the divide: diverse populations and cancer survivorship. Cancer. 2005;104(11 Suppl):2577–83.

Chapter 3
Patient and Family Tools to Aid in Education and Decision-Making About Oncofertility

Gwendolyn P. Quinn, Susan T. Vadaparampil, Ivana Sehovic, and Marla L. Clayman

When an adolescent or young adult (AYA) patient is facing cancer treatment, potential loss of fertility may not be the first thing on his or her mind. Patients often describe their immediate concern is "getting rid of the cancer" or wondering if they will survive. While these concerns are normal, addressing fertility preservation prior to the initiation of cancer treatment provides the most optimal options and opportunity for success. The majority of female AYA patients, based on recent literature, choose not to take steps to preserve fertility, but overwhelmingly appreciate being informed about potential loss of fertility [1]. The reasons for not using fertility preservation among females include financial costs, lack of a male partner, unwillingness to use donor sperm, and the perception of an inability to delay treatment [2, 3]. About 50 % of AYA males chose to bank sperm prior to cancer treatment and among those who do not, feelings of regret and remorse are often cited [4]. Males also report appreciation for the information, yet are more likely to recall they had not thought about and/or were embarrassed to discuss sperm banking and future children with their parents or healthcare professional.

How does a cancer patient make a decision about whether or not to pursue fertility preservation? The risk of potential fertility loss should be conveyed to patients by oncologists early in treatment planning, as suggested by the American Society for Clinical Oncology. When the oncologist is uncertain about the threat to fertility or what options may be available to the patient, ASCO also recommends that a referral be made to a reproductive endocrinologist or infertility specialist. However, receiving the medical information regarding potential fertility loss is just one component of the decision-making process. Decisions about fertility preservation

G.P. Quinn, Ph.D. (✉) • S.T. Vadaparampil, Ph.D. • I. Sehovic, M.P.H.
Department of Health Outcomes and Behavior, Moffitt Cancer Center, Tampa, FL, USA
e-mail: gwen.quinn@moffitt.org

M.L. Clayman, Ph.D., M.P.H.
Division of General Internal Medicine and Robert H. Lurie Comprehensive Cancer Center, Northwestern University, Chicago, IL, USA

T.K. Woodruff et al. (eds.), *Oncofertility Communication: Sharing Information and Building Relationships across Disciplines*, DOI 10.1007/978-1-4614-8235-2_3,

may be considered to have three components: risk appraisal, information integration, and long-term consideration.

In one component, the patient must appraise and comprehend the amount of risk associated with pursuing fertility preservation options. These risks may be cancer-related, such as the effect of treatment delay on cancer outcomes, as well as risks associated with the fertility preservation options themselves. The risk may also be psychological: how will the patient feel if she becomes infertile and did not take steps to preserve her fertility? It is also possible that for newer and more experimental options, patients may have to contend with an unknown or unappraisable likelihood of success. Based on this appraisal, the patient must decide if these risks and uncertain benefits are acceptable. To make these decisions, the patient must also consider present and future desire for a biological child. Added to this is the consideration of the patients' perception of mortality in light of the diagnosis and whether a limited life span has an impact on decisions about having a biological child. However, people tend to be poor forecasters of what they will want in the future [5]; this is especially true of teens and adolescents. A second component, which may occur concomitant with other decision-making processes, involves assessing information about the fertility preservation options, the medical procedures, the costs for the procedure and storage, the patient's current relationship status, health status, and religious, ethical, or moral concerns about these options. Steps one and two may not happen in a linear fashion and a patient may move back and forth between these components in the decision-making process.

The third component is one which is often not considered until years later, but we suggest it should be considered at the same time as the other two components. This component relates to retrieving the stored sperm, embryo, oocytes, or tissue. How will the patient feel about using assisted reproductive technology (ART) to become a parent? When will a patient be assessed for return of fertility posttreatment? If the patient regains fertility, will he or she continue to store gametes or embryos? How will long-term storage be financed? For men this may mean their female partner becomes the patient when stored sperm requires the use of ART for insemination. For women this may mean decisions about how long to store embryos, what to do with unused oocytes, or asking a partner to parent a child born from donor sperm or eggs. Thinking about these issues at the time of making fertility preservation decisions can be seen as analogous to the need to begin survivorship planning at the time of diagnosis.

The issues for decision making in fertility preservation among cancer patients are complex and intricate. As such, tools to support patients in this process, including decision aids, are limited. Decision support tools and decision-making strategies may be useful for the healthcare professional or researcher working with AYA cancer patients.

The criteria for what constitutes a patient decision aid are quite specific. According to the International Patient Decision Aid Standards (IPDAS) Collaboration, a decision aid prepares a patient for decision making by doing three things: (1) providing facts about the patients condition, options, and features (2) helping people to clarifying their values (the features that matter most to them) and

IPDAS Patient Decision Aid Checklist for Users

I. Content: Does the patient decision aid ...

Provide information about options in sufficient detail for decision making?

- describe the health condition 2.1
- list the options 2.2
- list the option of doing nothing 2.3
- describe the natural course without options 2.4
- describe procedures 2.5
- describe positive features [benefits] 2.6
- describe negative features of options [harms / side effects / disadvantages] 2.7
- include chances of positive / negative outcomes 2.8

Additional items for tests

- describe what test is designed to measure 2.9
- include chances of true positive, true negative, false positive, false negative test results 2.10
- describe possible next steps based on test result 2.11
- include chances the disease is found with / without screening 2.12
- describe detection / treatment that would never have caused problems if one was not screened 2.13

Present probabilities of outcomes in an unbiased and understandable way?

- use event rates specifying the population and time period 3.1
- compare outcome probabilities using the same denominator, time period, scale 3.2, 3.3, 3.6
- describe uncertainty around probabilities 3.4
- use visual diagrams 3.5
- use multiple methods to view probabilities [words, numbers, diagrams] 3.7
- allows the patient to select a way of viewing probabilities [words, numbers, diagrams] 3.8
- allow patient to view probabilities based on their own situation [e.g. age] 3.9
- place probabilities in context of other events 3.10
- use both positive and negative frames [e.g. showing both survival and death rates] 3.11

Include methods for clarifying and expressing patients' values?

- describe the procedures and outcomes to help patients imagine what it is like to experience their physical, emotional, social effects 4.1
- ask patients to consider which positive and negative features matter most 4.2
- suggest ways for patients to share what matters most with others 4.3

Include structured guidance in deliberation and communication?

- provide steps to make a decision 6.1
- suggest ways to talk about the decision with a health professional 6.2
- include tools [worksheet, question list] to discuss options with others 6.3

Fig. 3.1 IPDAS patient decision aid checklist. Permission from Anton Saarimaki, OHRI

(3) helping people share their values with their healthcare practitioner and others. The IPDAS has developed a set of criteria to determine the quality of patient decision aids. A "users' checklist" summarizes the standards that determine whether or not a decision aid is a source of reliable health information that can help in decision making [6]. The values clarification process may be particularly important with respect to fertility preservation, as there may be uncertainty surrounding disease outcome and survival as well as uncertainty about the success of fertility preservation techniques themselves (Fig. 3.1).

While the IPDAS provides recommended criteria for patient decision aids, the Ottawa Decision Support Framework (ODSF) offers a three-step process for a strategy to address the conflict experienced by patient in the medical decision-making process. Using concepts and theories from general psychology, social psychology, decision analysis, decisional conflict, values, social support, and self efficacy, the ODSF is an evidence-based theory for guiding patients in making health decisions [7, 8]. The three-step process assesses patient and practitioner determinants of decisions to identify decision support needs; provides decision support tailored to patient needs; and evaluates the decision-making process and outcomes (Fig. 3.2).

While IPDAS and ODSF provide structure for the design and development of patient decision aids and decision support strategies, Learner Verification (LV) is a framework that helps ensure the materials developed (e.g., decision aids, decision support strategies) are suitable for the intended audience and better matched to patients' learning needs [9]. LV provides an excellent framework for the health

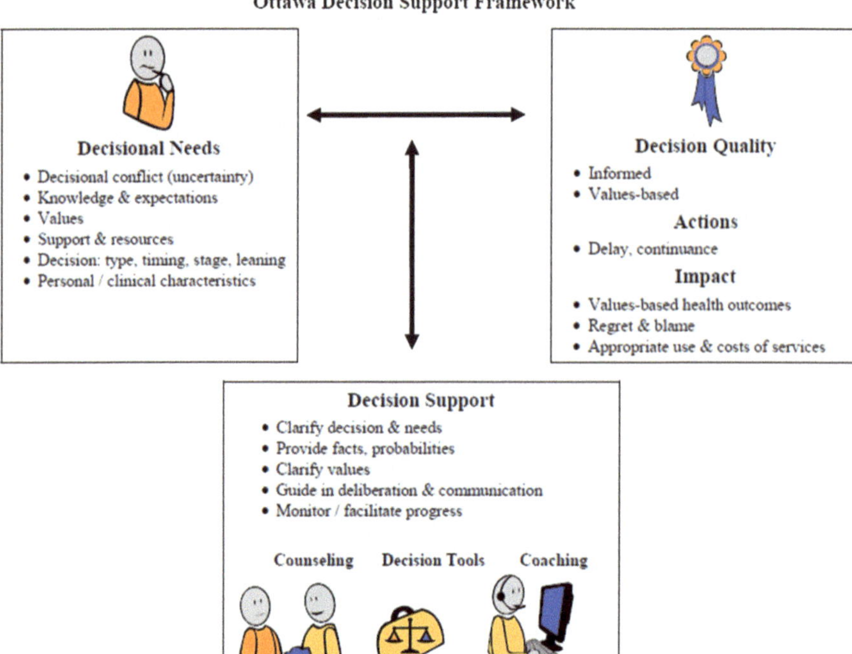

Fig. 3.2 Ottawa decision support framework. Permission from Anton Saarimaki, OHRI

communication challenge of developing materials with effective messaging [10]. LV is rooted in information processing theory, focusing on the persuasiveness of a health message and provides a systematic process for assessing the intended messages of a decision aid or educational materials [10]. Specific components of LV are typically assessed with the target audience (the specific group for whom the material is intended, e.g., AYA cancer patients considering fertility preservation). These components include Attractiveness, Comprehension, Cultural Acceptability, Self-efficacy, and Persuasion (4). LV is a quality control process and technique that helps ensure materials are suitable for the intended audience and better matched to patients' learning needs [9] (Table 3.1).

Examples of Oncofertility-Related Educational Materials and Decision Aids

As another chapter in this volume will present provider-oriented decision support, this section focuses on patient and family-oriented educational tools and decision aids. Institutions and healthcare professionals may wish to create their own educational materials or decision aids based on knowledge of their own patients or their

Table 3.1 Elements of learner verification assessed in study brochure

Elements of Learner Verification assessed	Questions from interview guide
Attraction (Does the material appeal to the target audience?)	What about the appearance of this brochure intrigued you? If you were sent this brochure in the mail, would you want to read it to find out more about breast cancer?
Comprehension (Does the target audience understand the material?)	Tell me in your own words what you think the purpose of this brochure is? Did this brochure help you to understand the purpose of genetic testing? Are there any risks in your family that would make you want to have genetic testing?
Self-efficacy (Does the target audience feel the message is doable for them?	After reading this brochure, would you want to participate in this study? (probes: If you wanted to participate would you be able to?) Did this brochure help you to understand why genetic testing is important to African American women with breast cancer?
Cultural acceptability (Does the target audience perceive the message to be salient and acceptable?)	How do feel about the phrase "Women of Color"? (probes: Do you think most African American women would feel the same way?; Do you think there is another term that African American women identify with?) Is there anything in this brochure that makes you feel uncomfortable about genetic testing? Do you relate to any of the women in this brochure?
Persuasion (does the message convince the target audience to take action?)	If you received this brochure in the mail, would you want to have a genetic test for *BRCA* ? Do you think your family and friends might have genetic counseling/testing if they received this brochure?

Permission from Dr. Susan Vadaparampil, MCC

institutions' policies, guideline, and resources. The following is a list of existing tools and strategies related to oncofertility that may serve as a guide for developing practice-specific tools. Practitioners may also choose to use these materials or modify them as allowed and applicable.

LiveStrong/Fertile Hope Brochure and Website [11]

This website includes a risk calculator, downloadable materials for healthcare professionals, different groups of cancer patients (male, female, pediatric) and provides links to the Sharing Hope program. This program provides need-based financial assistance to patients for using fertility preservation (Fig. 3.3).

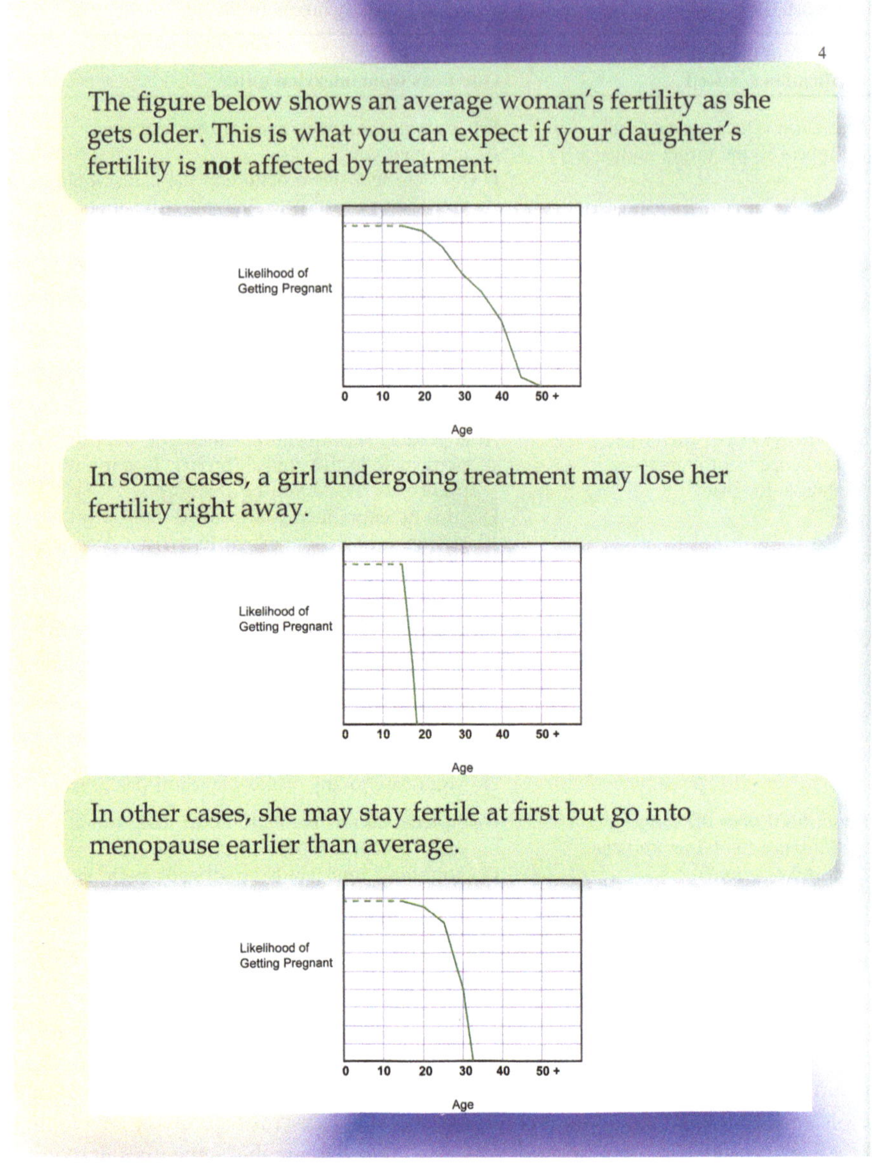

Fig. 3.3 FertileHope.org Website. Permission from Dr. Sarah Arvey, LIVESTRONG

Oncofertilty Website [12]

The Oncofertility Consortium maintains a website that has both provider and patient-oriented content. Patient content can be found at http://www.myoncofertility.org/printresources as well as http://oncofertility.northwestern.edu/patients/fertility-preservation-options-nu. In addition to information about fertility preservation,

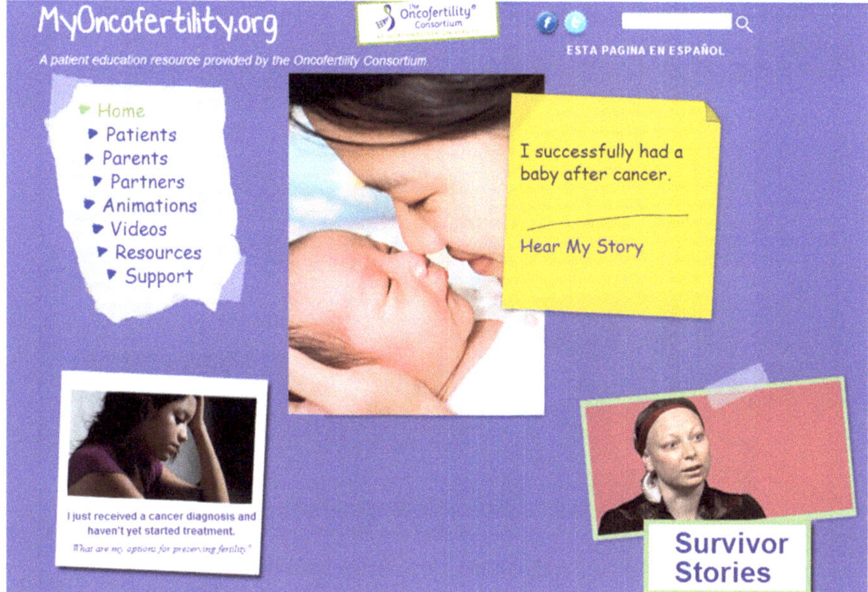

Fig. 3.4 MyOncofertility.org Website. Permission from Dr. Teresa Woodruff, NW

these resources include animated sequences that describe how and why fertility may be threatened by cancer treatment as well as the fertility preservation options. The website also includes testimonials by patients and providers. The website was developed as part of the Oncofertility Consortium's outreach efforts and has also been translated into Spanish (Fig. 3.4).

Web-Based Decision Aid [13]

This collaborative project between a reproductive endocrinologist, clinical psychologist, and oncology expert involves an interactive, web-based decision aid designed to be used in concert with fertility preservation counseling. The goal of the decision aid is to develop and make available a web-based tool that could be used for patients who do not have easy access to a full fertility preservation consultation with a reproductive endocrinologist (Fig. 3.5).

"A Young Person's Guide to Cancer and Fertility": Male and Female Brochure [14]

The majority of patient information on FP was designed by and for adults, and may not be appropriate for pediatric populations. These brochures were developed for a specific children's hospital after a review of available literature and existing

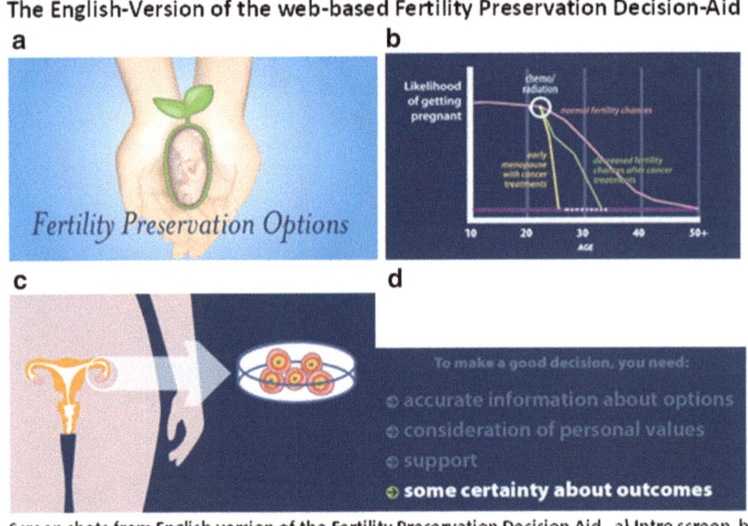

Fig. 3.5 Web-based fertility preservation decision aid. Permission from Dr. Jennifer Mersereau, UNC

educational materials. First, the research team designed a preliminary brochure outlining cancer-related infertility and the options available for pediatric patients. Due to the vast differences between female and male fertility issues and options, a separate male and female brochure was developed. The brochures were tested with three groups (patients and survivors aged 12-21 ($N=7$), their parents ($N=11$), and healthcare providers ($N=6$)). The final brochures were revised based on majority feedback and feasibility (Fig. 3.6).

Fertility-Related Choices: A Decision Aid for Younger Women with Early Breast Cancer [15]

This is a booklet for young women who have recently been diagnosed with early breast cancer. As chemotherapy and hormonal therapy may decrease fertility and reduce the chance of having children in the future, the information provided here is designed to help women decide which, if any, of the available fertility options are of interest to them. This booklet was specifically designed for the following patient characteristics: recently diagnosed with early breast cancer and reproductive age (having regular periods and no menopausal symptoms), and thinking of starting a family or having more children in the future (Fig. 3.7).

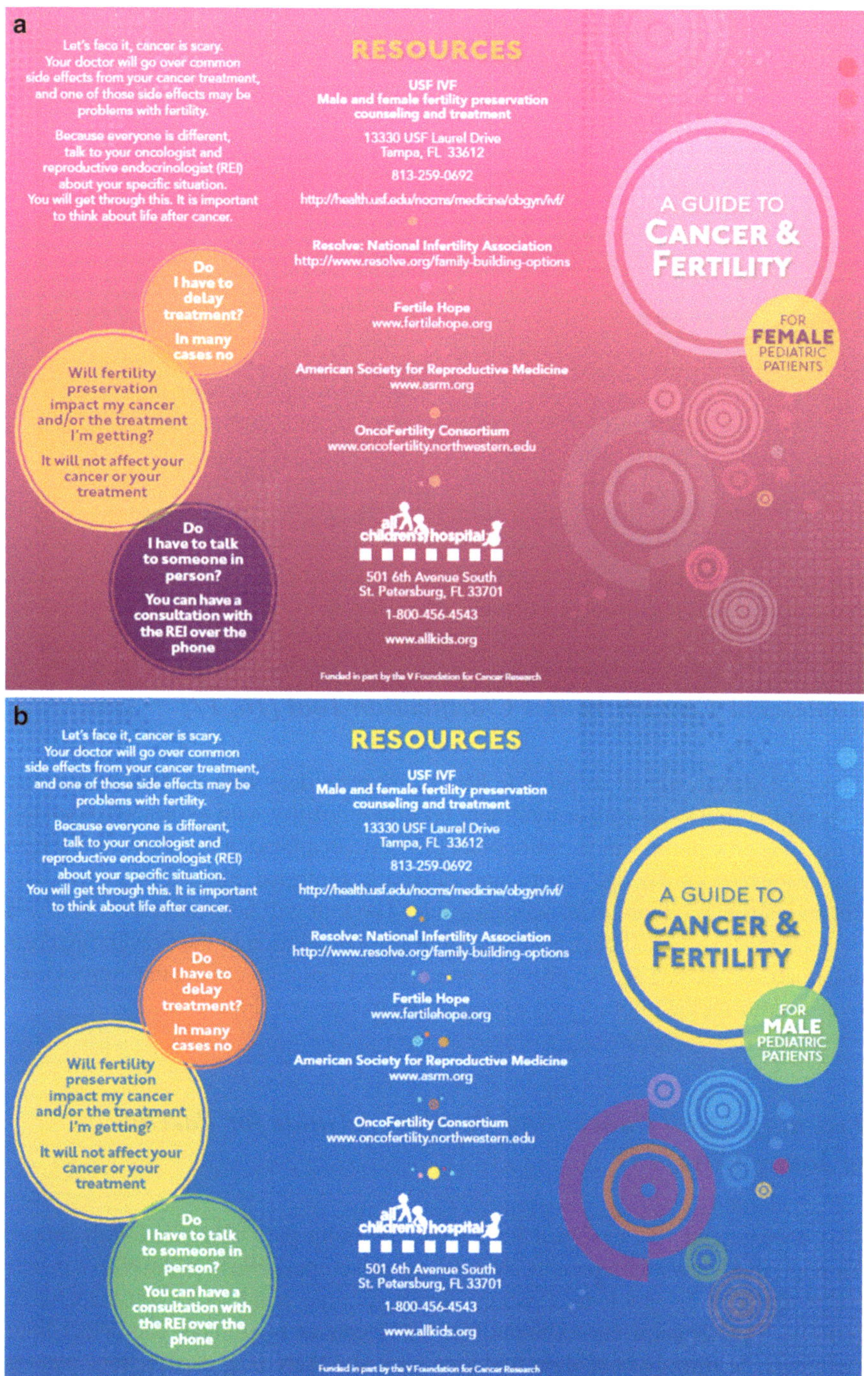

Fig. 3.6 A and B: A guide to cancer and fertility for female pediatric patients, a guide to cancer and fertility for male pediatric patients. Permission from Dr. Gwendolyn Quinn, MCC

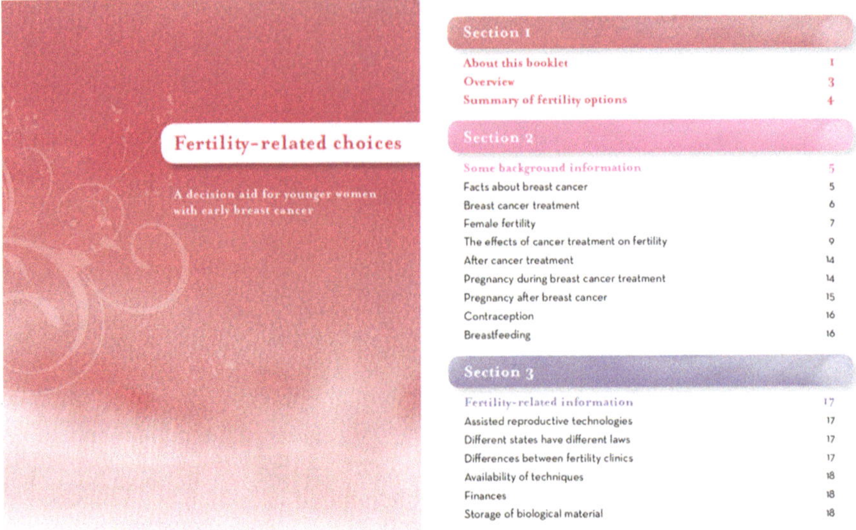

Fig. 3.7 Fertility-related choices: a decision aid for younger women with early breast cancer. Permission from Dr. Michelle Peate, UNSW

Adolescent Fertility Values Clarification Tool [16, 17]

This tool was designed to provide healthcare providers with a platform for discussing the impact of cancer treatment on future fertility with adolescent females. It discusses the preservation options and provides an approach for allowing the teen to consider her knowledge, desire, and value of parenthood. Since this is a tool, and not an instrument, there is no scoring guide. The tool will help practitioners assess the patient's values and understanding of fertility in relation to the cancer diagnosis and treatment plan. The tool provides examples of common coping techniques used by teens during the piloting and testing of the instrument (Fig. 3.8).

Learning About Cancer and Fertility: A Guide for Parents of Young Girls [18]

This decision aid was designed for parents of young girls diagnosed with cancer. Through interviews with parents ($N=20$), the developers chose to develop a paper-based tool that acknowledges parents' focus on their child's survival than future fertility. The decision aid explains that some cancer treatments can affect their daughter's fertility in both short and long term and there may be decisions parents

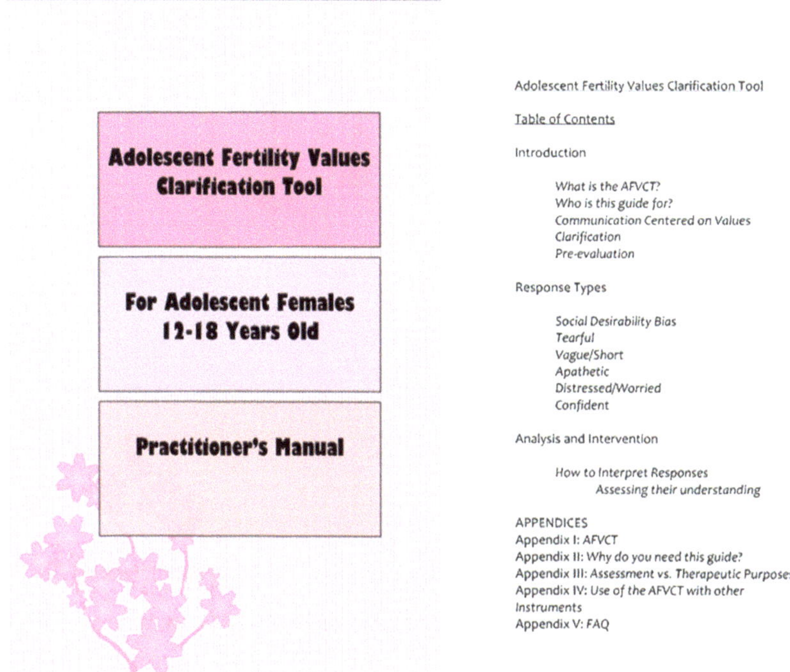

Adolescent Fertility Values Clarification Tool

Table of Contents

Fig. 3.8 Adolescent fertility values clarification tool. Permission from Dr. Gwendolyn Quinn, MCC

can make to preserve their daughter's fertility. Due to the age of the patients whose parents are the target of this decision aid, experimental options are also described. The focus of the tool is not just for making fertility preservation decisions but also serves as a guide to give parents information that will help them talk with their child's healthcare team now and in the future as she grows (Fig. 3.9).

This is not a comprehensive list of all tools and materials available on the topic of fertility preservation among AYA populations but serves as a sample of those that were developed with multidisciplinary teams and with a scientific approach. It is important for healthcare providers and researchers to explore decision aids and educational strategies that may improve the understanding of fertility preservation and its limitations. Healthcare professionals may consider which of these existing tools is appropriate for the institution and the population or if tailored tools should be developed based on unique characteristics of the patient population. Cancer survivors value the ability to make an informed decision about their future fertility preservation options. While decision aids, tools, and strategies are not a replacement for a discussion with a medical professional, they can assist patients and survivors with peace of mind about their choices.

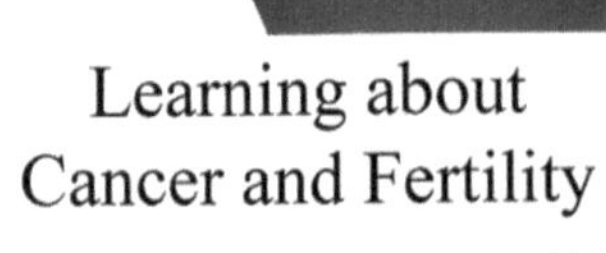

Right now, you are focused on your child and her survival. Thinking about her life after cancer may not seem like a priority in this moment.

However, some cancer treatments can affect your daughter's fertility.

This means that she may have trouble getting pregnant or having a healthy pregnancy when she is an adult.

There might be decisions you can make now to try to preserve her fertility.

Even if you cannot or do not want to use these options, this guide may give you information that will help you talk with your doctor now and talk with your child about this topic as she grows.

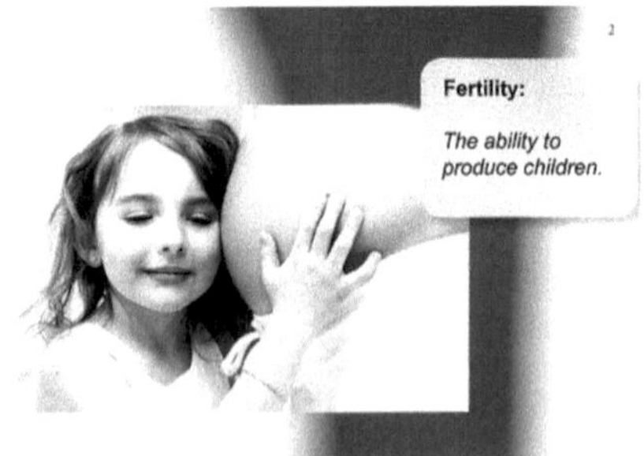

Can I do anything to protect my daughter's fertility?

Maybe.

First, not all cancer treatments affect fertility.
Second, even those that do are different in terms of how likely they are to affect fertility.

It is important to understand how cancer treatment affects fertility, and then you'll better decide if you can or if you want to take steps to protect your daughter's fertility. If you have questions about the short term and long term effects of cancer treatment on fertility, ask for a referral to a **fertility specialist**, such as a reproductive endocrinologist.

Fig. 3.9 Learning about cancer and fertility: a guide for parents of young girls. Permission from Dr. Marla Clayman, NW

References

1. Peddie V, Porter M, Barbour R, et al. Factors affecting decision making about fertility preservation after cancer diagnosis: a qualitative study. BJOG. 2012;119:1049–57.
2. Yee S, Abrol K, McDonald M, et al. Addressing oncofertility needs: views of female cancer patients in fertility preservation. J Psychosoc Oncol. 2012;30(3):331–46.
3. Quinn GP, Vadaparampil ST, Jacobsen PB, et al. Frozen hope: fertility preservation for women with cancer. J Midwifery Womens Health. 2010;55(2):175–80.
4. Knapp CA, Quinn GP, Murphy DM. Assessing the reproductive concerns of children and adolescents with cancer: challenges and potential solutions. J Adolesc Young Adult Oncol. 2011;1(1):31–5.
5. Quinn GP, Murphy DM, Knapp CA, et al. Who decides? Decision making and fertility preservation in teens with cancer: a review of the literature. J Adolesc Health. 2011;49(4):337–46.
6. IPDAS. Criteria for judging the quality of patient aids. 2005. Retrieved from http://www.ipdas.ohri.ca/IPDAS_checklist.pdf
7. O'Connor AM. Ottawa Decision Support Framework to Address Decisional Conflict. 2006. Retrieved from http://decisionaid.ohri.ca/docs/develop/ODSF.pdf
8. O'Connor AM, Stacey D, Jacobsen MJ. Ottawa decision support tutorial: improving practitioners' decision support skills Ottawa Hospital Research Institute: patient decision aids. 2011. Retrieved from https://decisionaid.ohri.ca/ODST/pdfs/ODST.pdf
9. Doak LG, Doak CC, Meade CD. Strategies to improve cancer education materials. Oncol Nurs Forum. 1996;23(8):1305–12.
10. Vadaparampil ST, Quinn GP, Gjyshi A, et al. Development of a brochure for increasing awareness of inherited breast cancer in black women. Genet Test Mol Biomarkers. 2011;15(1–2):59–67.
11. Fertile Hope. LiveStrong Foundation. 2013. Retrieved 31 Dec 2012. fertilehope.org

12. MyOncofertility.org. The Oncofertility Consortium. 2011. Retrieved on 31 Dec 2012. myoncofertility.org.
13. Web-based Fertility Preservation Decision-Aid: Fertility Preservation Options. Available at Oncofertilitydecision.org. Please contact author for more information: Mersereau JE: jennifer_mersereau@med.unc.edu
14. Murphy D, Sawczyn KK, Quinn GP. Using a patient-centered approach to develop a fertility preservation brochure for pediatric oncology patients: a pilot study. J Pediatr Adolesc Gynecol. 2012;25(2):114–21.
15. Peate M, Meiser B, Cheah BC, et al. Making hard choices easier: a prospective, multicentre study to assess the efficacy of a fertility-related decision aid in young women with early-stage breast cancer. Br J Cancer. 2012;106:1053–61.
16. Quinn GP, Murphy D, Wang H, et al. Having cancer does Not change wanting a baby: healthy adolescent Girls' perceptions of cancer-related infertility. J Adolesc Health. 2012;52(2):164–9.
17. Quinn G, Knapp C, Murphy D. Congruence of reproductive concerns among adolescents with cancer and their parents. Pediatrics. 2012;129:930–6.
18. Clayman ML. Learning about cancer and fertility: A guide for parents of young girls. Unpublished work 2012; please contact author for more information: m-clayman@nrthwestern.edu.

Chapter 4
Cancer-Related Infertility and Young Women: Strategies for Discussing Fertility Preservation

Karrie Ann Snyder and Alexandra Tate

Introduction

A cancer diagnosis is a life-altering event and since cancer treatment can impair future fertility capacity, cancer can also change a patient's parenting plans and family goals. There has been increased attention to the issue of cancer-related fertility impairment in recent years [1, 2], including the establishment of best practice guidelines from ASCO (American Society of Clinical Oncology) [3], ASRM (American Society for Reproductive Medicine) [4], and AAP (American Academy of Pediatrics) [5], as well as advocacy groups aimed at both patients and doctors to educate on the issue of fertility preservation (including Fertile Hope and the Oncofertility Consortium). There has even been increased coverage in entertainment and popular media on post-cancer parenthood, including notable high-profile cases such as Lance Armstrong. Despite these strides, there is continued concern that cancer patients are not always informed about potential impairment or available fertility preservation options that can help to safeguard their future fertility. Earlier studies in the growing field of oncofertility have indicated that many patients, particularly adolescent and pediatric patients [6], do not recall discussing fertility or fertility preservation options prior to beginning chemotherapy and/or radiation [1]. As a result, researchers are examining the barriers to the exchange of fertility-related discussions between patients and doctors (particularly oncologists) prior to potentially damaging cancer treatment (see [1] for review).

The exchange of fertility-related information between patients and oncologists becomes even more complicated when the patient is an adolescent, and parents (or other legal guardians) are the legal decision makers. Many ethical, legal, and

K.A. Snyder, B.A., M.A., Ph.D. (✉)
Department of Sociology, Northwestern University, Evanston, IL, USA
e-mail: karrie-snyder@northwestern.edu

A. Tate, B.A.
Department of Sociology, University of California, Los Angeles, Los Angeles, CA, USA

T.K. Woodruff et al. (eds.), *Oncofertility Communication: Sharing Information and Building Relationships across Disciplines*, DOI 10.1007/978-1-4614-8235-2_4,

practical issues arise as parents make treatment and fertility preservation decisions for their minor children [7, 8]. How do the parents begin to make a decision that has the potential to shape their child's ability to have biological children as adults? What if fertility preservation requires a delay of cancer treatment? What if the adolescents want to make a different choice regarding their future fertility than their parents? Even if the patients are just over 18 (or turn 18 during their treatment), parents may no longer be the legal decision maker; however, these "emerging adults," in the absence of partners or spouses, often rely heavily on their parents for input and support (including financial support and health insurance coverage) [9]. As oncofertility technologies and awareness grow, cancer care teams will increasingly need to help young patients, along with their families, navigate potential fertility impairment and possible treatment options, as well as provide information on the long- and short-term implications of their decisions. Thus, patient navigators with a concentration in fertility preservation would be invaluable resources for patients and cancer care teams.

In this chapter, we examine a series of focus groups with adult women who survived cancer during adolescence or early adulthood and connect their experiences to the possible role of a patient navigator specializing in fertility preservation. Two sets of themes emerged during these focus groups. One, participants shared their concerns at the time of their diagnosis. Often their main worries were not about fertility. Respondents instead focused on how cancer would affect their peer relationships and school experiences. It is important, however, to understand young women's concerns beyond fertility because these more pressing issues influence how they take in fertility-related information and make fertility preservation choices. Two, participants discussed their own experiences learning about fertility preservation as well provided feedback on current fertility preservation options. Respondents' experiences and feedback suggest strategies for patient navigators and cancer care teams to most effectively discuss fertility preservation with young women and teens facing cancer.

Methods

Data for this analysis comes from a series of retrospective focus groups conducted in 2010 with adult women who were diagnosed with various forms of cancer between the ages of 14 and 20 (see Table 4.1). Respondent #4 was initially diagnosed at 20 and several others had recurring cancer issues after turning 18. Therefore, some of the decision-making experiences discussed below are not instances where the respondent was a legal minor for the purposes of medical decision-making. Our aim here is not to compare decision-making when cancer patients are minors versus adults. Instead, our aim is to explore young women's experiences being diagnosed with cancer, and how they dealt with issues related to fertility during their diagnosis and treatment. We also examine their suggestions for improved strategies for communicating fertility preservation issues with newly diagnosed young

Table 4.1 Focus group respondent overview

	Diagnosis and age at diagnosis	Age at focus group
Focus Group 1		
Respondent #1	Non-Hodgkin's lymphoma at 17	Late 20s/Early 30s
Respondent #2	Hodgkin's lymphoma at 14 and breast cancer at 29	30
Respondent #3	Hodgkin's lymphoma at 17	31
Respondent #4	Hodgkin's lymphoma at 20	Late 20s/Early 30s
Focus Group 2		
Respondent #5	Ewing's sarcoma at 15	25
Respondent #6	Hodgkin's lymphoma at 16	34
Respondent #7	Ewing's sarcoma at 15	28
Respondent #8	Hodgkin's lymphoma at 16	29
Focus Group 3		
Respondent #9	Hodgkin's lymphoma at 15	35
Respondent #10	Hodgkin's lymphoma at 16	30

women with cancer. We find the experiences of women in our sample that occurred after the age of 18 illustrative, since these respondents were still dependent on their parents (e.g., a college student living at home part-time) and their parents, particularly mothers, remained quite involved (e.g., going to medical appointments, setting up consults) in their daughter's cancer care. Thus, while the adult children were legally making their own choices, parents were still intimately involved in the decision-making process, perhaps more so than in cases of older or partnered adults. Further, the experiences of emerging adults still shared many of the concerns and opinions of respondents diagnosed at earlier ages.

A moderator guided the focus groups, and discussion topics included diagnostic experiences, concerns during diagnosis and treatment, concerns regarding fertility and sexual health, and their parent's involvement in treatment decisions. Focus groups also included a presentation of the current fertility preservation options available to young women by a patient navigator from Northwestern University. Following this presentation, respondents were asked if and how they had learned of these options. Respondents gave feedback and suggestions for how patient navigators and medical personnel should broach these topics with young women (Note: Respondents were not necessarily treated at Northwestern University.).

The focus groups were audio-recorded and fully transcribed. Themes were coded inductively, meaning that we allowed the central themes to emerge through the process of analysis. We did not go into the data to test existing hypotheses or decision-making models. The setup of the focus groups allowed us to look at two general sets of issues: (1) concerns at the time of diagnosis and treatment including fertility preservation experiences and (2) suggestions for medical personnel and patient navigators on how to approach the issues of fertility impairment and fertility preservation. Through these two general sets of issues, other common feelings among this age group were reported that have been found in other studies, including the importance of control in the process, inclusion in decision-making, and concerns over feeling emotionally overwhelmed [6, 10]. Furthermore, we found, during respondents' discussions of sexual health during treatment, clear distinctions between sexuality and fertility were made, which is not uncommon for adolescents and emerging adults [11]. The transcripts were initially coded by one of the coauthors and were subsequently checked by the other coauthor.

The Experiences and Concerns of Young Women with Cancer

Primary Concerns at Diagnosis

Our sample's main concern mirrored that of many other studies looking at adolescents and emerging adults with cancer, where salient issues were survival, appearance, and alienation [12]. Respondent #3, who had been diagnosed at 17 with Hodgkin's lymphoma: "I think my big concern at the time was knowing whether it was going to be treatable or curable." Beyond survival, respondents thought about issues such as hair loss and whether they could attend school during their treatment:

> I'm sure I was worried about losing my hair, "Am I going to be missing school, am I going to be able to finish school, graduate with people I'm in school with ..." and all that stuff. It was a year worth of chemo and I was in the hospital basically for a whole week at a time every month when I had to go in and I missed a lot of school. And I was a really good student too so for me, not being there and also missing.
> Respondent #7, diagnosed with Ewing's Sarcoma at 15

The impact that cancer would have on their peer relationships and social lives was a prominent theme throughout the focus groups. Respondents felt that cancer can heighten all of the sensitive social issues adolescents already face:

> When you find out you have cancer, you're like, "Ugh, am I going to die ..." and I remember my hair being a big issue because I was a junior in high school and just imagine the social awkwardness that you worry about, who you're going to go to prom with ..., and then no hair adds to just all that awkwardness.
> Respondent #8, diagnosed with Hodgkin's Lymphoma at 16.

Similarly, Respondent #10 worried about fitting in with her friends and issues of disclosure:

> Ya, I think I was concerned about the hair too. Just like being a girl, high school, you're 16, that's like the biggest deal in the world. Um, and taking that a step further, just like having something that someone could recognize as you having cancer ... Ya know, it's pretty obvious when someone doesn't have hair, that they're sick. So the loss of the hair being a statement of being sick and then, ya know, just how this whole thing was going to fit into being a 16 year old. Ya know, like I wanted to still go to dances and do well in school, participate in sports and it's pretty much from the get go.
> Respondent #10, diagnosed with Hodgkin's Lymphoma at 16.

Like other studies on fertility preservation and adolescents [6], our respondents believe that there is a need for improved communication on the issue of fertility preservation. However, for most focus group respondents, issues of fertility were not at the forefront of their concerns when diagnosed and as they went through treatment, unlike studies of older cohorts of women in their later 20s and 30s [13].

> I remember I was like, "Am I going to die and am I going to lose my hair?" That was the important thing to me. I was a sophomore in high school and those were important things to me looking back. The hair thing was crucial, but I don't even think I thought about [fertility]
> Respondent #5, diagnosed with Ewing's Sarcoma at age 15

> I was younger so I didn't really … I just wanted to be done with the cancer. I wasn't thinking about fertility the first time.
> Respondent #2, diagnosed with Hodgkin's Disease at 14 and Breast Cancer at 29

Several participants noted that while fertility itself, or the biological ability to bear children, may not have been central at the time, the broader issue of how cancer may influence or change their future adult lives was a concern:

> I remember thinking, because it was my senior year, was I going to be able to go to college? Was I going to get a job? Was I ever going to get married? I had a lot of scar concerns because there are some up here and they're humongous. Ya know, was I ever going to be normal and in that came, will I ever have a family? It wasn't specific enough about fertility.
> Respondent #3, diagnosed with Hodgkin's Lymphoma at 17

> [B]ut it wasn't much about the end result of the baby, it was more about kind of what I said earlier, about the loss of the family or that stage of life. So I think it was indirectly, but not exactly, "Will I be able to have a kid?"
> Respondent #4, diagnosed with Hodgkin's Lymphoma at 20

At the time, more pressing issues of friends and school were more relevant or significant to respondents, but as they got older issues of fertility became increasingly important for many respondents:

> [T]hey mentioned [fertility preservation], but I was 15. I was like, "I'm 15, why the hell would I be thinking about babies right now?" Ya, I was like 15 and like, "We don't need to think about that right now." I mean as I got older, when I was in college I was like, "Oh I might not be able to have children," but I don't let things faze me very often.
> Respondent #9, diagnosed with Hodgkin's Lymphoma at age 15

Missing information about Fertility Preservation

Fertility issues may not have been forefront, but as Respondents #4 and #9 convey, being able to become a parent in the future was important and most respondents had thought on some level about having biological children prior to their diagnosis. In order to most effectively preserve fertility, best practice guidelines outline that fertility preservation needs to be discussed prior to treatment in order for the patient to have the most effective options available [3]. Unfortunately, the respondents' experiences mirror much research in oncofertility that finds young people are not consistently discussing the issue with their cancer care teams or are receiving spotty information at best [1, 6]:

> I think my first time, my first go at it … I don't ever remember them saying anything, that that would be a problem and then after that, I got my period so I don't think that first year

> of chemo affected me, but then on the relapse, honestly I don't really even remember them discussing it.
> Respondent #7, diagnosed with Ewing's Sarcoma at age 15

> [I remember] a lot of vague, random statements. I hear a lot of other people saying that too about fertility or sexual health and they're just kind of these clouds of information and what you need are the details and I remember them saying vague cloudy things about … [fertility]. And I didn't know what to do with that either.
> Respondent #3, diagnosed with Hodgkin's Lymphoma at 17

Some respondents found out more about fertility impairment during their treatment or soon after, and most have learned much more about the issue since their cancer. However, our respondents felt that the onus was on them to seek out additional information, including through advocacy groups like Gilda's Club. In some cases, parents were described as being the ones taking in the more detailed information at the time of diagnosis on treatment options and related fertility issues. However, few respondents recalled in-depth conversations regarding fertility and most were not given options like egg retrieval or ovarian cryopreservation. None of the sample underwent fertility preservation, which may have been due to several factors, including the technologies that were available at the time for adolescent women as well as the lack of detailed information given to respondents and their parents. Nevertheless, a few respondents' parents made treatment choices that were intended to minimize the potential for fertility impairment, such as choosing a certain chemotherapy regime thought to cause less fertility damage. Overall, however, respondents and their families were not well informed on the topic of fertility.

Role in Decision-Making

As respondents discussed how they did or did not learn about cancer-related infertility, they also discussed their role in decision-making, both for cancer treatment and fertility-related issues. Most respondents did not feel that they were excluded from important discussions, but saw their parents as the primary decision makers:

> … in that instant moment you're like, "Ok, I don't want to die. What do I have to do not to die?" That's why I'm really lucky because I think the doctors talked to my mom and my mom was better able to understand. At that point I was 16 and what do you care? So my mom was the one really concerned about that and really took initiative. So I'm lucky because my mom was really active as well.
> Respondent #8, diagnosed with Hodgkin's at age 16

All respondents believe that fertility preservation needs to be directly addressed with detailed information available to young women facing cancer. However, there was some variation in terms of how involved respondents wanted to be in the decision-making process when they were diagnosed. Respondent #8 was comfortable with her parents being the decision makers in terms of overall treatment but also fertility: "it was pretty much like I wanted them to handle it." Like Respondent #8, others also felt they were not fully capable because of age or emotional distress to fully comprehend what was going on and to make sense of all of the information they were presented with. Most were comfortable with parents making key decisions, and similar to studies of adult patients [14], respondents were also comfortable trusting medical experts, their doctors, to make the final decisions. A few respondents did voice a desire to have greater control in treatment decisions, including Respondent #5 who tearfully explained how she wished she could have made decisions regarding fertility preservation, but was not given any options: "I wasn't given that option and I think it's really important for teenage girls to have that option and to have that discussion at diagnosis. I think being a teenager, I could have made the decision on my own ..."

Sexual Health: More Missed Opportunities

Most discussions of cancer-related infertility and adolescents have focused on whether these patients and their parents learned about fertility preservation and made treatment decisions. Almost no research has looked at broader discussions of sexual health between adolescent women and healthcare workers in the context of a cancer diagnosis. Some evidence suggests that young people with a history of cancer may erroneously be under the assumption that they cannot get pregnant and forgo birth control (for further discussion, see [15]), but a fuller understanding of sexual health in this context of a cancer diagnosis is missing. Beyond fertility issues, sexual health includes issues of pain or discomfort during sex, being able to be intimate, feeling desirable, being able to address sexual needs, and building romantic relationships. Most respondents did not recall any discussion of such larger sexual health issues:

> When the oncologist would leave after every time I saw her she would be like, "Don't smoke and don't get pregnant," and that was it and I was 20. Maybe I don't remember, but I think I would have remembered. Those were her 2 things. I didn't know why. I mean, I knew it wasn't a good time in my life to get pregnant, but I didn't understand everything that would have complicated it. I just knew not to smoke and not to get pregnant.
> Respondent #4, diagnosed with Hodgkin's Lymphoma at 20

For Respondent #4, not only was there a lack of dialog on the issue, sexual health was very narrowly defined as becoming pregnant while young and in treatment. Respondent #10 had a similar experience:

> I just assumed that they thought that I was having sex even though I wasn't. I don't know why, but I just would assume that. There was a time, about a year and half after I started getting my treatment that I stopped getting my period and they were really worried about it and they were like, "Are you pregnant," and I was like, "No," and so that was when there was an issue and so they changed birth control pills and it was fine.
> Respondent #10, diagnosed with Hodgkin's Lymphoma at age 16

For Respondent #6 as well, sexual health was only brought up because she was on birth control. Respondent #6 found the exchange to be awkward and partly because the topic was broached in front of her parents:

> "I had sex once and when I got a pill that said it was a prophylactic and my parents joked that I was too young for prophylactics and they knew I'd had sex and they mentioned it, I thought I am dying but I'm going to die of embarrassment."
> Respondent #6 diagnosed with Hodgkin's Lymphoma at age 16

Respondents' experiences reveal an interesting dynamic. Fertility preservation was presented as an issue that would affect their lives down-the-road, or well into survivorship, whereas immediate sexual issues were only about avoiding pregnancy. Fertility in the future and fertility in the present were treated as very separate issues and neither was presented in the context of a respondent's sexual health overall (for further reading, see [16]).

Respondents differed in their sexual experience and relationship status at the time of diagnosis and treatment, and thus diverged on how important issues of sexual health were to them as teens or young adults. The experiences of Respondent #3 show, however, that issues of sexuality can be significant, and frank discussions in the healthcare setting could benefit some young cancer patients:

> I remember it being a huge deal for me at that time, but because I'd been sexually active before the diagnosis, it had been a part of keeping me normal. I don't even remember talking about it with my friends so I don't think it's that kind of social "keeping me normal," but I didn't feel attractive in any way, I didn't feel comfortable—everything was painful or uncomfortable and it was this time where that didn't matter. I remember, and my parents aren't the strictest people in the world, but I remember that they'd go out, not overnight, but they'd go out and leave me with my boyfriend and we weren't always intimate, but they were trusting and treating me like an adult and acknowledging how important it was for it to be just the two of us to spend time together.
> Respondent #3, diagnosed at Hodgkin's Lymphoma at 17

Strategies for Fertility Preservation Counseling

As part of the focus group, respondents also gave feedback on how fertility preservation can best be discussed. One strategy talked about during the focus groups was the use of patient navigators. Patient navigators are specialized healthcare workers that assist patients and families throughout the cancer process, including support group referrals, setting up appointments, and helping with insurance issues [17]. Northwestern University and some other cancer care centers have used patient navigators specializing in fertility preservation as a way to inform patients about fertility preservation, discuss options, and help coordinate care. The feedback from respondents on the use of patient navigators coupled with their experiences described above suggest strategies that would be useful for a range of healthcare providers (including oncologists and oncology nurses) to help young female patients and their families learn about and make fertility preservation decisions.

The Importance of Information

All of the following issues and strategies addressed in this chapter rely on patients having a fundamental knowledge of fertility preservation and cancer-related infertility. Research in oncofertility (see [1, 3, 6]) and the experiences of our respondents clearly show that fertility-related discussions may not always happen with oncologists (or only "vague" information is relayed as in the case of Respondent #3 above). A variety of healthcare providers from patient navigators to oncologists can be a way to integrate detailed information into the diagnostic and treatment processes. All respondents agreed that fertility preservation information must be provided—especially more detailed information such as costs and experimental options. This information should also be age-appropriate. For example, a very young teen may require more background on women's reproductive health than an older teen.

Many respondents also asserted that there should be separate discussions between a healthcare provider and an adolescent patient on the topic, and also discussions where parents can be involved. Issues of sexuality and fertility are sensitive topics, and not all young women will be comfortable raising questions and concerns in front of parents or other medical personnel, as exhibited by Respondent #6's experiences where she described being embarrassed by a discussion of her being on birth control.

Moreover, while not all young women will desire a more broad discussion of sexual health beyond the details of fertility preservation, meetings between a patient navigator and a young patient could be an opportunity for sexual health discussions or referrals to appropriate resources. The experience of Respondent #1 illustrates well the need for the opportunity for more frank discussions regarding sexuality among this population:

> I was not sexually active at that time although I did have a long-term boyfriend and I just knew that was something important, my parents were always very open about that aspect of being a human being, being a person who is a sexual being. I don't know if I was necessarily thinking about it actively at the time, but it saddens me that it never was discussed. I just think it should be apart of a conversation even if it's a nurse practitioner and not maybe the male doctor. I know you have to connect with the person who you have the conversation with, ya' know, even if they send you to a gynecologist to have that discussion. It's a doctor you need to be seeing anyway at that time, especially if you're a cancer patient.
> Respondent #1, diagnosed with Non-Hodgkin's Lymphoma at 17

Another issue that became very apparent during focus group discussions was that not many respondents were concerned with their future fertility at the time of diagnosis. Survival and social issues related to school and friends were more prominent and parenting was seen more as an event that may happen well into their adult lives rather than a pressing concern. As young patients are counseled, it is important that issues related to fertility are not pushed onto younger patients who are not interested and may be emotionally overwhelmed with a cancer diagnosis. Rather, framing the topic of fertility preservation as one that may be significant to them in the future or bringing up future goals more generally may be effective ways to begin a discussion on the topic. Also, presenting the goal of fertility preservation as not about having biological children per se, but as helping individuals reach parenting and family goals in the future, and that fertility preservation can help to broaden their options. Based on our findings, these may be more effective strategies to start a dialogue about fertility with a patient population for whom parenting plans may not be an immediate goal.

Empowering Young Women

Overall, respondents seemed comfortable with the level of involvement they had in their cancer treatment decisions with parents often being the primary decision makers.

But many respondents also described that cancer itself felt like something was happening to them that was out of their control. Being informed is a way to feel empowered, or in control, over one's health. While most respondents were happy letting parents and doctors make treatment decisions, other young patient may seek a more central role in the decision-making process. Respondent #10 shared how making choices helped her feel like a "normal" teenager:

> I mean, I was pretty actively involved in the decisions. I decided when I was going to start treatment, when the cycles were going to happen ... Going back to the point of being a typical teenager, ya know, I scheduled my chemo and radiation around my social schedule and as bad as that sounds, my oncologist at the time said, "Let her do her thing, she needs ownership over her life and her body and if she needs to go to a dance and if it happens to fall on a day that she starts her chemo rounds, we'll just push it back a day, no biggie ..."

Issues of control may also arise during fertility preservation consultations and healthcare providers involved in these consultations should be aware of the need for many adolescent patients to feel empowered. Being informed about treatments and fertility preservation, and even assisting in such decisions, may be vital to a young person's sense of control. Previous studies on patient empowerment bolster the claim that patients who employ shared decision-making with their physician during cancer care have more positive attitudes about their treatment [18].

Experiential Support

Respondent #10's concerns above over fitting in her old teenage life with her new diagnosis were echoed many times throughout the focus groups. Many respondents voiced a desire to be able to talk to others who have insight or experience with cancer. Other research on younger adult women with cancer has found similar unmet needs in terms of "experiential support," defined as emotional support and insight from those who have gone through a similar medical crisis [19]. Experiential support may be particularly important for young adults and teens facing cancer because they are forced to contend with a serious health issue—something that most of their friends will not have experienced and may not be able to relate to. In addition to cancer, survivors of adolescent cancer may also have to contend with issues of infertility far before their peers as well. Knowing from an early age that infertility may be an issue later on is yet another experience that may isolate an adolescent or young adult cancer survivor from friends and peers [12, 20]. As fertility preservation is discussed, issues of normalcy, peer relationships, romantic relationships, and feeling different may surface. Similar to issues of sexual health, healthcare providers who deal with fertility preservation should be prepared to address experiential support needs to some degree and have resources available where adolescent patients can seek out desired experiential support, including support groups for adolescent patients and peer-to-peer social networking sites (like myoncofertility.com).

Conclusion

Following this analysis, it is clear that even a few focus groups allow us to shed light on a previously ignored area of oncologic care. We are grateful that there has been increased attention to the issue of cancer-related fertility impairment in recent years; however, the attention paid to adolescents and emerging adults with cancer and cancer-related fertility issues is still lacking. Unlike their older counterparts, younger cancer patients face unique complexities related to peer group isolation, sexual health, appearance, parental involvement, fertility, and empowerment. Having healthcare providers available, including potential patient navigators specializing in fertility preservation, who are knowledgeable and prepared to discuss the topic, would have been undoubtedly an effective and much utilized resource for the women in our sample.

Our aim by examining the retrospective accounts of women who confronted a cancer diagnosis during this unique time in their life course is to call for more stringent best practice guidelines for healthcare professionals working with this group so that the aforementioned complexities, and, most importantly, future fertility options, are directly addressed to each patient undergoing treatment. We hope that in examining these case studies, it has become clear that the treatment processes and psychosocial situations confronted by female adolescents and emerging adults are part of an elaborate puzzle requiring specialized knowledge and empathy.

Acknowledgement This work was supported by the Oncofertility Consortium NIH 5UL1DE019587.

References

1. Snyder KA, Pearse W. Discussing fertility preservation options with patients with cancer. JAMA. 2011;306(2):202–3.
2. Jeruss JS, Woodruff TK. Preservation of fertility in patients with cancer. N Engl J Med. 2009;360(9):902–11.
3. Lee SJ, Schover LR, Partridge AH, Patrizio P, Wallace WH, Hagerty K, Beck LN, Brennan LV, Oktay K. American Society of Clinical Oncology recommendations on fertility preservation in cancer patients. J Clin Oncol. 2006;24(18):2917–31.
4. Ethics Committee of the American Society for Reproductive Medicine. Fertility preservation and reproduction in cancer patients. Fertil Steril. 2005;83(6):1622–8.
5. Fallat ME, Hutter J. American academy of pediatrics committee on bioethics; American Academy of Pediatrics Section on Hematology/Oncology; American Academy of Pediatrics Section on Surgery. Preservation of fertility in pediatric and adolescent patients with cancer. Pediatrics. 2008;121(5):e1461–9.
6. Quinn GP, Vadaparampil ST. Fertility preservation and adolescent/young adult cancer patients: physician communication challenges. J Adolesc Health. 2009;44(4):394–400.
7. Gracia CR, Gracia JJE, Chen S. Ethical dilemmas in oncofertility: an exploration of three clinical scenarios. In: Woodruff TK, Zoloth L, Campo-Engelstein L, Rodriguez S, editors. Oncofertility: ethical, legal, social, and medical perspectives. New York: Springer; 2010. p. 195–208.

8. Galvin KM, Clayman ML. Whose future is it? Ethical family decision making about daughters' treatment in the oncofertility context. In: Woodruff TK, Zoloth L, Campo-Engelstein L, Rodriguez S, editors. Oncofertility: ethical, legal, social, and medical perspectives. New York: Springer; 2010. p. 429–46.
9. Arnett J. Emerging adulthood: the winding road from the late teens through the twenties. New York: Oxford University Press; 2006.
10. Kyngäs H, Mikkonen R, Nousiainen EM, Rytilahti M, Seppänen P, Vaattovaara R, Jämsä T. Coping with the onset of cancer: coping strategies and resources of young people with cancer. Eur J Cancer Care (Engl). 2001;10(1):6–11.
11. Morgan S, Davies S, Palmer S, Plaster M. Sex, drugs, and rock 'n' roll: caring for adolescents and young adults with cancer. J Clin Oncol. 2010;28(32):4825–30.
12. Hedström M, Skolin I, von Essen L. Distressing and positive experiences and important aspects of care for adolescents treated for cancer. Adolescent and nurse perceptions. Eur J Oncol Nurs. 2004;8(1):6–17; discussion 18–9.
13. Gardino SL, Emanuel LL. Choosing life when facing death: understanding fertility preservation decision-making for cancer patients. In: Woodruff TK, Zoloth L, Campo-Engelstein L, Rodriguez S, editors. Oncofertility: ethical, legal, social, and medical perspectives. New York: Springer; 2010. p. 447–60.
14. Mendick N, Young B, Holcombe C, Salmon P. The ethics of responsibility and ownership in decision-making about treatment for breast cancer: triangulation of consultation with patient and surgeon perspectives. Soc Sci Med. 2010;70(12):1904–11.
15. Laurence V, Rousset-Jablonski C. Contraception and cancer treatment in young persons. Adv Exp Med Biol. 2012;732:41–60.
16. Katz A. The sounds of silence: sexuality information for cancer patients. J Clin Oncol. 2005;23(1):238–41.
17. National Cancer Institute. What are patient navigators? [Internet.] [updated 2009 Jul 23; cited 2013 Jan 2.] Available from http://crchd.cancer.gov/pnp/what-are.html.
18. Gattellari M, Butow PN, Tattersall MH. Sharing decisions in cancer care. Soc Sci Med. 2001;52(12):1865–78.
19. Snyder KA, Pearse W. Crisis, social support, and the family response: exploring the narratives of young breast cancer survivors. J Psychosoc Oncol. 2010;28(4):413–31.
20. Enskär K, von Essen L. Prevalence of aspects of distress, coping, support and care among adolescents and young adults undergoing and being off cancer treatment. Eur J Oncol Nurs. 2007;11(5):400–8.

Chapter 5
Fertility Communication and High-Risk Patients

Natalia C. Llarena and Jacqueline S. Jeruss

Introduction

Due to improved genetic screening and cancer risk assessment among families, many women are now aware that they have an increased risk of developing breast or ovarian cancer at a young age. This cohort of young women, termed "previvors," faces unique concerns related to childbearing and cancer risk reduction. They must make decisions regarding prophylactic therapy and how, or whether, to balance preventive treatment with childbearing and breastfeeding. Often, interventions that effectively reduce cancer risk must be undertaken during the reproductive years, and may pose a permanent or temporary threat to fertility. The emergence of oncofertility has empowered these patients—who may have a high-risk family history of breast or ovarian cancer or carry deleterious genetic mutations—to take a proactive approach to both cancer prevention and fertility preservation. Fertility preservation may benefit high-risk patients who (1) are at increased risk of developing premenopausal breast or ovarian cancer and (2) may require a risk-reducing intervention prior to menopause that poses a threat to future fertility. In this chapter, we present the topics discussed during a high-risk consultation followed by case examples that illustrate effective communication about fertility preservation to patients at high risk for developing breast or ovarian cancer.

N.C. Llarena, B.A. • J.S. Jeruss, M.D., Ph.D. (✉)
Department of Surgery, Feinberg School of Medicine, Northwestern University, 300 E Chicago Ave, Chicago, IL 60611, USA
e-mail: natalia-llarena@fsm.northwestern.edu; j-jeruss@northwestern.edu

T.K. Woodruff et al. (eds.), *Oncofertility Communication: Sharing Information and Building Relationships across Disciplines*, DOI 10.1007/978-1-4614-8235-2_5,

Who Are High-Risk Patients?

Women with a genetic predisposition to breast or ovarian cancer develop malignancies at a higher rate and younger age than the general population, indicating that preventive therapy could be undertaken before menopause. Because prophylactic interventions may temporarily or permanently compromise young patients' ability to have children, women at high risk for breast or ovarian cancer are in a unique position to benefit from fertility preservation options.

Approximately 10 % of breast cancer and 15 % of ovarian cancer patients have a heritable form of the disease, most commonly attributed to a mutation in the BRCA1 or BRCA2 gene. Women with germline BRCA1 or BRCA2 mutations tend to develop breast and ovarian cancer at a higher rate and earlier age than the baseline population. Female carriers of BRCA1 and BRCA2 mutations have a 45–65 % lifetime risk of developing breast cancer and an 11–39 % lifetime risk of developing ovarian cancer (Table 5.1) [1–3]. Although BRCA1 and BRCA2 mutations are most commonly implicated in hereditary breast cancer, other autosomal dominant cancer syndromes are also associated with an increased risk of breast cancer, including Li–Fraumeni syndrome (linked to TP53 mutations) and Cowden syndrome (related to PTEN mutations). In addition, ovarian cancer is associated with Lynch syndrome, cell nevus syndrome, and multiple endocrine neoplasia type 1 (MEN1) [4].

Women without a known genetic mutation but who have a strong family history of breast or ovarian cancer are also at increased risk for cancer. A review of 38 studies showed that the pooled estimate of relative risk of breast cancer in women with an affected first-degree relative was 2.1, and risk increased with each additional first-degree relative diagnosed with cancer [5]. Similarly, in a meta-analysis of 15 studies, the relative risk of ovarian cancer among women with at least one first-degree relative with disease was 3.1 [6].

Patients with a history of atypical ductal or lobular hyperplasia (ADH, ALH) or lobular carcinoma in situ (LCIS) represent another group at increased risk for breast cancer. Proliferative lesions with atypia (those with excessive growth of abnormal cells in the ducts or lobules of the breast tissue) confer a breast cancer risk four to five times that of an average-risk woman [7–9].

Table 5.1 Breast and ovarian cancer risk in BRCA mutation carriers

	Breast CA risk by age 70 (%)	Ovarian CA risk by age 70 (%)	References
General population	12	1.4	[1]
BRCA1	55–65	39	[2, 3]
BRCA2	45–47	11–17	[2, 3]

CA cancer

Prophylactic Interventions for High-Risk Patients

Prophylactic interventions are available to reduce the risk of developing breast and ovarian cancer; however, these approaches, which are often undertaken prior to menopause, have the potential to compromise a young patient's fertility. Guidelines for BRCA1/2 mutation carriers suggest that women consider prophylactic bilateral salpingo-oophorectomy (BSO) and prophylactic mastectomy after age 35 or as soon as they are finished having children; however, women with a strong family history of very early-onset cancer may also wish to pursue surgical interventions at a younger age. In the absence of prophylactic mastectomy, annual mammography and MRI screening are recommended; usually they are staggered every 6 months. Additionally, antiestrogen treatment with tamoxifen is recommended for breast cancer chemoprevention.

The therapeutic benefits of tamoxifen for high-risk patients are considerable; treatment can reduce the risk of developing invasive cancer by nearly 50 % [10]. However, tamoxifen is a teratogen, and pregnancy should be avoided during the recommended duration of therapy, which could extend up to 10 years [11]. At the dose used to treat breast cancer patients, tamoxifen generally does not cause cessation of ovulation. However, tamoxifen use may be associated with irregular or missed menses in some women, particularly when it is prescribed following cytotoxic chemotherapy. A significantly increased risk of amenorrhea at 1 year posttreatment was found among patients older than age 40 who were taking tamoxifen [12]. Additionally, there is a reported 15 % decrease in the odds of continuing menstrual cycles after the first 1–2 years of tamoxifen therapy, though some studies have also found this effect to be reversible and temporary [13–16]. As fertility begins to decline substantially after the age of 35, the considerable length of recommended tamoxifen therapy may be a critical deterrent for young, high-risk women.

Preventive interventions for women at high risk for ovarian cancer are particularly critical, as there are currently no effective screening algorithms for detecting early-stage ovarian cancer. Although clinical outcomes are good for early-stage ovarian cancer, 80 % of ovarian cancers are identified only after metastasis to the pelvic organs, abdomen, or beyond, at which point cure rates are low [17]. Prophylactic BSO dramatically reduces the risk of both breast and ovarian cancer in BRCA mutation carriers (by 50 % and 96 %, respectively) [18], but permanently eliminates the possibility of having biologic children if the patient's oocytes or embryos have not been preserved prior to oophorectomy. Oral contraceptives and tubal ligation have also been shown to reduce ovarian cancer risk [19], but these are not as effective as BSO. Unlike oophorectomy, however, they do allow for the possibility of a future pregnancy, as patients who have had tubal ligation may become pregnant through assisted reproductive technologies.

The decision to pursue prophylactic surgery is complex; often it is influenced by concerns about fertility, as well as worries about appearance, menopausal side effects, and sexuality. Despite these concerns, a survey of BRCA mutation carriers who have undergone prophylactic BSO found that approximately 97 % of patients would pursue the surgery again and would recommend the surgery to other BRCA mutation carriers. Survey respondents also stated, however, that they would have benefitted from additional information about the impact of BSO on sexuality and cardiovascular health prior to undergoing the surgery [20]. Fertility is one of many concerns that physicians must address with high-risk patients considering BSO as an approach to cancer risk reduction.

Pregnancy and Cancer Risk

One topic that is highly relevant to the dialogue about fertility and cancer risk is the possible impact a pregnancy would have on cancer risk. Most large studies of BRCA1 and BRCA2 mutation carriers have shown that parity and number of live births positively correlate with a reduced breast cancer risk [21]. Additionally, fertility treatment has not been associated with an increased risk of breast cancer in BRCA mutation carriers. A case–control study of 1,380 pairs of BRCA1 and BRCA2 mutation carriers did not find an increased risk of breast cancer in women who had undergone fertility treatment compared to controls [22].

Communicating with High-Risk Patients

During the initial consultation with a high-risk patient of childbearing age, the objectives to be met include cancer risk assessment and discussion of strategies for cancer risk management. The approach to cancer risk reduction should take into account the patient's level of comprehension and concern about the risk of developing cancer, as well as the patient's childbearing goals. Typically, patients are referred for cancer risk assessment because of a strong family history of cancer or the identification of a deleterious genetic mutation. The patient's family cancer history is often discussed at the beginning of the encounter. A detailed family history includes affected relatives, types of cancer, cases of bilateral cancer, age at diagnosis, treatment procedures, and treatment outcomes. Any familial history of genetic testing is reviewed, and patients with a strong family history of cancer who have not yet had genetic testing are referred to a genetic counselor. The patient's personal medical history is also reviewed in detail. This includes prior illnesses and hospitalizations, medications, a review of prior breast imaging or biopsies, and an evaluation of hormone use including oral contraceptives and fertility treatments [23].

Focusing the discussion on how the patient's past medical history, family history, and mutation status affect the patient's personal risk of developing cancer helps to facilitate both patient and physician understanding of the patient's risk of developing cancer. This discussion also helps ensure that the patient is sufficiently informed and can actively participate in decision-making about preventive therapy. Risk assessment tools such as the Gail model, a breast cancer risk assessment tool, are often used to

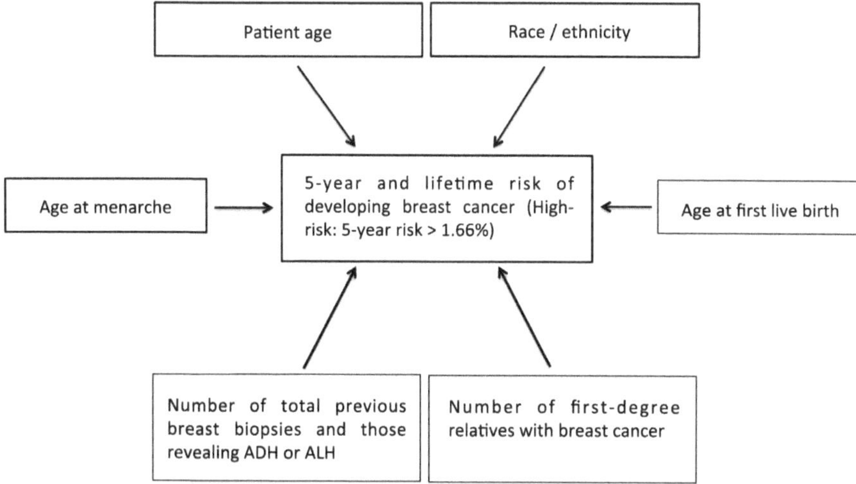

Fig. 5.1 Estimating 5-year and lifetime breast cancer risk using the Gail model. The Gail model is a risk assessment tool that estimates a patient's 5-year and lifetime risks of developing breast cancer. The model takes into account patient age, age of menarche, age at first birth or nulliparity, family history of breast cancer in a primary relative (mother, sister, daughter), race/ethnicity, number of prior breast biopsies, and number of prior biopsies yielding atypical hyperplasia [24]

help patients understand their risk relative to that of the general population. The Gail model estimates a woman's 5-year and lifetime risk of developing breast cancer (Fig. 5.1). The model accounts for patient age, age of menarche, age at first birth or nulliparity, family history of breast cancer in a primary relative (mother, sister, daughter), race/ethnicity, number of prior breast biopsies, and number of prior biopsies yielding atypical hyperplasia [24].

During the review of the patient's medical history, the patient's childbearing and lactation history are discussed, and it is at this time that the topic of fertility preservation may be introduced [23]. Having witnessed their relatives experience the impact of cancer treatment at a young age, many patients with a strong family history of cancer will prioritize their fertility concerns. To aid in the discussion of fertility preservation, often a basic question—such as, "Were you thinking about having a child?" or "Were you planning to have any more children?"—can help initiate the conversation [23]. Patients at high risk for breast or ovarian cancer face unique concerns related to fertility and cancer risk management, and it is critical that providers attempt to elicit and understand these concerns.

At this point, the consultation typically focuses on strategies for cancer prevention that take into account the patient's individual risk, her childbearing goals, and the patient's level of concern about her risk of developing cancer. When the strategies under consideration for cancer prevention pose a fertility threat, a discussion of available options for fertility preservation can be included in the high-risk consultation (Fig. 5.2). One of the advantages of discussing fertility preservation with high-risk patients (as opposed to patients who have already been diagnosed

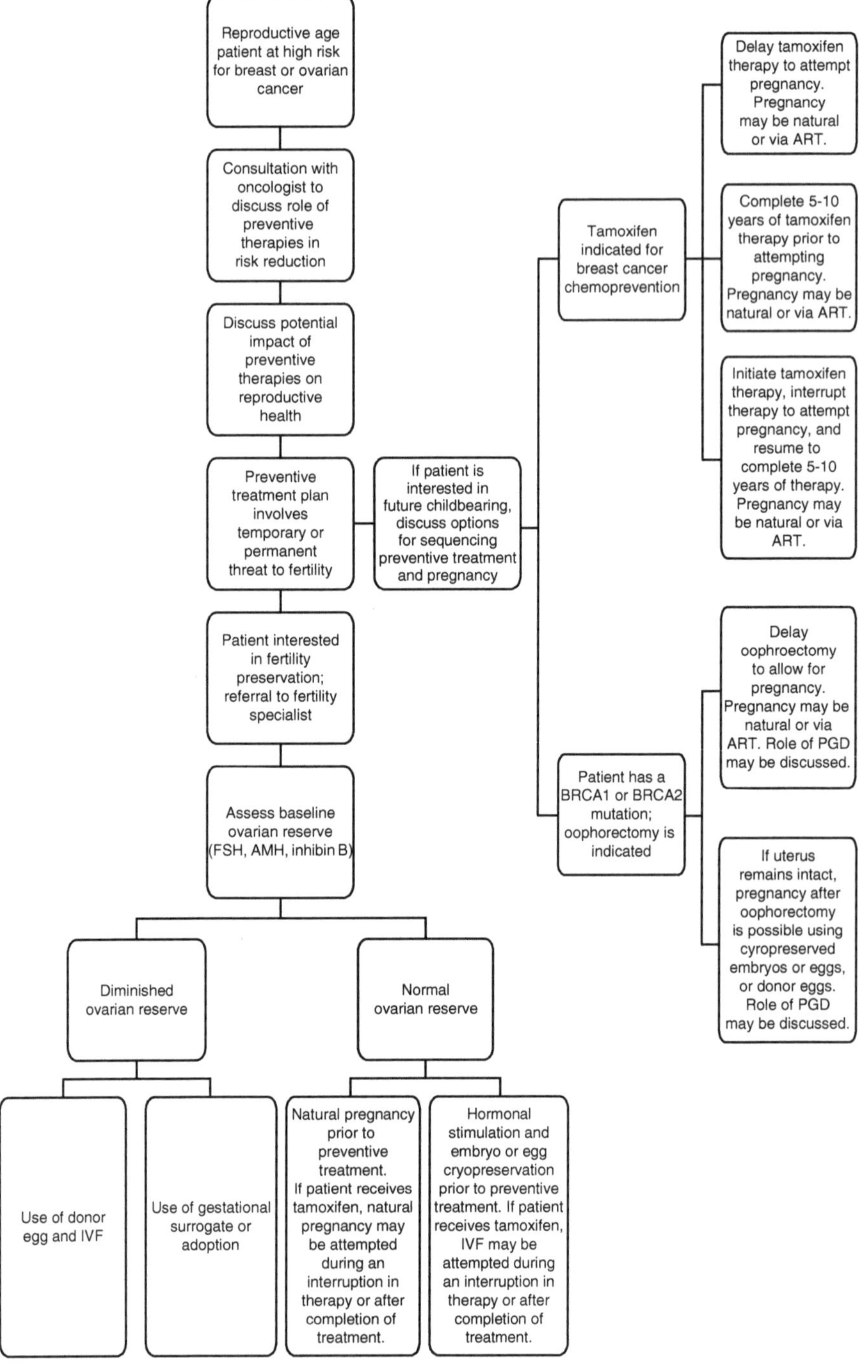

Fig. 5.2 Treatment guidelines for fertility preservation in young women at high risk for breast or ovarian cancer. A discussion about fertility as it pertains to preventive cancer treatment is an integral part of care for young patients at increased risk of breast and ovarian cancer. Referral to a

with cancer) is that there is ample time for the patient to consider her options without the time pressure imposed by the need for immediate cancer treatment. Ideally, the patient is referred for independent fertility preservation counseling with a fertility preservation specialist following the high-risk oncologic consultation. A second consultation with a fertility specialist ensures that the high-risk patient receives information about fertility preservation in a balanced and unbiased manner.

The following case examples explore the challenges that young patients face regarding the prioritization of preventive cancer therapy and reproductive goals. Case 1 describes a high-risk breast cancer patient who declined fertility preservation and suggests an alternative strategy for supporting fertility goals while managing cancer risk. Case 2 illustrates an approach to integrating fertility preservation into the preventive treatment plan for a BRCA1 mutation carrier.

Case #1: A High-Risk Breast Cancer Patient Who Declined Fertility Preservation

A 37-year-old woman presented for cancer risk assessment and preventive treatment. She had a personal history of atypical ductal hyperplasia and a family history of breast cancer, diagnosed in her mother at age 41. The patient's ADH had been diagnosed 2 years earlier by needle core biopsy and managed surgically by excision of the lesion. She had been receiving annual screening mammograms since the time of her ADH diagnosis but no other preventive therapy, and she expressed concern about her risk of developing breast cancer. The patient's 5-year Gail model risk score was calculated to be 2.5 %, compared to 0.4 % for an average-risk person. Patients with a 5-year predicted risk of breast cancer greater than 1.66 % are considered to be at high risk for breast cancer and are candidates for prophylactic tamoxifen therapy [10]. A 5-year course of tamoxifen was recommended for chemoprevention, along with annual screening mammography and a breast exam every 6 months. The patient

fertility specialist ensures that the patient receives accurate, unbiased information about fertility preservation. The fertility specialist can obtain information about the patient's premenopausal status by inquiring about menstrual history and measuring follicle stimulating hormone (FSH) on an early day in the menstrual cycle. Strategies for fertility preservation are determined based on the patient's ovarian function, preference, and decisions about preventive treatment. Patients receiving tamoxifen for breast cancer chemoprevention may attempt pregnancy naturally or via assisted reproductive technologies (ART) prior to initiating 5–10 years of therapy, during an interruption in a 5- to 10-year course of therapy, or after the completion of 5–10 years of treatment. BRCA mutation carriers may attempt pregnancy naturally or via ART prior to oophorectomy. It is possible for patients who retain an intact uterus to become pregnant after oophorectomy using ART. Preimplantation genetic diagnosis may be offered to BRCA mutation carriers who wish to reduce the risk of transmitting the mutation to offspring. AMH denotes antimullerian hormone, ART denotes assisted reproductive technologies, PGD denotes preimplantation genetic diagnosis, and IVF denotes in vitro fertilization. This figure was adapted from Fig. 2, Jeruss JS, Woodruff TK. Preservation of fertility in patients with cancer. The New England journal of medicine. 2009;360(9):902–11. Epub 2009/02/28 expressed concern about the possibility of experiencing menopausal side effects from tamoxifen but was reassured that menopausal symptoms are usually well tolerated. The patient agreed to initiate tamoxifen.

Because pregnancy is contraindicated during tamoxifen therapy and the patient would be at least 42 years of age at the conclusion of therapy, the issue of fertility preservation was discussed with the patient at the end of her initial consultation. The patient, who had a 5-year-old child, declined an oncofertility consultation and stated that she was not planning on having additional children. Nine months after initiating therapy, the patient returned to the clinic for a breast exam and expressed a desire to stop tamoxifen as she was now planning to have another child. She was again offered a fertility preservation consultation, but declined and stated that she wished to stop treatment to pursue a natural pregnancy and then resume tamoxifen therapy postpartum. The patient's individual high-risk status and the effect of stopping tamoxifen prematurely on this risk were reviewed. The patient was then advised to wait 8 weeks after stopping tamoxifen before attempting pregnancy; based on the half-life of tamoxifen, a 2-month "washout" period is recommended prior to becoming pregnant [25]. Eight months after stopping tamoxifen, the patient became pregnant. She resumed tamoxifen 6 months postpartum after she was finished breastfeeding and completed 4 additional years of therapy.

This case highlights the challenges that young high-risk patients face regarding how to balance preventive cancer treatment, childbearing, and breastfeeding. When a patient's childbearing plans change during her course of treatment, appropriate counseling should be provided and, within the context of the patient's treatment plan, effort should be made to support the patient's reproductive goals. Although treatment with at least a 5-year course of tamoxifen is recommended for chemoprevention, indirect evidence from the Early Breast Cancer Trialists' Collaborative Group (EBCTCG) suggests that antiestrogen therapy with tamoxifen can be delayed to allow for pregnancy [16, 26, 27]. Another study of patients who delayed initiation of tamoxifen therapy for 2 years and then completed a 5-year course showed a significantly improved disease-free survival rate (35 % reduction in recurrence risk) compared with the control group who did not take tamoxifen [28, 29]. Results from the Wisconsin Tamoxifen Study, where tamoxifen treatment was delayed 7–8 years, also showed a benefit for patients in the treatment versus control group [28, 30]. Together, these data support the potential for a tailored delay in tamoxifen therapy to allow for pregnancy, with the expectation that the patient is counseled to ultimately complete 5–10 years of therapy.

Case #2: A High-Risk Patient with a BRCA1 Mutation Who Desired Fertility Preservation

A 35-year-old woman with a family history of breast and ovarian cancer presented for cancer risk assessment and preventive treatment. Her sister was diagnosed with ovarian cancer at the age of 39, her mother was diagnosed with breast cancer at the age of 42, and her maternal grandmother died from ovarian cancer at the age of 51.

The patient was referred for genetic counseling and found to have a deleterious mutation in the BRCA1 gene. Preventive approaches discussed with her included breast cancer screening every 6 months with staggered MRI and mammograms, ovarian cancer screening with serum CA-125 and twice annual transvaginal ultrasound, BSO, and prophylactic mastectomy. The patient was interested in prophylactic mastectomy and considering risk-reducing BSO, but was concerned about the associated loss of fertility. She strongly desired a child, but did not currently have a partner and was unsure about the time in her life when she would be ready to conceive.

After consultation with a gynecological oncologist regarding BSO, the patient met with an oncofertility patient navigator and a reproductive endocrinologist. The reproductive endocrinologist discussed the patient's options for fertility preservation, including embryo cryopreservation with donor sperm and oocyte cryopreservation. Although oocyte cryopreservation has previously been offered on an experimental basis, recent guidelines from the American Society for Reproductive Medicine (ASRM) indicate that the procedure should no longer be considered experimental. Based on an examination of nearly 1,000 studies, the ASRM reports that pregnancy rates for in vitro fertilization and intracytoplasmic sperm injection (IVF/ICSI) are similar with cryopreserved versus fresh oocytes. Additionally, available data show no increase in chromosomal abnormalities or birth defects among children born from cryopreserved oocytes compared with those born from IVF/ICSI with fresh oocytes or the general population [31]. Ovarian tissue cryopreservation for BRCA1 mutation carriers would be considered experimental, however, with the majority of the resected ovarian tissue sent for pathologic analysis. A fraction of the ovarian tissue could be preserved for potential oocyte extraction with the hope of implementing currently developing technologies for in vitro oocyte growth and maturation, but none of the tissue would be intended for future reimplantation given the persistent risk of malignant transformation.

The patient also expressed concern about passing the BRCA mutation down to her future children and was advised that preimplantation genetic diagnosis (PGD) could be performed on her embryos to minimize the risk. She opted for oocyte cryopreservation and completed successful ovarian stimulation and oocyte harvest. Shortly after completing fertility preservation, the patient underwent risk-reducing BSO and prophylactic mastectomy. Six months after surgery, the patient stated that she was very satisfied with her decision to pursue risk-reducing BSO and felt more at ease about her risk of developing breast and ovarian cancer. The patient expressed that preserving her fertility had allowed her to pursue surgery without significant regret and served as a great source of comfort to her as she experienced the effects of surgical menopause. Three years later, the patient is married and she and her husband are considering having a child using the patient's banked oocytes.

Fertility concerns are a major factor for high-risk patients when making decisions about cancer risk management. The options for fertility preservation have the potential to influence patients' selection of risk-reducing strategies and when to pursue risk reduction. Thus, it is critical for patients to be educated about their options for fertility preservation early on in the process of cancer risk management. Oocyte and embryo cryopreservation are options for high-risk women who do not have a partner or who plan to undergo risk-reducing BSO prior to completing their families. For

BRCA mutation carriers concerned about passing the mutation on to their children, PGD offers a means to minimize this risk. Several studies have shown that high-risk patients often do not receive adequate information from their physicians about fertility preservation and PGD, and many are not aware of PGD as an option [32–34]. This information gap for high-risk women highlights the need for more effective education about fertility preservation and PGD and the importance of the referral to an oncofertility specialist for this patient population.

Conclusions

Patients at high risk for breast and ovarian cancer face complex decisions about how to prioritize preventive treatment, childbearing, and breastfeeding. Fertility preservation offers the possibility for high-risk patients—many of whom wish to initiate prophylactic therapy at a young age—to maintain the ability to have biologic children. It is critical that physicians who care for high-risk patients take time to approach the issues unique to this patient population with sensitivity and empathy. Interventions for cancer risk reduction should take into account patients' reproductive goals. Educating patients about fertility preservation early on in the discussion about prevention strategies allows patients the opportunity to receive appropriate counseling, consider the available options, and then incorporate fertility preservation into their risk reduction plans if desired.

It is an ongoing challenge for physicians to ensure that the high-risk patient has an accurate understanding of her cancer risk compared with the general population, and is sufficiently informed to actively participate in decision-making about preventive treatment and fertility preservation. Additionally, the physician should ensure that plans for fertility preservation complement the approach to cancer risk reduction and do not cause significant delays in the initiation of risk-reducing therapy. Given that high-risk patients are healthy and working to take a preemptive role in the preservation of good health, it follows that these patients would also be motivated to protect their fertility if given the option. Fertility preservation services are currently available to all high-risk patients under the age of 45 and to those who convey interest.

Acknowledgements This work was supported by the Oncofertility Consortium NIH 5UL1DE019587 and the Specialized Cooperative Centers Program in Reproduction and Infertility Research NIH U54HD076188.

References

1. Antoniou A, Pharoah PD, Narod S, et al. Average risks of breast and ovarian cancer associated with BRCA1 or BRCA2 mutations detected in case Series unselected for family history: a combined analysis of 22 studies. Am J Hum Genet. 2003;72:1117–30.
2. National Cancer Institute. PDQ genetics of breast and ovarian cancer. Bethesda, MD: National Cancer Institute; 2012.

3. Chen S, Parmigiani G. Meta-analysis of BRCA1 and BRCA2 penetrance. J Clin Oncol. 2007; 25:1329–33.
4. Lindor NM, McMaster ML, Lindor CJ, Greene MH. Concise handbook of familial cancer susceptibility syndromes—second edition. J Natl Cancer Inst Monogr. 2008;1–93.
5. Pharoah PD, Day NE, Duffy S, Easton DF, Ponder BA. Family history and the risk of breast cancer: a systematic review and meta-analysis. Int J Cancer. 1997;71:800–9.
6. Stratton JF, Pharoah P, Smith SK, Easton D, Ponder BA. A systematic review and meta-analysis of family history and risk of ovarian cancer. Br J Obstet Gynaecol. 1998;105:493–9.
7. Hartmann LC, Sellers TA, Frost MH, et al. Benign breast disease and the risk of breast cancer. N Engl J Med. 2005;353:229–37.
8. Ashbeck EL, Rosenberg RD, Stauber PM, Key CR. Benign breast biopsy diagnosis and subsequent risk of breast cancer. Cancer Epidemiol Biomarkers Prev. 2007;16:467–72.
9. American Cancer Society. Breast cancer facts & figures 2011–2012. Atlanta, GA: American Cancer Society; 2011.
10. Dunn BK, Ford LG. Breast cancer prevention: results of the National Surgical Adjuvant Breast and Bowel Project (NSABP) breast cancer prevention trial (NSABP P-1: BCPT). Eur J Cancer. 2000;36 Suppl 4:S49–50.
11. Davies C, Pan H, Godwin J, et al. Long-term effects of continuing adjuvant tamoxifen to 10 years versus stopping at 5 years after diagnosis of oestrogen receptor-positive breast cancer: ATLAS, a randomised trial. Lancet. 2013;381(9869):805–16.
12. Abusief ME, Missmer SA, Ginsburg ES, Weeks JC, Partridge AH. The effects of paclitaxel, dose density, and trastuzumab on treatment-related amenorrhea in premenopausal women with breast cancer. Cancer. 2010;116:791–8.
13. Port ER, Montgomery LL, Heerdt AS, Borgen PI. Patient reluctance toward tamoxifen use for breast cancer primary prevention. Ann Surg Oncol. 2001;8:580–5.
14. Ruddy K, Mayer E, Partridge A. Patient adherence and persistence with oral anticancer treatment. CA Cancer J Clin. 2009;59:56–66.
15. McCowan C, Shearer J, Donnan PT, et al. Cohort study examining tamoxifen adherence and its relationship to mortality in women with breast cancer. Br J Cancer. 2008;99:1763–8.
16. Hulvat MC, Jeruss JS. Fertility preservation options for young women with breast cancer. Curr Opin Obstet Gynecol. 2011;23:174–82.
17. Bast Jr RC, Hennessy B, Mills GB. The biology of ovarian cancer: new opportunities for translation. Nat Rev Cancer. 2009;9:415–28.
18. Rebbeck TR, Lynch HT, Neuhausen SL, et al. Prophylactic oophorectomy in carriers of BRCA1 or BRCA2 mutations. N Engl J Med. 2002;346:1616–22.
19. Narod SA, Risch H, Moslehi R, et al. Oral contraceptives and the risk of hereditary ovarian cancer. Hereditary Ovarian Cancer Clinical Study Group. N Engl J Med. 1998;339:424–8.
20. Campfield Bonadies D, Moyer A, Matloff ET. What I wish I'd known before surgery: BRCA carriers' perspectives after bilateral salipingo-oophorectomy. Fam Cancer. 2011;10:79–85.
21. Cullinane CA, Lubinski J, Neuhausen SL, et al. Effect of pregnancy as a risk factor for breast cancer in BRCA1/BRCA2 mutation carriers. Int J Cancer. 2005;117:988–91.
22. Kotsopoulos J, Librach CL, Lubinski J, et al. Infertility, treatment of infertility, and the risk of breast cancer among women with BRCA1 and BRCA2 mutations: a case-control study. Cancer Causes Control. 2008;19:1111–9.
23. Jeruss JS. Discussing fertility preservation with breast cancer patients. Cancer Treat Res. 2010;156:461–6.
24. Gail MH, Brinton LA, Byar DP, et al. Projecting individualized probabilities of developing breast cancer for white females who are being examined annually. J Natl Cancer Inst. 1989;81:1879–86.
25. Braems G, Denys H, De Wever O, Cocquyt V, Van den Broecke R. Use of tamoxifen before and during pregnancy. Oncologist. 2011;16:1547–51.
26. Hershman DL, Kushi LH, Shao T, et al. Early discontinuation and nonadherence to adjuvant hormonal therapy in a cohort of 8,769 early-stage breast cancer patients. J Clin Oncol. 2010;28:4120–8.

27. Grunfeld EA, Hunter MS, Sikka P, Mittal S. Adherence beliefs among breast cancer patients taking tamoxifen. Patient Educ Couns. 2005;59:97–102.
28. Gradishar WJ, Hellmund R. A rationale for the reinitiation of adjuvant tamoxifen therapy in women receiving fewer than 5 years of therapy. Clin Breast Cancer. 2002;2:282–6.
29. Delozier T, Switsers O, Genot JY, et al. Delayed adjuvant tamoxifen: ten-year results of a collaborative randomized controlled trial in early breast cancer (TAM-02 trial). Ann Oncol. 2000;11:515–9.
30. Love RR, Olsen MR, Havighurst TC. Delayed adjuvant tamoxifen in postmenopausal women with axillary node-negative breast cancer: mortality over 10 years. J Natl Cancer Inst. 1999;91:1167–8.
31. Practice Committees of American Society for Reproductive Medicine; Society for Assisted Reproductive Technology. Mature oocyte cryopreservation: a guideline. Fertil Steril. 2012;99(1):37–43.
32. Quinn GP, Vadaparampil ST, Tollin S, et al. BRCA carriers' thoughts on risk management in relation to preimplantation genetic diagnosis and childbearing: when too many choices are just as difficult as none. Fertil Steril. 2010;94:2473–5.
33. Quinn G, Vadaparampil S, Wilson C, et al. Attitudes of high-risk women toward preimplantation genetic diagnosis. Fertil Steril. 2009;91:2361–8.
34. Vadaparampil ST, Quinn GP, Knapp C, Malo TL, Friedman S. Factors associated with preimplantation genetic diagnosis acceptance among women concerned about hereditary breast and ovarian cancer. Genet Med. 2009;11:757–65.

Chapter 6
Incorporating Partners and Spouses in Oncofertility Communication

Megan Johnson Shen and Hoda Badr

Regardless of gender, patients undergoing the diagnosis and treatment of cancer list their future fertility as an important concern [1]. Seventy-six percent of cancer patients without a child have expressed a desire to have children in the future [2]. Reproductive age female cancer survivors rate concerns about children and family as second only to fears of cancer recurrence [3], and many report that fertility issues played a role in altering their cancer treatment decisions [4, 5]. Fertility preservation is also important to men diagnosed with cancer. Fifty-eight percent in one study reported that cryopreserving their sperm helped them in the emotional battle against cancer [6]. Despite the fact that fertility issues and fertility preservation are personal issues, most patients face the issue of how to incorporate their partner (spouse or significant other) into oncofertility discussions with very little guidance or support. Almost 80 % of young female patients of cancers and treatments known to affect their fertility report having a partner [7]. These women cite their partner as their most commonly used (66 %) and most helpful fertility discussion partner [7]. In fact, discussing fertility issues with one's partner was rated as more helpful to patients than discussing fertility issues with one's oncologist. At the same time, decision-making about fertility treatment options has been shown to contribute to marital distress among couples who are not affected by cancer [8]. Actively involving partners in oncofertility discussions may thus help patients cope with oncofertility issues, promote shared decision-making, and reduce potential marital distress.

To date, oncofertility communication research has focused on communication between patients and their physicians [1] or on how to involve parents of children

M.J. Shen, Ph.D.
Department of Psychiatry and Behavioral Sciences, Memorial Sloan-Kettering Cancer Center, 641 Lexington Ave., 7th Floor, New York, NY 10022, USA
e-mail: shenm@mskcc.org

H. Badr, Ph.D. (✉)
Department of Oncological Sciences, Mount Sinai School of Medicine, One Gustave L Levy Place, Box 1130, New York, NY 10128, USA
e-mail: hoda.badr@mssm.edu

T.K. Woodruff et al. (eds.), *Oncofertility Communication: Sharing Information and Building Relationships across Disciplines*, DOI 10.1007/978-1-4614-8235-2_6,

and adolescents diagnosed with cancer into oncofertility discussions [9]. No studies have addressed the issue of communication about this very sensitive issue between patients and their partners. Thus, the focus of this chapter will be on better understanding the impact of fertility preservation and infertility on couples and the communication needs of adult cancer patients and their partners.

Issues for couples to consider when approaching oncofertility communication include:

- What is the impact of potential infertility on cancer patients, their partners, and the couple's relationship?
- What are the fertility preservation options available to women and men and how might these options affect the couple?
- What are the ethical and legal concerns of fertility preservation faced by couples?
- How should partners be involved in oncofertility communication and decision-making?
- How can couples' communication surrounding fertility preservation and potential infertility be improved in order to promote shared decision-making and reduce marital distress caused by fertility issues related to cancer treatment?

In this chapter, we will discuss these challenges and suggest potential ways to actively involve partners and improve couples' communication surrounding the fertility issues that arise as a result of cancer and its treatment.

Impact of Potential Infertility on Cancer Patients, Their Partners, and the Couple's Relationship

One issue that cancer patients and their partners face is the distressing effect that potential infertility can have on the couple's relationship. Although little research has examined the impact of this on couples in which one partner is battling cancer, there is an extensive literature on the effects of infertility on healthy couples. We draw from this literature to examine the potential effects of cancer-related infertility on patients, their partners, and the couple's relationship.

Infertility and Psychological and Marital Distress

Among non-cancer populations, infertility has been shown to exacerbate distress (depression and anxiety symptoms) in both members of the couple [8, 10], and infertile couples report higher levels of depression than those who are fertile [11]. The stress associated with the threat of infertility is only compounded by the stress of cancer [12], and it can wear on couples' relationships in the following ways: (1) feeling loss of control over one's life or ability to reproduce [8], (2) the perceived loss of femininity and masculinity due to the inability to conceive [12], and (3) the perceived loss of attractiveness or self-esteem of the cancer patient [8, 12]. Indeed, the loss of control over one's life can be one of the most difficult emotional outcomes of infertility [13]. This loss could be compounded by cancer, which could also be perceived as having a loss of control over one's life. Although confronting this sense of loss of control is important to ensure that fertility issues do not become the focal centerpiece of the couple's relationship [8], a key challenge for couples coping with cancer is that they can become so consumed with "fighting the cancer" that they neglect to consider fertility preservation options.

Infertility and Sexual Dissatisfaction

Infertility has been shown to lead to decreases in sexual and marital satisfaction in both men and women [14–16]. It has also been associated with decreases in marital satisfaction and intimacy [14], and increases in social isolation and divorce [8, 10]. Compounding these challenges, cancer and its treatments often result in decreased sexual functioning and satisfaction—particularly in cancers known to affect the sexual/reproductive system such as prostate cancer [17] and gynecologic cancers [18].

There is emerging evidence to suggest that couples coping with cancer find it difficult to talk about sexual dysfunction resulting from the disease and its treatment. For example, a cross-sectional study of prostate cancer patients and their partners found that when patients had poor sexual functioning, their partners were more likely to report that the couple avoided open spousal discussions [19]. This lack of openness about discussing sexual issues was associated with partners' marital distress. However, couples who engaged in high levels of mutual constructive communication—a positive couple's communication technique—reported greater marital adjustment, regardless of their sexual satisfaction [19]. Although studies have yet to investigate the specific communication challenges couples encounter when discussing oncofertility concerns, they are likely to be similar given that fertility problems are often closely tied to the sexual problems that arise as a result of cancer and its treatment. Given this, working with couples to help facilitate open, supportive, and constructive discussions about sexual dysfunction and infertility may help to alleviate marital distress.

Summary

The stress of infertility can lead to marital distress and divorce [8, 10] as well as decreases in marital and life satisfaction and intimacy [14]. Additionally, other cancer-related fertility issues such as loss of control over one's life, loss of masculine or feminine identity, decreases in self-esteem [8, 12], and sexual dysfunction [19] contribute to distress in couples. The increases in marital distress and decreases in marital and sexual satisfaction due to infertility most likely effect couples' ability to communicate. Given that teaching effective communication and conflict management skills has been shown to reduce marital distress [20], it is important to understand how to improve couples' communication about fertility issues and the distress surrounding these issues. In order to understand how to improve communication, however, it is important to consider the fertility preservation options available to men and women and how these options might affect the couple.

Fertility Preservation Options and the Couples' Issues Surrounding Them

Women's Fertility Preservation Options

Fertility preservation in both women and men centers on the concept of gamete storage and future utilization [21]. The most established and highly recommended technique for fertility preservation in women is embryo cryopreservation [22]. In this technique, eggs are harvested, fertilized in vitro, and then the resulting embryos are frozen for later implantation [22]. This could be a preferred method of fertility preservation among women with partners because it requires a partner or donor sperm. Alternatively, women can opt for oocyte cryopreservation in which unfertilized eggs are harvested and frozen [22]. This technique, however, leads to fewer successful outcomes. Both of these methods generally take 2–5 weeks to complete, potentially causing a delay in cancer treatment [21].

To circumvent the issue of time involved in the above-mentioned procedures, women can opt for ovarian cryopreservation and transplantation in which ovarian tissue is frozen and reimplanted after cancer treatment is completed [22]. This procedure can be completed in a single day through an outpatient surgical procedure. Although most women utilizing this technique have had their endocrine function later restored, few women later deliver healthy babies [21]. Additionally, there is a risk of reintroducing aggressive cancer cells because the ovarian tissue is leukocyte-rich [21].

As an alternative to attempting to preserve embryos, oocytes, or ovarian tissue, women can also opt to shield or protect existing tissue from radiation or chemotherapy treatment. First, women can utilize gonadal shielding during radiation therapy which helps reduce the dose of radiation delivered to their reproductive organs [22]. Second, women can utilize ovarian transposition in which the ovaries are surgically repositioned [22]. Both of these procedures can be done quickly within a day's time. Finally, women can opt for ovarian suppression with a gonadotropin releasing hormone (GnRH) analogs or antagonists [22].

Men's Fertility Preservation Options

Fortunately, fertility preservation options for men are less time-consuming than most options for women. The most established technique for fertility preservation in men is sperm cryopreservation in which sperm is obtained through masturbation and then frozen to be utilized later [22]. Other forms of fertility preservation for men are similar to those of women. For instance, men can also choose to have gonadal shielding during radiation therapy [22]. Alternatively, men can have testicular tissue cryopreservation in which testicular tissue is frozen and then later reimplanted posttreatment [22]. Finally, men can choose to have testicular suppression with GnRH analogs or antagonists in which, similarly to women, hormonal therapies are used to protect testicular tissue during radiation therapy or chemotherapy [22]. All of these fertility preservation options for men are done in a single day through an outpatient procedure.

Couples' Issues Involved in Fertility Preservation Options

Given the wide variety of fertility preservation options available, couples face the difficult task of navigating these options and making an informed decision about the choice that is best for them. Sometimes couples face a tradeoff between risking the effectiveness of the fertility preservation technique and risking the delay in treatment of cancer. This issue is more of a concern for women but less of a concern for men because most fertility preservation options for men can be completed within a day's time [22]. Moreover, even though delays in treatment to preserve fertility may not have any adverse medical consequences in terms of fighting the cancer, such delays can be emotionally taxing for both patients and their partners. The most effective fertility preservation options for women include embryo and oocyte cryopreservation, but each of these options can take 2–5 weeks to complete, which could cause a delay in cancer treatment [21]. Shorter procedures, including ovarian cryopreservation and transplantation and shielding of reproductive tissues, can be completed in just a single day but often lead to less successful fertility outcomes [21, 22]. The main risk associated with some forms of fertility preservation in men is that testicular tissue cryopreservation (like ovarian tissue cryopreservation) can later reintroduce aggressive cancer cells when reimplanted [21].

As couples make decisions about their fertility preservation options, it is important to determine to what degree the couple deems it important to treat the cancer immediately versus choosing a more effective mode of fertility preservation. A recent survey of cervical cancer patients showed that women who opted for fertility preservation experienced a decrease in distress [23]. Despite this, the delays in cancer treatment that are caused by some fertility preservation options may exacerbate patient and partner distress. Indeed, patients and partners may differ in terms of the level of risk they are willing to take to preserve future fertility. For example, a female cancer patient may view preserving her ability to reproduce as paramount, whereas her partner may view seeking immediate treatment and prolonging life as factors that take precedence over future fertility concerns. Because open, supportive communication may help to decrease marital distress [20], it is important to help couples communicate about their potentially differing priorities about preserving fertility. Similar to the risk of delaying treatment, couples must also agree on the degree of risk they are willing to take when pursuing actual reproductive options later in the future. For instance, a risk associated with auto-transplantation of ovarian cortical strips is the possibility of reintroducing malignant cells that were stored in the tissue that was preserved earlier [24].

In order for couples to communicate effectively about fertility preservation options, it is important that they understand the risks and benefits associated with each of the preservation options that are available to them. Unfortunately, cancer patients frequently report deficits in knowledge and information about fertility preservation [25]. Providing informational and communication support for cancer patients and their partners has been shown to effectively facilitate cancer treatment decision-making and reduce levels of distress [26]. Healthcare professionals who provide this type of support may also facilitate fertility preservation decision-making and reduce the distress associated with making these decisions.

Summary

The various risks associated with fertility preservation options can heighten couple distress during an already stressful time (e.g., at diagnosis, before treatment commences). In addition to choosing a mode of fertility preservation, couples must also grapple with the potentially distressing [27] ethical and moral issues surrounding fertility preservation such as whether they want to create fertilized embryos. These issues will be discussed in the following section.

Ethical and Legal Concerns of Fertility Preservation

Ethical Concerns

One ethical concern for couples is that the patient and his or her partner may not agree on the mode of fertility preservation they would like to pursue. If couples do not agree, physicians may need to consider the rights of the patient to make his or her own decisions about future fertility apart from his or her partner. The possibility of the premature death of the patient is another ethical concern. For instance, what are the ethical implications of reproducing when one of the partners (the cancer survivor) may have a shortened lifespan, leaving the child with only a single parent? Although this concern has been raised, the Ethics Committee of the American Society for Reproductive Medicine determined that the possibility of being raised in a single parent home is, "not a sufficient reason to deny cancer patients assistance in reproducing" [28]. The risk and potential burden of becoming a single parent early in one's child's life, however, could be an area of great distress for the partner. Thus, discussion about this risk prior to reproducing posttreatment is an important issue for couples to consider. Finally, couples may have differing values, morals, and beliefs that influence their willingness to pursue certain fertility preservation options. For instance, some patients opt not to create or store embryos for ethical, religious, or personal reasons [29]. If a cancer patient and his or her partner do not hold the same ethical, religious, or moral views on the various modes of fertility preservation, extreme conflict could occur, potentially causing strain on the couple's relationship. Ultimately, if this distress and conflict are not handled appropriately, it could prevent one or both partners from obtaining the fertility preservation option they prefer.

Legal Concerns

Very little research has focused on the unique legal issues associated with couples' rights in fertility preservation and later reproduction. One issue is the legal rights to any resulting gametes (e.g., sperm or eggs) created during this fertility preservation stage [30]. Although gametes and tissue remain the sole possession of the person they were removed from, individuals may choose to leave their gametes to their partners through planned gamete donation [30]. As such, it is imperative that cancer patients leave written documents with detailed directions for the disposition of remaining tissue and/or donation of gametes to one's partner for posthumous reproduction [31]. In the case of posthumous reproduction, it is recommended that the surviving partner wait a minimum of 1 year to allow for proper grieving to occur before using the gametes [30].

A more complicated legal issue involves the legal rights to any resulting embryos created. Rights to embryos is a more complicated legal issue than rights to gametes or tissue because both the egg and sperm donor technically have legal rights to the embryo [30], which in this case is likely to be the patient and his or her partner. Conflict over the rights to embryos is likely to occur if the patient and his or her partner disagree about the later use of embryos such as might be the case in separation, divorce, or even death [30]. Changes in the status of a donor (egg or sperm), such as in cases of divorce, can make the ownership of the resulting embryos legally complicated [32]. Unfortunately, there is still much legal ambiguity surrounding this issue. To help address this problem, some infertility clinics have started to create contracts which specify how embryos will be managed should the parties divorce, die, or disagree on the future use of embryos [30]. This can be an important step in avoiding later legal battles and confusion surrounding the rights to the resulting embryos. Some clinics go so far as to suggest that the woman fertilize half her eggs with her partner's sperm and the other half with donor sperm to avoid the legal battles that could ensue in the case of separation or divorce [30]. Because partners are one of the primary sources of social support for cancer patients during this stressful time of cancer diagnosis and treatment [33], forcing couples to plan for a scenario in which they would later be divorced or separated may be distressing or even unimaginable for the couple. As such, contracts instructing how to handle future embryos may be the best solution to this legal issue.

Summary

Because the rights of two parties to stored tissue, gametes, or embryos are involved, couples face more complicated ethical and legal issues than single individuals. For instance, couples must reconcile potentially differing beliefs, morals, or ethics surrounding various modes of fertility preservation. Moreover, couples also face unique legal issues such as who will have legal rights to the resulting preserved embryos and whether or not there can be posthumous reproduction. In some instances, couples may need to provide legal documentation as to the rights of gametes and embryos. Due to the need for this legal documentation, it is important for an expert to communicate the ethical and legal issues involved in fertility preservation to couples so that they may make an informed decision together.

In reviewing all barriers and issues involved in couples' oncofertility discussions, it is apparent that partners' involvement in oncofertility discussions is crucial. Previous research has indicated that improving couple's communication among cancer patients and their partners has reduced marital distress [20], yet little research has examined how improving couple's communication could reduce distress related to fertility preservation decision-making and potential infertility due to cancer treatment. In the next section, we discuss areas for future research that can be examined to better understand the barriers to oncofertility communication that couples experience. Additionally, we provide recommendations on how to improve couples' oncofertility communication based on the literature of couples' psychosocial adaptation to cancer.

Need to Develop Models for Involving Partners in Oncofertility Communication

Research Agenda

Marital distress. As noted earlier, an important area of potential research is the impact of cancer patients' fertility issues on marital functioning. Although we know that most couples experience infertility as a stressful experience [8], we still do not know if the cancer experience compounds or exacerbates this. Additionally, infertility related to cancer treatment may lead to decreases in relationship and sexual satisfaction given the established associations between infertility and decreases in sexual and marital satisfaction in healthy couples (i.e., those not afflicted with cancer) [14–16]. Given this, the compounding effects of cancer, sexual problems, and infertility may lead to high levels of sexual dissatisfaction marital distress.

Another issue that may further decrease sexual satisfaction is the struggle with masculine or feminine identity that many cancer patients experience once discovering the potential infertility cancer may cause [12]. Both men and women view the ability to reproduce as a strong part of their masculine and feminine identities, and cancer treatment's potential to lead to infertility may cause a threat to this identity [34]. Additionally, the impact that loss of control over one's life has on distress should also be examined in future research. Past research indicates that both being unable to reproduce [8] and a life-threatening event like cancer [35] can cause a loss of control over one's life. Future research could examine if these two combined effects compound to create an even greater sense of loss of control of one's life. This loss of control over one's life, in turn, may lead to increases in distress.

Couple's communication and decision-making. Increases in marital distress and decreases in sexual and relationship satisfaction may contribute to the larger issues of communication, coping, and decision-making difficulties surrounding fertility preservation. Because the relationship can be an important resource for partners to draw upon to facilitate emotional and psychological adaptation to cancer [36], it is important to determine ways to cope with these issues. Interventions aimed at improving couples' communication, reciprocal understanding, and intimacy have been the most successful at reducing distress and improving relationship functioning among cancer patients and their partners [37]. Interventions based on similar principles may also help to ameliorate the marital and psychological distress that accompanies the fertility challenges and decisions associated with cancer and its treatment. Below we discuss promising avenues for clinical interventions designed to improve couples' communication regarding fertility preservation and potential infertility based on the literature on couples' coping and adjustment to cancer.

Clinical Agenda

Involving partners in oncofertility discussions. Because cancer patients identify their partners as the most used and most helpful fertility discussion partner [7], and infertility related to cancer treatment may carry with it feelings of regret or anger about the fertility preservation decision made, it is crucial to involve partners in oncofertility discussions as early as possible. One way to do this is for healthcare professionals to discuss available options with both patients and their partners, together. Given the deficits in knowledge regarding fertility preservation reported by cancer patients [25], it is apparent that patients and their partners are in need of more information regarding the risks, benefits, and ethical and legal issues associated with each of their fertility preservation options. A multidisciplinary team could be helpful in navigating patients and partners through the process of making fertility preservation decisions [24]. For example, a team of providers, including a medical oncologist, a reproductive endocrinologist, a pathologist, a psychologist, and a legal expert, could work with patients and their partners throughout the fertility preservation process as well as later with the reproductive process. These specialists could be utilized to present patients and their partners with all of their fertility preservation options, discuss the risks and benefits of each option, and discuss the ethical and legal issues associated with choosing a mode of fertility preservation. Once patients and partners have been adequately informed about fertility preservation options, a psychologist could be utilized to improve communication between patients and their partners as well as ultimately help them make a decision together. Finally, a legal expert from this team could guide couples in how to create the necessary legal documents to ensure that their intended fertility preservation decisions are carried out. Improving information and communication support has been shown to be effective in both improving cancer treatment decision-making [26] and reducing distress and improving relationship functioning among cancer patients and their partners [37]. Similarly, providing the informational and communication support for couples discussed in this section regarding fertility preservation options may also aid in the decision-making process and improve relationship outcomes.

Improving couples' communication. Because negative couples' communication can have adverse effects on adjustment and can increase distress [36], interventions that teach and facilitate adaptive communication regarding oncofertility issues are needed. Helping patients and their partners learn how to engage in healthy communication (e.g., open, supportive, mutually constructive) could help cancer patients cope with potential cancer treatment-related infertility and to make the fertility preservation decision that is the most appropriate for their needs/goals as a couple. Couples may also benefit from utilizing approaches that have been shown in the couples' cancer literature to be effective [37]. For example, one of the most harmful tactics to engage in is protective buffering, in which individuals attempt to protect their partner from being upset or burdened by avoiding conflicts by yielding to one's partner, concealing worry, or hiding concerns [38]. Prior research demonstrates that protective buffering among cancer patients and their partners was negatively associated with marital satisfaction [39]. In contrast, active engagement, which involves including partners in discussions and using constructive problem solving to deal with cancer-related problems [38], has been positively associated with marital satisfaction [39].

Other helpful ways to improve communication include mutual expression of feelings, expressing support and understanding for one's partner's views, resolving problems or disagreements as a team (e.g., joint problem solving), and negotiating solutions [40]. In order to increase the effectiveness of interventions designed to improve these forms of communication, couples should be taught how to engage in these problem-solving skills, how to build teamwork, how to communicate better, and how to approach the issues of fertility preservation and potential infertility as a team [37]. Each of these tactics has been associated with higher levels of marital satisfaction [37, 40]. Avoiding discussion of the issue [41] and forcing one's partner to discuss issues while he/she becomes passive or withdrawn [42] have both been associated with lower marital satisfaction. Similarly, openly discussing fertility concerns as well as concerns about various fertility preservation options rather than avoiding the topic could help benefit couples in dealing with fertility preservation options as well as potential future infertility.

Although most counseling and guidance will be needed pretreatment, patients and their partners may need guidance in decision-making after treatment has ended as well. For instance, when couples are ready to attempt to reproduce, they may face infertility despite efforts to preserve their fertility. Infertility can cause increases in marital distress and decreases in marital satisfaction, intimacy, and sexual satisfaction [8, 14–16]. In the case that infertility occurs, cancer patients and their partners may need clinical interventions to help them cope with infertility.

Summary

This chapter has reviewed the limited research available on couples' issues in oncofertility and the need to involve partners in oncofertility communication. More importantly, however, it has brought an important area to light in the research on oncofertility communication. Namely, the partners of cancer patients also need to be involved in oncofertility communication. Couples bring with them a unique set of issues to the topic of fertility preservation and potential infertility in cancer patients. As such, this area needs to be examined so that clinical interventions can be developed to involve partners in oncofertility communication and, ultimately, to improve couples' communication surrounding oncofertility issues. Our hope is that this chapter has brought this need to light and that researchers will begin to examine these important questions to advance the new but quickly growing field of oncofertility.

Acknowledgement Dr. Shen's work on this project was supported by a cancer prevention fellowship from the National Cancer Institute (5R25CA081137, Guy Montgomery, Ph.D., Principal Investigator) and by the Oncofertility Consortium NIH 5UL1DE019587.

References

1. Mersereau J. Communication between oncofertility providers and patients. In: Gracia C, Woodruff TK, editors. Oncofertility Medical Practice. New York: Springer; 2012. pp. 149–160. Available at: http://link.springer.com/chapter/10.1007/978-1-4419-9425-7_11. Accessed 3 Dec 2012.
2. Schover LR, Rybicki LA, Martin BA, Bringelsen KA. Having children after cancer. Cancer. 1999;86(4):697–709.
3. Connell S, Patterson C, Newman B. Issues and concerns of young Australian women with breast cancer. Support Care Cancer. 2006;14(5):419–26.
4. Fallowfield L, McGurk R, Dixon M. Same gain, less pain: potential patient preferences for adjuvant treatment in premenopausal women with early breast cancer. Eur J Cancer. 2004; 40(16):2403–10.
5. Partridge AH, Gelber S, Peppercorn J, et al. Web-based survey of fertility issues in young women with breast cancer. J Clin Oncol. 2004;22(20):4174–83.
6. Saito K, Suzuki K, Iwasaki A, Yumura Y, Kubota Y. Sperm cryopreservation before cancer chemotherapy helps in the emotional battle against cancer. Cancer. 2005;104(3):521–4.
7. Tschudin S, Bunting L, Abraham J, Gallop-Evans E, Fiander A, Boivin J. Correlates of fertility issues in an Internet survey of cancer survivors. J Psychosom Obstet Gynecol. 2010;31(3):150–7.
8. Cousineau TM, Domar AD. Psychological impact of infertility. Best Pract Res Clin Obstet Gynaecol. 2007;21(2):293–308.

9. Galvin KM, Clayman ML. Whose future is it? Ethical family decision making about daughters' treatment in the oncofertility context. In: Woodruff TK, Zoloth L, Campo-Engelstein L, Rodriguez S, editors. Oncofertility. Cancer Treatment and Research. New York: Springer; 2010. pp. 429–445. Available at: http://link.springer.com/chapter/10.1007/978-1-4419-6518-9_33. Accessed 6 Dec 2012.
10. World Health Organization. Progress report in reproductive health research, No. 23. Geneva, Switzerland; 2003.
11. Greil AL. Infertility and psychological distress: a critical review of the literature. Soc Sci Med. 1997;45(11):1679–704.
12. Schover LR. Psychosocial aspects of infertility and decisions about reproduction in young cancer survivors: a review. Med Pediatr Oncol. 1999;33(1):53–9.
13. Heffner L. Advanced maternal age—how old is too old? N Engl J Med. 2004;351:1927–9.
14. Andrews FM, Abbey A, Halman LJ. Stress from infertility, marriage factors, and subjective well-being of wives and husbands. J Health Soc Behav. 1991;32(3):238.
15. Daniluk JC. Gender and infertility. In: Leiblum SR, editor. Infertility, psychological issues and counseling strategies. New York: John Wiley & Sons; 1997. p. 103–25.
16. Edelmann RJ, Humphrey M, Owens DJ. The meaning of parenthood and couples' reactions to male infertility. Br J Med Psychol. 1994;67(3):291–9.
17. Gritz ER, Wellisch DK, Wang H-J, Siau J, Landsverk JA, Cosgrove MD. Long-term effects of testicular cancer on sexual functioning in married couples. Cancer. 1989;64(7):1560–7.
18. Jensen PT, Groenvold M, Klee MC, Thranov I, Petersen MA, Machin D. Longitudinal study of sexual function and vaginal changes after radiotherapy for cervical cancer. Int J Radiat Oncol Biol Phys. 2003;56(4):937–49.
19. Badr H, Carmack Taylor CL. Sexual dysfunction and spousal communication in couples coping with prostate cancer. Psychooncology. 2009;18:735–46.
20. Markman HJ, Renick MJ, Floyd FJ, Stanley SM, Clements M. Preventing marital distress through communication and conflict management training: a 4- and 5-year follow-up. J Consult Clin Psychol. 1993;61(1):70–7.
21. Woodruff TK. The oncofertility consortium—addressing fertility in young people with cancer. Nat Rev Clin Oncol. 2010;7(8):466–75.
22. Lee SJ, Schover LR, Partridge AH, et al. American Society of Clinical Oncology recommendations on fertility preservation in cancer patients. J Clin Oncol. 2006;24(18):2917–31.
23. Carter J, Rowland K, Chi D, et al. Gynecologic cancer treatment and the impact of cancer-related infertility. Gynecol Oncol. 2005;97(1):90–5.
24. Patrizio P, Butts S, Caplan A. Ovarian tissue preservation and future fertility: emerging technologies and ethical considerations. J Natl Cancer Inst Monogr. 2005;2005(34):107–10.
25. Tschudin S, Bitzer J. Psychological aspects of fertility preservation in men and women affected by cancer and other life-threatening diseases. Hum Reprod Update. 2009;15(5):587–97.
26. Davison B, Goldenberg S, Gleave M, Degner L. Provision of individualized information to men and their partners to facilitate treatment decision making in prostate cancer. Oncol Nurs Forum. 2003;30(1):107–14.
27. Domar AD, Seibel MM. Emotional aspects of infertility. In: Infertility: a comprehensive text. East Norwalk, CT: Appleton & Lange; 1990. p. 23–35.
28. Ethics Committee of the American Society for Reproductive Medicine. Fertility preservation and reproduction in cancer patients. Fertil Steril. 2005;83(6):1622–8.
29. Noyes N, Porcu E, Borini A. Over 900 oocyte cryopreservation babies born with no apparent increase in congenital anomalies. Reprod Biomed Online. 2009;18(6):769–76.
30. Shah DK, Goldman E, Fisseha S. Medical, ethical, and legal considerations in fertility preservation. Int J Gynecol Obstet. 2011;115(1):11–5.
31. Robertson JA. Cancer and fertility: ethical and legal challenges. J Natl Cancer Inst Monogr. 2005;2005(34):104–6.
32. Chian R-C, Huang JY, Tan SL, et al. Obstetric and perinatal outcome in 200 infants conceived from vitrified oocytes. Reprod Biomed Online. 2008;16(5):608–10.
33. Manne S. Couples coping with cancer: research issues and recent findings. J Clin Psychol Med Settings. 1994;1(4):317–30.

34. Gardino S, Rodriguez S, Campo-Engelstein L. Infertility, cancer, and changing gender norms. J Cancer Surviv. 2011;5(2):152–7.
35. Taylor SE. Adjustment to threatening events: a theory of cognitive adaptation. Am Psychol. 1983;38(11):1161–73.
36. Manne S, Badr H. Intimacy and relationship processes in couples' psychosocial adaptation to cancer. Cancer. 2008;112(S11):2541–55.
37. Badr H, Carmack CL, Milbury K, Temech M. Psychosocial interventions for couples coping with cancer: a systematic review. In: Carr BI, Steel J, editors. Psychological aspects of cancer. New York: Springer; 2012. p. 177–98.
38. Coyne JC, Smith DAF. Couples coping with a myocardial infarction: contextual perspective on patient self-efficacy. J Fam Psychol. 1994;8(1):43–54.
39. Hagedoorn M, Kuijer RG, Buunk BP, Majella G, Wobbes T, Sanderman R. Marital satisfaction in patients with cancer: does support from intimate partners benefit those who need it most? Health Psychol. 2000;19(3):274–82.
40. Heavey CL, Larson BM, Zumtobel DC, Christensen A. The communication patterns questionnaire: the reliability and validity of a constructive communication subscale. J Marriage Fam. 1996;58(3):796.
41. Christensen A, Heavey CL. Gender and social structure in the demand/withdraw pattern of marital conflict. J Pers Soc Psychol. 1990;59(1):73–81.
42. Christensen A, Shenk JL. Communication, conflict, and psychological distance in nondistressed, clinic, and divorcing couples. J Consult Clin Psychol. 1991;59(3):458–63.

Chapter 7
Genetic Counselors: Bridging the Oncofertility Information Gap

Allison Goetsch, Amber Volk, and Teresa K. Woodruff

Introduction

Approximately 1,660,290 new cancer cases will be diagnosed in 2013, 805,500 of which will be in women [1]. Approximately 10 % of those cancer diagnoses will occur in individuals younger than 45 years, and thus still within their reproductive years [2]. Additionally, the 5-year relative survival rate for all cancers diagnosed between 2002 and 2008 is 68 %, up from 49 % between 1975 and 1977 [1]. The increase in survival rate can be attributed to progress in earlier diagnosis and improvements in treatment. With an increase in cancer survival, we can expect that more young women diagnosed with cancer will be seeking information about fertility preservation prior to cancer treatment. In fact, approximately 75 % of young adult cancer survivors who have not previously had children express a desire for children in the future [2].

The goal of oncofertility is to balance life-preserving cancer treatments with fertility preserving options. Three main gaps have created an unmet need for preserving fertility in patients with cancer: an information gap, a data gap, and an option gap. The information gap, in particular, involves a lack of cancer patient understanding regarding the effects of cancer treatment on fertility and the option of fertility preservation. Many cancer patients do not recall ever discussing the impact of cancer treatment on fertility with their physician; because of this,

A. Goetsch, B.S., M.S. (✉)
Center for Genetic Medicine, Northwestern University, 676 N St. Clair, Chicago IL 60611, USA
e-mail: allisongoetsch2014@u.northwestern.edu

A. Volk
Department of Medical Genetics, Mayo Clinic, Rochester, MN, USA

T.K. Woodruff, Ph.D.
Department of Obstetrics and Gynecology, Feinberg School of Medicine, Northwestern University, Chicago, IL, USA

T.K. Woodruff et al. (eds.), *Oncofertility Communication: Sharing Information and Building Relationships across Disciplines*, DOI 10.1007/978-1-4614-8235-2_7,

multidisciplinary care that includes fertility treatment is especially valuable for bridging the information gap. In particular, genetic counselors, who are specifically trained to deliver options and facilitate decision making while also focusing on psychosocial issues, are an untapped resource for educating cancer patients about fertility impairment and fertility preservation options. Genetic counselors have the skills necessary to bridge the oncofertility information gap.

The Oncofertility Information Gap

Advances in cancer diagnostics and treatments have redefined the previous treatment-based approach to a broader perspective including survivorship and quality of life [3]. This new longer-term perspective on cancer care has revealed gaps in clinician–patient education, communication, and decision support with regard to fertility preservation that need to be addressed.

Lack of Oncofertility Patient Education and Communication

As part of their care, oncology healthcare providers should not only focus on the short-term goal of treatment and survival but also help cancer patients to preserve the best possible quality of life, including the possibility of having children [4]. If women are not informed of the risk that cancer treatment poses to their fertility, they may lose the opportunity to preserve their fertility prior to cancer treatment [5]. Even women who choose not to become parents value the opportunity to preserve their fertility [6]. Fertility preservation is especially important in adolescent and young adult patients with cancer, and unfortunately it is one of the most underprescribed and least implemented services in their cancer care [7]. The National Comprehensive Cancer Network (NCCN) guidelines for young adults with cancer state that fertility preservation should be an essential part of cancer management, and the risk of infertility associated with cancer therapy should be discussed at the time of diagnosis [7]. Yet, up to 75 % of young women express interest in the opportunity to have children after a cancer diagnosis, but as few as 34 % of reproductive-age women treated for cancer recall having a discussion about the effects of cancer treatment on fertility [5]. The lack of patient education about fertility preservation is associated with the desire of the healthcare provider to start cancer treatment immediately, a lack of adequate knowledge regarding fertility preservation by the cancer care team, and insufficient provider–patient communication skills.

Many oncologists leave little time to discuss future fertility or options for fertility preservation with their patients because the immediate focus is on cancer treatment [8]. In their recent survey of women with cancer and healthcare professionals involved in cancer care, Peddie et al. reported that few women were afforded the opportunity to discuss the benefits and limitations of fertility preservation options available to them [8]. The clinical staff felt justified in withholding fertility information from women and guiding their decision making because of their belief that treatment was urgently needed, fertility preservation techniques were not effective or useful, or that fertility would not be affected by first-line chemotherapy.

In addition to their focus on the immediate need to start treatment, healthcare providers may not have adequate knowledge or sufficient communication skills to counsel concerned patients in a timely and supportive manner [9]. Physicians rarely ask about patients' concerns and questions in the oncology setting [10]. Some oncologists cite that lack of discussion is due to the perception that if a patient did not raise the issue themselves, then they were not interested [5].

Patient communication involves not only the transfer of information but also the provision of psychological and emotional support. Emotional support for young women with cancer is especially important because they experience greater distress and less emotional well-being than older women [3]. Without proper training in patient counseling, however, oncology providers may find it challenging to offer psychological and emotional support to their patients. Counseling requires the ability to take into account a patient's individual background, provide information and support in a timely and accurate manner, and address the patient's emotional needs [9]. In a recent study by Kirkman et al., young women with cancer reported that their psychosocial needs were not met and staff numbers in psychology and counseling were inadequate [6]. In another study, women cancer survivors reported that fertility was a vital concern because they wanted to preserve not only quality of life after cancer but also protect their mental and emotional health [4]. Patients also report wanting healthcare providers who are honest, compassionate, and patient [11]. We believe that healthcare providers with proper training in counseling are better equipped to provide emotional support to cancer patients and therefore facilitate discussions of fertility preservation and post-cancer quality of life.

To address psychosocial and behavioral issues, the NCCN provides a detailed list of support healthcare workers who can provide counseling to young adults with cancer. These patients need healthcare providers who are able to assess cognitive function, emotional issues, and evaluate other psychiatric symptoms, depression, and anxiety. Additionally, healthcare providers offering psychosocial support to young adult cancer patients need to be able to take into consideration patient existential/spiritual issues, personal relationships, decision-making preferences, and communication preferences that may affect cancer treatment and fertility preservation decisions [7].

Lack of Oncofertility Patient Decision Support

A lack of support for patient decision making also contributes to the oncofertility information gap. Patients value fertility preservation and those healthcare providers who recognize that child bearing is a future option [6]. Patients want healthcare providers to offer options—including a discussion of the off-target effects of cancer treatment—and to support the decision to try for pregnancy after cancer treatment [6]. Patients can be particularly troubled when their fertility concerns are not well managed. In the Kirkman et al. study, some women reported feeling excluded from discussions and decision making about their own fertility [6]. They were given minimal information and regret not being treated with consideration, especially when unwarranted assumptions were made about their fertility plans.

Healthcare providers should not assume that they understand patient fears, priorities, or preferences related to their cancer treatment and fertility preservation. Doing so may influence the quality of the information a provider gives to a patient [8]. Alternatively, healthcare providers should be supportive of patient decisions and implement the use of the shared decision-making model, discussed in more detail below.

Multidisciplinary Care

The oncofertility information gap can be addressed with multidisciplinary care. Kirkman et al. identified this team approach to cancer care as especially valuable in their qualitative study of the significance of fertility and motherhood after a cancer diagnosis [6]. Multidisciplinary team members should be experienced in cancer care as well as sensitive to fertility concerns. Cancer patients report a desire for referral to fertility specialists, psychological support, and counseling, emphasizing the importance of a multidisciplinary approach to cancer care that includes fertility preservation [6].

Multidisciplinary care also mitigates the need for the integration of the sensitive topic of fertility into an already overwhelming oncology consultation. Patients are given a lot of information at their first oncology visit and are also at their most vulnerable [8]. A discussion of fertility and fertility preservation may not be beneficial or realistic immediately after a cancer diagnosis. Research suggests that recruiting the help of healthcare workers who have special training to address fertility issues in the confusing period of time just after a cancer diagnosis can be helpful [12].

The Role of the Genetic Counselor

Genetic counselors are medical professionals who have undergone extensive graduate level human genetics and psychosocial coursework. They possess the necessary skill sets to deliver options and facilitate decision making while also focusing on psychosocial issues. The four critical domains that genetic counselors demonstrate competency in are communication, critical thinking, psychosocial assessment, and professional ethics and values [13]. A typical genetic counseling session for a patient with cancer may involve the following components: pedigree analysis, risk assessment, genetic testing options, genetic testing results interpretation, facilitation of medical management decision making, and discussion of risk for family members.

Genetic counseling practice is guided by the ethical principle of nondirectiveness [14]. A nondirective counseling approach allows genetic counselors to support client autonomy and facilitate informed patient decision making [15]. Additionally, psychosocial training gives genetic counselors the necessary skill set to provide emotional support to patients as well as make mental health referrals when needed. Genetic counselors who work in cancer clinics are in the unique position of being able to utilize their skill sets to discuss fertility preservation options with patients in that sensitive window of time prior to cancer treatment or prophylactic surgery.

Nondirectiveness

The guiding ethical principle of genetic counseling—nondirectiveness—is an active counseling strategy used by genetic counselors to promote patient autonomy. The goal of this approach is to increase patient self-esteem and enable patients to make independent, informed decisions free from coercion [16]. Nondirective counseling techniques employed by genetic counselors leave patients with greater sense of control over their lives and decisions [14]. The nondirective approach used by genetic counselors differs from the typical healthcare provider content-oriented approach. Nondirectiveness is person-oriented, meaning that it places emphasis on what facts and information mean to a patient as well as the intrapsychic and interpersonal consequences of these meanings [16]. In order to implement a nondirective counseling approach, genetic counselors begin by identifying their own personal biases and intentions [16]. This is done in order to direct the process of genetic counseling but not direct the outcome.

Decision Making

Important medical decisions that affect quality of life, such as whether to pursue fertility preservation prior to cancer treatment, should follow the shared decision-making model. With this approach, healthcare providers are respectful of their patients' perspectives and take into consideration patient values and self-efficacy. Patients should be informed of all relevant options, including the corresponding risks and benefits, in order to make informed medical decisions [17]. Genetic counselors facilitate informed medical decision making by patients for genetic testing, screening, and treatment, including chemoprevention and risk-reducing surgery. They are able to provide relevant information, reduce anxiety, and empower patients to make decisions through nondirective counseling.

Shared decision making has four key principles. The first is that two participants are involved—the patient and the healthcare provider. Genetic counselors take steps to develop a partnership with their patient. The second principle is the sharing of information. Genetic counselors first establish and review patients' preferences for receiving information and then respond to ideas, concerns, and expectations. A decision being made is the third principle. To do this, genetic counselors identify choices and evaluate available evidence, then present the evidence and help the patient reflect upon and assess the impact of alternatives in the context of their values and lifestyle. The fourth principle of the shared decision-making model is both parties agreeing to the decision. Genetic counselors use their skills to manage conflicts that arise from the decision. They also agree upon an action plan and arrange for follow up [18].

Psychosocial training allows genetic counselors to assess which phase of the decision-making process a patient is in: identify, contemplate, resolve, and engage. Once a genetic counselor has assessed the stage of the decision-making process, they can use the appropriate counseling techniques to reach the goal of a firm decision.

Psychosocial Skills

Genetic counselors undergo extensive psychosocial training that allows them to provide emotional support to cancer patients, assess patient psychosocial situations, and provide the appropriate mental health referrals. Examples of techniques genetic counselors use to gather and assess psychosocial information from patients include reflective listening, assessment of patient understanding, and empathy.

Reflective listening is a patient-centered approach that involves more listening than talking [9]. Genetic counselors respond to personal statements that patients make, rather than to impersonal, distant, or abstract thoughts. The technique of restating and clarifying what a patient has said is commonly used by genetic counselors to assess the emotional state of patients. Reflective listening allows understanding of the feelings involved in what a patient is saying, not just the facts or ideas [9].

Another technique genetic counselors use to provide psychosocial and emotional support is eliciting the patient's understanding and evaluation of the provided information [9]. Additionally, genetic counselors use acceptance and empathy when responding to patients.

Genetic counselors can reduce patient anxiety, enhance the patient's sense of control and mastery over life circumstances, increase patient understanding of the genetic disease and options for testing and disease management, and provide the individual and family with the tools required to adjust to potential outcomes [13]. The unique skill set of genetic counselors can be used to address the effects of cancer treatment on fertility as well as fertility preservation techniques for women with a personal or family history suggestive of a hereditary or familial cancer.

Genetic Counselors and Fertility Preservation

Volk et al. conducted a research study to estimate genetic counselors' attitudes, knowledge, and discussion of fertility preservation in referred breast and ovarian cancer patients, including *BRCA1* and *BRCA2* mutation-positive patients [19]. A total of 218 genetic counselors participated in the research study, citing an average of 15.5 breast or ovarian cancer patients per month and 2.4 *BRCA* mutation-positive patients per month. Of these, more than 50 % had a basic understanding of embryo cryopreservation, egg cryopreservation, ovarian tissue cryopreservation, and emergency IVF, and were aware of fertility preservation research. Several study themes emerged, including the general belief that fertility preservation discussions are important and part of the role of the genetic counselor. The study also identified barriers that prevent genetic counselors from discussing fertility preservation with their breast and ovarian cancer patients; the primary obstacle was the timing of cancer treatment.

Genetic Counseling for Breast and Ovarian Cancer

In the general population, approximately 12 % of women will develop breast cancer and 1.4 % will develop ovarian cancer in their lifetime [1]. It is estimated that 29 % of all new female cancer diagnoses in 2013 will be breast cancer and 3 % of all new female cancer diagnoses will be ovarian cancer [1]. Approximately 3–7 % of women with early-stage breast cancer are under the age of 40 at diagnosis [1], and therefore may be interested in learning how cancer treatment can affect fertility as well as fertility preservation options.

Between 5 and 10 % of breast and ovarian cancers are associated with a hereditary predisposition [20, 21]. Deleterious mutations in the *BRCA1* and *BRCA2* genes cause 80 % of hereditary breast cancer and 90 % of hereditary ovarian cancer [20]. The average age of hereditary breast or ovarian cancer diagnosis in women is lower than that in the general population. For women with the *BRCA1* mutation, the average age at diagnosis is 39.9–44.1 years for breast cancer and 49–53 years for ovarian cancer; for women with a *BRCA2* mutation, the average age of diagnosis is 42.2–47.3 years for breast cancer and 55–58 years for ovarian cancer. By comparison, in the general population, the average age of diagnosis is 61 years for breast cancer and 63 years for ovarian cancer [22].

Female *BRCA* mutation carriers have much higher lifetime risk of ovarian cancer, between 15 and 60 %, compared to the general population risk of 1–2 %. Even with current screening options—CA-125 testing and transvaginal ultrasound—ovarian cancer is difficult to detect at an early, treatable stage.

Therefore, the NCCN and the American College of Obstetricians and Gynecologists (ACOG) recommend that *BRCA* mutation-positive women consider undergoing risk-reducing prophylactic bilateral salpingo-oophorectomy (BSO) between 35 and 40 years of age, or when childbearing is complete [11, 22, 23]. Prophylactic BSO at ages younger than 35 may be recommended based on family history [11]. Greater than 80 % of women with a *BRCA* mutation who are eligible for prophylactic BSO will pursue surgery [11]. Campfield et al. found that of 98 female *BRCA* carriers, 85 % pursued PBSO after learning of their *BRCA* status and 48 % were premenopausal at the time [11]. Additionally, 70.4 % of the study participants had discussed their surgery with a genetic counselor, while another 11.8 % would have liked their healthcare providers to refer them to a genetic counselor and direct them to other resources or programs for additional information [11].

Women with *BRCA* gene mutations may have additional concerns about passing on hereditary cancer to future children [24]. Preimplantation genetic diagnosis (PGD) is one option for parents who want to prevent this possibility. Since 2006, PGD has been used in conjunction with in vitro fertilization (IVF) to screen for specific genetic or chromosomal abnormalities, including *BRCA* gene mutations [24]. Genetic counselors can discuss the possibility of PGD with women who have hereditary breast or ovarian cancer and are considering fertility preservation.

Individuals with a personal or family history suggestive of a hereditary or familial cancer should be referred for further counseling and risk assessment [25], whether to genetic counselors or other healthcare professionals who are trained to do so. For patients who have a personal or family history suggestive of a hereditary or familial cancer, a genetic counseling session to discuss breast and ovarian cancer treatment, *BRCA1/BRCA2* mutation testing, and prophylactic surgery provides an opportune time to discuss the effect of cancer treatment on fertility and fertility preservation options.

Genetic Counselor Attitudes Towards Fertility Preservation

Almost all (98.7 %) of the participating genetic counselors in the Volk et al. study agreed or strongly agreed that breast and ovarian cancer patients should be told of the risk to fertility associated with cancer treatments [19]. In addition, the majority (95.4 %) agreed that patients should be offered a fertility preservation referral prior to cancer treatment, and (85.9 %) agreed if one was not offered prior to treatment, a referral should be offered after cancer treatment. Approximately 70.2 % of genetic counselors believed that discussing fertility preservation with their breast and ovarian cancer patients is part of their role as genetic counselors. A majority (61 % and 65.4 %, respectively) also stated that both cancer and *BRCA* mutation-positive patients have asked about the potential threats to their fertility caused by treatment. In fact, most genetic counselors stated that fertility options were a major concern for all of their cancer patients (51.7 %) as well as *BRCA* mutation-positive patients (63.8 %).

Fertility preservation was a major concern for those *BRCA* mutation-positive patients who were considering prophylactic BSO; 85.5 % of genetic counselors agreed that *BRCA* mutation-positive patients should be offered a fertility referral prior to undergoing this procedure, and 71.1 % reported that they have had patients inquire about the associated fertility complications of BSO.

The majority of genetic counselors in the study stated that cancer patients have asked about fertility problems associated with both surgical and nonsurgical treatment options, *BRCA* mutation-positive patients have asked about problems associated with prophylactic oophorectomy, and in general, fertility is a major concern for both breast and ovarian cancer patients as well as *BRCA* mutation-positive patients. They also believe that fertility preservation should involve a multidisciplinary team of health care professionals, including oncologists, reproductive endocrinologists, and fertility preservation specialists, as well as obstetrician/gynecologists, surgeons, radiation oncologists, and social workers and genetic counselors.

Inconsistencies in Genetic Counselor Attitudes and Actions

Despite believing that genetic counselors should discuss fertility preservation with their breast and ovarian cancer patients, including those who are *BRCA* mutation-positive, only 17.9 % said that they often or always discuss egg or embryo cryopreservation with these patients. Even fewer genetic counselors (8.5 %) discuss ovarian tissue cryopreservation. The same trend is seen in genetic counselor patient referrals to fertility specialists: 98.7 % of genetic counselors believe cancer patients should be offered a referral prior to treatment, yet only 11.1 % of genetic counselors often or always refer cancer patients to a fertility specialist prior to treatment. These numbers are slightly higher for *BRCA* mutation-positive patients, with 33 % of genetic counselors expressing the belief that fertility preservation should be considered prior to prophylactic treatment and 23.1 % of genetic counselors often or always discussing embryo or egg cryopreservation. For referrals to a fertility specialist, 16.7 % of genetic counselors often or always refer their *BRCA* mutation-positive patients and 35.2 % refer when the patient is considering a prophylactic BSO.

Barriers to Discussions of Fertility Preservation by Genetic Counselors

The major barrier that prevents more frequent discussion of fertility preservation in genetic counseling sessions is the fact that breast and ovarian cancer patients are seeing genetic counselors after cancer treatment (reported by 79.7 % in the Volk et al. study). Only 29.5 % of genetic counselors reported seeing breast and ovarian cancer patients prior to cancer treatment [19]. Ideally, discussion of fertility preservation should occur before cancer treatment. When genetic counseling sessions are held prior to cancer treatment, genetic counselors can integrate fertility preservation into the cancer treatment options discussion and facilitation of patient decision making.

Genetic counselors also cited timing as the number one barrier to discussing fertility preservation with *BRCA* mutation positive patients. Genetic counselors can discuss management options such as prophylactic BSO with their *BRCA* mutation-positive patients; again, this would be an optimal time for discussing fertility preservation options. While the majority of genetic counselors (78.5 %) reported that *BRCA* mutation-positive patients choose not to undergo prophylactic treatment, including prophylactic BSO, for those that do select this procedure prior to completing their family, genetic counselors can use their unique skill set to integrate fertility preservation information into genetic counseling sessions prior to surgery.

Conclusion: Genetic Counselors Can Bridge the Oncofertility Information Gap

The goal of oncofertility is to balance life-preserving cancer treatments with fertility preservation options. Gaps in information, data, and options have led to an unmet need for preserving fertility in patients with cancer. The information gap, in particular, involves a lack of cancer patient education about fertility impairment associated with cancer treatment and fertility preservation options. As few as 34 % of reproductive-age women treated for cancer recall discussing the effect of cancer treatment on fertility [5], yet NCCN guidelines for young adults with cancer state that fertility preservation should be an essential part of cancer management and the effects of treatment on fertility should be discussed at the time of diagnosis [7]. The oncofertility information gap can be attributed to the healthcare provider's desire to start treatment immediately, lack of adequate knowledge regarding fertility preservation, and insufficient communication and counseling skills.

The oncofertility information gap can be addressed with the implementation of a multidisciplinary approach to fertility preservation. Many patients have emphasized the importance of having access to not only fertility specialists and oncologists, but also psychological support and counseling [6]. Meeting this need has led to recommendations for a healthcare worker with special training to address the sensitive topic of fertility preservation separate from the often overwhelming initial oncology consultation [12].

According to Volk et al., genetic counselors believe that fertility preservation discussions are important and that they are a part of the genetic counselor's role in cancer care [19]. Genetic counselors possess the necessary skills to bridge the oncofertility information gap with their patients—those who have a personal of family history suggestive of familial or hereditary cancer. The four critical domains that genetic counselors contribute to the cancer care team are communication skills, critical thinking skills, psychosocial assessment training, and professional ethics and values [13]. Unlike the traditional treatment-based discussions with patients, genetic counselors use a nondirective, patient-centered counseling approach to facilitate shared decision making.

The NCCN guidelines for young adult cancer recommend a genetic and familial risk assessment within the first 2 months after the start of treatment [7]. However, because timing of cancer treatment is identified as the number one barrier to genetic counselors' ability to discuss potential threats to fertility and fertility preservation options, healthcare providers should refer young women diagnosed with cancer to a genetic counselor prior to cancer treatment. Genetic counselors have a unique skill set that allows them to discuss options, facilitate decision making, and make valuable psychosocial assessments that may underlie cancer treatment and subsequent fertility preservation. Genetic counselors can use their skill set to effectively bridge the oncofertility information gap for patients with a personal or family history suggestive of a hereditary or familial cancer.

Acknowledgements This work was supported by the Oncofertility Consortium NIH 5UL1DE019587 and the Specialized Cooperative Centers Program in Reproduction and Infertility Research NIH U54HD076188.

References

1. American Cancer Society. Cancer facts & figures 2013. Atlanta, GA: American Cancer Society; 2013.
2. Jeruss JS, Woodruff TK. Preservation of fertility in patients with cancer. N Engl J Med. 2009;360:902–11.
3. Hershberger PE, Finnegan L, Pierce PF, Scoccia B. The decision-making process of young adult women with cancer who considered fertility cryopreservation. J Obstet Gynecol Neonatal Nurs. 2013;42:59–69.
4. Yee S, Abrol K, McDonald M, Tonelli M, Liu KE. Addressing oncofertility needs: views of female cancer patients in fertility preservation. J Psychosoc Oncol. 2012;30:331–46.
5. Letourneau JM, Ebbel EE, Katz PP, Katz A, Ai WZ, Chien AJ, Melisko ME, Cedars MI, Rosen MP. Pretreatment fertility counseling and fertility preservation improve quality of life in reproductive age women with cancer. Cancer. 2012;118:1710–7.
6. Kirkman M, Stern C, Neil S, Winship I, Mann GB, Shanahan K, Missen D, Shepherd H, Fisher JR. Fertility management after breast cancer diagnosis: a qualitative investigation of women's experiences of and recommendations for professional care. Health Care Women Int. 2013; 34:50–67.
7. Coccia PF, Altman J, Bhatia S, Borinstein SC, Flynn J, George S, Goldsby R, Hayashi R, Huang MS, Johnson RH, Beaupin LK, Link MP, Oeffinger KC, Orr KM, Pappo AS, Reed D, Spraker HL, Thomas DA, von Mehren M, Wechsler DS, Whelan KF, Zebrack BJ, Sundar H, Shead DA. Adolescent and young adult oncology. Clinical practice guidelines in oncology. J Natl Compr Canc Netw. 2012;10:1112–50.
8. Peddie V, Porter M, Barbour R, Culligan D, MacDonald G, King D, Horn J, Bhattacharya S. Factors affecting decision making about fertility preservation after cancer diagnosis: a qualitative study. BJOG. 2012;119:1049–57.
9. Tschudin S, Bitzer J. Psychological aspects of fertility preservation in men and women affected by cancer and other life-threatening diseases. Hum Reprod Update. 2009;15:587–97.
10. Hayat Roshanai A, Lampic C, Ingvoldstad C, Askmalm MS, Bjorvatn C, Rosenquist R, Nordin K. What information do cancer genetic counselees prioritize? J Genet Couns. 2012;21:510–26.
11. Campfield Bonadies D, Moyer A, Matloff ET. What I wish I'd known before surgery: BRCA carriers' perspectives after bilateral salipingo-oophorectomy. Fam Cancer. 2011;10:79–85.

12. Lee MC, Gray J, Han HS, Plosker S. Fertility and reproductive considerations in premenopausal patients with breast cancer. Cancer Control. 2010;17:162–72.
13. Bennett RL, Hampel HL, Mandell JB, Marks JH. Genetic counselors: translating genomic science into clinical practice. J Clin Invest. 2003;112:1274–9.
14. Uhlmann WR, Schuette JL, Yashar BM. A guide to genetic counseling. Hoboken, NJ: Wiley; 2009.
15. Weil J. Psychosocial genetic counseling. New York: Oxford University Press; 2000.
16. Veach PM, LeRoy BS, Bartels DM. Facilitating the genetic counseling process: a practice manual. New York: Springer; 2003.
17. Clayman ML, Galvin KM, Arntson P. Shared decision making: fertility and pediatric cancers. In: Woodruff TK, Snyder KA, editors. Oncofertility. New York: Springer Science+Business Media, LLC.; 2007.
18. Elwyn G, Gray J, Clarke A. Shared decision making and non-directiveness in genetic counselling. J Med Genet. 2000;37:135–8.
19. Volk A, Aufox S, Fallen T, Beaumont J, Woodruff TK. Genetic Counselor attitudes, knowledge, and discussions of fertility preservation in the hereditary breast and ovarian cancer clinic. [unpublished manuscript]; 2012.
20. Berliner JL, Fay AM. Practice Issues Subcommittee of the National Society of Genetic Counselors' Familial Cancer Risk Counseling Special Interest G. Risk assessment and genetic counseling for hereditary breast and ovarian cancer: recommendations of the National Society of Genetic Counselors. J Genet Couns. 2007;16:241–60.
21. Wevers MR, Hahn DE, Verhoef S, Bolhaar MD, Ausems MG, Aaronson NK, Bleiker EM. Breast cancer genetic counseling after diagnosis but before treatment: a pilot study on treatment consequences and psychological impact. Patient Educ Couns. 2012;89:89–95.
22. Miesfeldt S, Lamb A, Duarte C. Management of genetic syndromes predisposing to gynecologic cancers. Curr Treat Options Oncol. 2013;14:34–50.
23. Domchek SM, Friebel TM, Neuhausen SL, Wagner T, Evans G, Isaacs C, Garber JE, Daly MB, Eeles R, Matloff E, Tomlinson GE, Van't Veer L, Lynch HT, Olopade OI, Weber BL, Rebbeck TR. Mortality after bilateral salpingo-oophorectomy in BRCA1 and BRCA2 mutation carriers: a prospective cohort study. Lancet Oncol. 2006;7:223–9.
24. Quinn G, Vadaparampil S, Wilson C, King L, Choi J, Miree C, Friedman S. Attitudes of high-risk women toward preimplantation genetic diagnosis. Fertil Steril. 2009;91:2361–8.
25. Shulman LP, Dungan JS. Cancer genetics: risks and mechanisms of cancer in women with inherited susceptibility to epithelial ovarian cancer. In: Woodruff TK, Zoloth L, Campo-Engelstein L, Rodriguez S, editors. Oncofertility ethical, legal, social, and medical perspectives. New York: Springer Science+Business Media, LLC.; 2010.

Chapter 8
Communicating Oncofertility to Children: A Developmental Perspective for Teaching Health Messages

Ellen Wartella, Alexis R. Lauricella, and Lisa B. Hurwitz

Introduction

Oncofertility is a new discipline that focuses on the intersection of oncology and fertility [1]. People often think about cancer as a disease that occurs in aging populations. While this is true, there are a number of cancers that affect children and younger adults, resulting in a population of cancer patients and survivors whose cancer treatment may impact their future fertility. With young cancer patients, especially children, communicating about cancer is undeniably an arduous task, which makes communication about the impact that cancer and its treatment may have on their future fertility even more complex.

Communicating health information generally, and information about sexuality and health more specifically, requires an understanding of what is developmentally appropriate for children to comprehend. Research shows that children under age 7 struggle with abstract concepts and hypothetical reasoning [2]. Further, American children know very little about their bodies or their reproductive system [3]. Given that children have a poor understanding of their own bodies, explaining health- and fertility-related issues of cancer often requires education about their bodies in general and then education about oncofertility-related issues, or they may be left to rely on largely abstract ideas and concepts.

For children with cancer, communicating about oncofertility is a new concept and one that has not yet been well researched. In this chapter, we provide a

E. Wartella, Ph.D. (✉)
School of Communication, Northwestern University (not the hospital), 2240 Campus Drive, 2-148 Frances Searle Building, Evanston, IL 60208, USA
e-mail: ellen-wartella@northwestern.edu

A.R. Lauricella, Ph.D., M.P.P. • L.B. Hurwitz, B.A.
Department of Communication Studies, Northwestern University (not the hospital), 2240 Campus Drive, 2-147 Frances Searle Building, Evanston, IL 60208, USA
e-mail: alexislauricella@gmail.com; lisa.hurwitz@u.northwestern.edu

T.K. Woodruff et al. (eds.), *Oncofertility Communication: Sharing Information and Building Relationships across Disciplines*, DOI 10.1007/978-1-4614-8235-2_8,

developmental perspective about what children already know about their bodies and reproductive systems. Next, we discuss the use of various types of media to communicate health messages to children in a general audience as well as to specific populations of children, particularly patients in hospital settings. We conclude with recommendations for how oncofertility experts can use media to educate young audiences.

Developmental Progression of Health Concepts and Body Knowledge

Research indicates that there is a developmental progression in children's sexual knowledge and that there are cultural differences in children's understanding of procreation, birth, and sexual activity [3–5]. Investigations of very young children's sexual knowledge focused on their understanding of gender identity and genital differences [3]. Volbert found that by age 2 or 3, children can identify themselves as either boys or girls and by age 4 or 5, they are able to identify gender-appropriate genitalia [3]. According to Gordon, Schroeder, and Abrams, before middle childhood (approximately age 7), children have very little understanding of the sexual functions of genitalia; children typically only understand that they are involved in making babies [6]. Up to age 7, children have a rudimentary understanding of pregnancy and gestation in the mother's "stomach," but little understanding of birth or adult sexual behavior [3]. In cross-cultural research with 6-year-old children in the USA, England, the Netherlands, and Sweden, Caron and Ahlgrim found that American children lagged behind those of the other countries in understanding conception and birth [4]. Moreover, children from the Netherlands and Sweden (both countries with progressive attitudes toward sexual education) showed greater understanding of sexuality, procreation, and birth than children in the other countries [4].

More recent research on sixth-grade middle school students found that, when allowed to ask questions anonymously, children asked about sexual activity (e.g., "If you have anal sex, is it still sex?"), the female anatomy (e.g., "How big is the vagina?"), reproduction (e.g., "Does reproduction hurt?"), and puberty (e.g., "What is the latest age a person can get puberty?") [7]. These findings suggest that, even with middle school students, there is some confusion and uncertainty about reproduction and sexual activity. This is consistent with the American Academy of Pediatrics Committee on Public Education [8], which has pointed out that much of children and adolescents' knowledge about sexuality comes from popular television and movies, which provide little information about birth control and how to protect against HIV or other sexually transmitted diseases [8]. By the time children reach adolescence, puberty and sexual development lead them to a much better understanding of their bodies, sexual behavior, and reproduction. Along with hormonal changes associated with puberty and increased interest in sexuality comes increased risk-taking and increased influence of peers as adolescents explore their own sexuality and identity, often via media portrayals [9].

Just as children's understanding of sexuality and reproduction improve as they grow older, so too does children's understanding of health and illness. Bibace and Walsh conducted the most complete age-related systematic studies of children's understanding of illness and its causes [10, 11]; their study has become the classic reference for how children's understanding of health concepts and illness is related to their development of logical reasoning and their ability to differentiate between themselves and others. Bibace and Walsh [10, 11] identify six stages in children's development of an understanding of illness and its causes between ages 4 and 12: (1) phenomenism explanations—whereby illness is understood as an external phenomenon separate from the person; (2) contagion type explanations offered by 4-year-olds who understand illness can be caused by objects or people around the child; (3) contamination type explanations in which illness is understood to be related to physical contact with people who are sick; (4) internalization explanations whereby illness is understood as a process of internalizing elements such as breathing in bacteria; (5) physiologic explanations whereby illness is understood as a process such as people getting colds from a virus that gets into the body; and (6) psychophysiologic explanations in which the child (typically by age 11 or 12) understands that psychological factors can also influence health status. Doctors generally are cognizant of this developmental progression and use language consistent with children's understanding about health when discussing illness with young patients.

Overall, as children develop, they learn and understand more about health, illness, and their bodies, but again, Americans know less than children in other countries. This disparity may exist due to aspects of American culture in which we avoid communication and conversation with young children about their bodies or sexuality. When children have a lack of understanding of basic bodily functions, it makes communicating about complex health and illness issues even more challenging, especially for parents who are uncomfortable talking to their children about health and sexuality.

Communicating with General Audiences Through Mass Media

Forty years of research has demonstrated that children can learn from educational, curriculum-based television programs [12, 13], but they can also learn from entertainment-based media [14]. Research on learning from mass media has focused primarily on social-emotional and academic skill learning for younger children [15] and less on specific health issues and outcomes. However, there is considerable research about how teens learn health information from mass media [16], specifically information about sexual health [14, 17], and there are a few examples of programs created specifically to teach younger children health information.

There are fewer educational curriculum-based programs dedicated to teaching young children about health. *Fizzy's Lunch Lab*, a PBS online website, provides an opportunity for children to learn more about healthy eating through online videos, games, and activities. *Doc McStuffins* is a Disney preschool program about a child who pretends to be a doctor to her stuffed animals to help them feel better. Neither program has been assessed for its effectiveness in teaching young children health information. *Sesame Street* recently began its Healthy Habits for Life initiative, which includes videos, books, PSAs, and outreach materials to promote health and healthy practices, both in the USA and around the world [18]. Abroad, *Sesame Street* co-productions have had success in educating mass audiences about health concepts like HIV/AIDS and malaria. Specifically, *Takalani Sesame* in South Africa, *Kilimani Sesame* in Tanzania, and *Jalan Sesam* in Indonesia focus on teaching and educating young children and families about specific area-related health messages.

In South Africa in 2001, there was a very high rate of HIV infection: nearly 11 % of the population was affected [19], and a considerable stigma was associated with the disease. *Takalani Sesame* was created to communicate both academic and health messages to preschool children. One of the primary aspects of this project was the creation of an HIV-positive character, named Kari, who taught young children basic health and social information about HIV/AIDS [20]. Multiple studies have demonstrated the vast success that *Takalani Sesame* has had on educating young children about HIV/AIDS in South Africa [21]; specifically, there was improvement in children's basic knowledge of HIV/AIDS, blood safety, destigmatization, and coping with the illness [21].

Mass media, and television specifically in the USA, has been a successful tool used to educate teens about certain health-related behaviors, primarily sexual health. While entertainment television in the USA often depicts sexual content [22], it can occasionally provide positive information about sexuality. Recent data suggest that online media currently outranks parents and health professionals as the primary source of information about sex for teenagers [23]. Teens also report that they rely on television as a source of information about birth control, menstruation, pregnancy, and sexually transmitted diseases [23]. One study found that 67 % of teens who watched the *Friends* episode about condom failure recalled that the condom failure resulted in pregnancy and 10 % of viewers spoke with an adult about condom efficacy as a result of the show [14]. Also, social network sites like Twitter have been used by the World Health Organization to provide updates to mass audiences about diseases such as the H1N1 influenza [24]. For teens, social networking sites may be a particularly appropriate and comfortable environment for youth to receive and learn about health information [25].

Some television shows work with organizations like the National Campaign to Prevent Teen Pregnancy and the Media Project to incorporate health messages into their television shows. In the past, *Dawson's Creek*, *Felicity*, *ER*, and *Beverly Hills 90210* developed episodes in which the characters dealt with teen sexual health to provide information for viewers [26]. While there are few studies on the effectiveness of these episodes, viewer's knowledge of emergency contraception increased by 17 % after an *ER* show depicted a date rape victim taking an emergency contraceptive [27]. More recently, a study of a particular episode of *Grey's Anatomy* found that viewers learned that with proper treatment an HIV+ mother can give birth to a healthy baby; the study also found that this information was retained for 6 weeks after viewing the episode [28]. These studies provide some evidence that even through traditional media, such as entertainment television, health messages can be communicated and positively influence adolescent health knowledge.

For some health issues, information needs to be presented to both the parent and child simultaneously. Oncofertility is a new concept for parents and children alike, and both audiences are learning about the consequences of cancer and its treatment on fertility together. An example of how to successfully communicate to the adults and children simultaneously comes from Sesame Workshop. As a result of the long wars in Iraq and Afghanistan, the Workshop created a toolkit of videos and information for military families to help them cope with military transitions that included deployment, homecoming, and changes [29]. Sesame Workshop uses friendly, child-like characters, and child-appropriate language in their videos to educate children about issues related to such transitions, and also provides activities and information that can help educate parents about best practices and ways for them to continue the conversation with their children. This method of addressing both the child and parent together can increase parent–child interaction and communication around sensitive topics, and can also help the parent provide the child with concrete examples to enhance their understanding of what is going on. For example, a parent could say, "Remember in the video how Rosita's father was in a wheelchair? Well when we see Daddy at the hospital, he will be in a wheelchair like Rosita's daddy." For young children, these explicit, concrete examples can help them understand and process the messages being presented.

Media to Communicate with Special Audiences

To communicate health information in hospital settings, medical practitioners have used, created, and advocated for a variety of media- and non-media-based tools/interventions, including printed leaflets, hospital tours, medical play sessions, puppet shows, instructional videos, and computer-based multimedia demonstrations [30–32]. Large numbers of health researchers first began advocating for the use of educational puppet shows and videos in the mid-1970s [31, 33]. Staff have used these tools with children who are preparing for surgery [31], with children about to undergo dental procedures [34, 35], and with healthy children who may be unfamiliar with or frightened by the hospital or various illnesses [36]. Many health practitioners and researchers believe that children can learn about illness, hospitalization, and medical procedures [30, 32, 37], and have developed child-friendly educational tools to encourage the acquisition of health knowledge and ease anxiety about health issues.

Educational interventions involving puppets and dolls have been used to target preschool- and school-aged children [38]. Puppetry "is active and immediate, and it engages a child at once verbally and physically" [36], p. 129. Puppets are "likeable, trustworthy, and interesting enough to command attention" [39], p. 33, for many children. To ensure that puppet-based interventions are effective, it is important that the puppets are used in ways that are as realistic as possible [39]. These interventions have effectively taught children health-related information [38]. Additionally, by talking to a puppet or about a puppet show, children can work through tough emotions—such as fear and anger—about health issues [36].

To communicate health-related information to children, many practitioners alternatively opt for instructional videos, including filmed puppet shows [36] and filmed enactments of various medical procedures with child actors serving as model patients [34, 35]. Media-based interventions offer several distinct advantages for medical staff over live demonstrations with puppets and dolls. First, healthcare providers can show a filmed puppet show if they themselves lack facility with puppets or the time to enact a long show in front of children [36, 39]. Second, the use of media-based tools can standardize the transmission of educational information in hospitals, ensuring that every family is given the same information [40]. Finally, these tools can be dispersed widely, potentially reaching multiple hospitals and children in need of learning health-related information outside the hospital setting [32].

Indeed, films have successfully imparted topical information about health and reduced children's anxiety in health settings [34, 35]. Through the use of imagery, films help make health-related ideas and concepts more concrete for young children [30]. In particular, tapes that star child actors have been demonstrated to be more educationally efficacious than tapes that simply feature doctors describing medical procedures [35]. When appropriate, children who have been encouraged to act out behavior modeled in health videos (e.g., practicing breathing while sitting in a dental chair prior to a procedure), have demonstrated less fear and greater gains in knowledge compared to children who viewed similar videos that did not prompt their participation [34].

More recently, practitioners have advocated for the use of computer-based educational tools with children; these tools can simultaneously display written and pictorial information to enhance learning [35, 40]. Nelson and Allen [32] demonstrated that children learned and became less fearful after exploring a hospital-created computer demonstration, and children who engaged with these demonstrations were more satisfied with their learning experience than children who viewed static slideshows. Many scholars are particularly enthusiastic about computer-based interventions because they can easily be shared across the Internet [30, 32]. Nevertheless, experts have identified a need for further evaluation of the efficacy of such computer-based tools [30].

In a survey of healthcare providers at a children's hospital in the UK, respondents identified a lack of age-appropriate educational resources as a major barrier in serving adolescents, a finding those researchers believe reflects an international problem [41]. Further, only a limited number of studies have examined media-based health interventions/tools designed for adolescents [42]. Nonetheless, the existing research indicates that health media targeted to adolescents can be educationally efficacious. For instance, in a review of sexual health interventions with adolescents and young adults, a panel of experts identified 30 interventions they deemed particularly promising for implementation across the nation, 17 of which included educational video components [43]. Prior published evaluations of all of these programs demonstrated that participants adopted healthy sexual behaviors, such as increased condom use, in response to each intervention. Similarly, in a study with adolescents and young adults, youth who played a video game specifically created to teach about cancer and its treatment improved their knowledge about these areas, perhaps in part because the video game stimulated participants' topical interest [42].

Although ground-level health practitioners are sometimes unfamiliar with research demonstrating the efficacy of various educational tools such as instructional videos, increasingly, hospitals are relying on media-based educational aids [33]. For example, the GetWellNetwork provides on-demand, health-themed educational television programming to 28 children's hospitals nationally [44].

The Potential for Media to Convey Challenging Messages: Recommendations

Children's developmental needs are sometimes an afterthought in the planning and execution of hospital-based educational interventions [30]:

> In a sociocultural climate where detailed medical information provision is a legal requirement, information is generally provided to parents and children but often without much consideration as to how children of different ages will understand and respond to the information (p. 137).

That said, experts have offered suggestions on choosing and tailoring the aforementioned techniques depending on the ages of the children being targeted.

Aspects of the information need to be simplified for very young audiences. Jaaniste and colleagues [30] recommend "using [age-appropriate] terminology consistent with the child's own spontaneous language production" (p. 134). They also propose using displays and demonstrations that are fairly concrete, straightforward, and focused on external and sensory descriptions for preschool-age children. Creators should select out a few topics to teach the child, rather than providing them with too much complicated material to process all at once. For example, since children know very little about reproduction and the human body [3], initial media presentations should focus on these key aspects of the body before bringing in details about the effects of treatment on future fertility.

Additionally, Morrison and researchers [38] advocate incorporating tactile components if possible when designing interventions for very young children. Therefore, a simple video that focuses on one aspect of oncofertility (e.g., sadness an adult may feel when learning about cancer-related fertility issues) that comes with a related physical display or dolls for the child to play may work well with preschool-age children. Further, if possible, interactive technologies, like computers or touch screens, in which the child can interact and help the characters on the screen express or display their emotions may be an effective way for young children to strongly engage and learn about oncofertility.

Older children may be receptive to more complex interventions. Elementary school-age children, who have greater symbolic processing abilities, may learn more from puppet shows or videos featuring models than younger children [30, 39]. Accordingly, video demonstrations of puppets or children interacting with cancer patients may be well received by school-aged children and may be sufficient to teach them about the basic concepts of oncofertility. As elementary school-aged children know more about their bodies [3] and have a better understanding of abstract ideas and concepts as they get older [2], videos and media that communicate the range of issues that may arise as a result of cancer treatment may still be informative and helpful for these children. However, for all young audiences, creators of educational media and experts who communicate with young children should understand Bibace and Walsh's six stages of children's understanding of illness [10, 11].

Keller and Brown [26] make recommendations that mass media be used to teach responsible sexual behavior to teens as it is successfully done in other countries. If teens have already received information about sexual behavior and reproduction via mass media, oncofertility communication can delve into the more complex aspects of how cancer and treatment can influence fertility now and in the future. Adolescents are capable of processing multifaceted informational interventions describing internal bodily functions and future states [30]. Likewise, more so than younger children, adolescents may have an "appreciation of situations in which there are competing plausible explanations or approaches" [30], p. 131, which is important for understanding health and illness information. Therefore, adolescents may be capable of understanding thorough and complex explanations about oncofertility—or other health issues—that feature unanswered questions and various potential outcomes associated with cancer treatment.

It is also important to note that parents often participate in hospital-based, multimedia educational interventions with their children [33, 36]. Both adults and children can learn from media-based educational offerings. For instance, parents who participated in a multimedia consent process demonstrated a stronger understanding of the procedure their children were about to undergo compared to parents who participated in a traditional consent process without media aids [40]. In some cases, parents who participated in these interventions felt less anxious prior to their children's procedures [31].

Conclusions

Oncofertility is a new interdisciplinary approach to understanding and preparing patients and their families for potential fertility issues during and after cancer treatment. When these patients are children and adolescents, special communication practices are necessary. To provide an understanding of promising strategies for educating youth about oncofertility, this chapter has examined broadly how children and adolescents develop an understanding of sexuality, health, and illness. In particular, previous research indicates that cognitive developmental changes in children's abilities to comprehend abstract concepts and causality can impact children's understanding of their own sexuality, procreation, and childbirth. Medical practitioners should take into account the differences among preschoolers, elementary school children, and adolescents in the ways in which they explain oncofertility to pediatric patients. Media-based tools may aid these conversations. Indeed, research on how media productions are used in conveying health information to youth demonstrates the potential of media outlets (especially videos and online website information) for educating children and adolescents about health-related topics, such as oncofertility, in ways that are sensitive to young people's needs and sensibilities.

Acknowledgements This work was supported by the Oncofertility Consortium NIH 5UL1DE019587 and the Specialized Cooperative Centers Program in Reproduction and Infertility Research NIH U54HD076188.

References

1. Woodruff TK. The emergence of a new interdiscipline: oncofertility. In: Woodruff TK, Snyder KA, editors. Oncofertility preservation for cancer survivors. New York: Springer; 2007.
2. Piaget J. Play, dreams and imitation in childhood. New York: Norton; 1962.
3. Volbert R. Sexual knowledge of preschool children. J Psychol Hum Sex. 2000;12(1–2):5–26.
4. Caron SL, Ahlgrim CJ. Children's understanding and knowledge of conception and birth: comparing children from England, the Netherlands, Sweden, and the United States. Am J Sex Educ. 2012;7(1):16–36.
5. Goldman RJ, Goldman JDG. How children perceive the origin of babies and the roles of mothers and fathers in procreation: a cross-national study. Child Dev. 1982;53:491–504.
6. Gordon BN, Schroeder CS, Abrams M. Age and social-class differences in children's knowledge of sexuality. J Clin Child Psychol. 1990;19:33–43.
7. Charmaraman L, Lee AJ, Erkut S. What if you already know everything about sex? Content analyses of questions from early adolescents in a middle school sex education program. J Adolesc Health. 2012;50:527–30.
8. American Academy of Pediatrics. Media education. Pediatrics. 1999;104:341–3.
9. Strausburger VC, Wilson B, Jordan A. Children, adolescents, and the media. Los Angeles, CA: Sage; 2008.
10. Bibace R, Walsh M. Development of children's concepts of illness. Pediatrics. 1980;66: 912–7.
11. Bibace R, Walsh M. Children's conceptions of illness. New Dir Child Adolesc Dev. 1981;1981:31–48.
12. Ball S, Bogatz GA. First year of Sesame Street: an evaluation; a report to the Children's Television Workshop. Princeton, NJ: Educational Testing Service; 1970.
13. Fisch SM, Truglio RT. "G" is for growing: thirty years of research on children and Sesame Street. Mahwah, NJ: Lawrence Erlbaum Associates Publishers; 2001.
14. Collins RL, Elliot MN, Berry SH, Kanouse DE, Hunter SB. Entertainment television as a healthy sex educator: the impact of condom-efficacy information in an episode of *Friends*. Pediatrics. 2003;112:1115–21.
15. Mares M, Woodard EH. Positive effects of television on children's social interactions: a meta-analysis. Media Psychol. 2005;7:301–22.
16. Strausburger VC, Jordan AB, Donnerstein E. Children, adolescents, and the media: health effects. Pediatr Clin North Am. 2012;59:533–87.

17. Gavin J. Television teen drama and HIV/AIDS: the role of genre in audience understandings of safe sex. J Media Cult Stud. 2001;15:77–96.
18. Cole CF, Kotler J, Pai S. "Happy healthy muppets": a look at Sesame workshop's health initiatives around the world. In: Gaist PA, editor. Igniting the power of community: the role of CBO's and NGO's in global public health. New York: Springer Science+Business Media, LLC; 2010.
19. UNAIDS. United Nations General Assembly Special Session on HIV/AIDS: HIV/AIDS Global Crisis-Global Action. 2001 June 25–27. http://www.unaids.org/fact_sheets/ungass/pdf/Fscomplet_en/pdf
20. Segal L, Cole CF, Flud J. Developing an HIV/AIDS education curriculum for *Takalini Sesames*, South Africa's Sesame Street. Early Educ Dev. 2002;13:363–78.
21. Khulisa Management Services. Impact assessment of "Takalani Sesame" Season II Programme. Johannesburg, South Africa; 2005.
22. Kunkel D, Biely E, Eyal K, Cope-Farrar K, Donnerstein E, Fanrich R. Sex on TV3: a biennial report to the Kaiser family foundation. Santa Barbara, CA: Kaiser Family Foundation; 2003.
23. Boyer R, Levine D, Zensius N. TECHsex USA—youth sexuality and reproductive health in the digital age. Oakland, CA: ISIS; 2011.
24. McNab C. What social media offers to health professions and citizens. Bull World Health Organ. 2009;87:566.
25. Moreno MA, Kolb J. Social networking sites and adolescent health. Pediatric Clin North Am. 2012;59:601–12.
26. Keller SN, Brown JD. Media interventiosn to promote responsible sexual behavior. J Sex Res. 2002;39:67–72.
27. Brodie M, Foehr U. Communicating health information through the entertainment media. Health Aff. 2001;20:192–200.
28. Rideout V. Television as a health educator: a case study of Grey's Anatomy. Menlo Park, CA: Kaiser Family Foundation; 2008.
29. Sesame Workshop (n.d.). Kilimani Sesame Focuses on Malaria Prevention. http://supportus.sesameworkshop.org/site/c.nlI3IkNXJsE/b.4334103/k.3538/Kilimani_Sesame_Focuses_on_Malaria_Prevention.htm?auid=3973718. Accessed 10 Dec 2012.
30. Jaaniste T, Hayes B, Von Baeyer CL. Providing children with information about forthcoming medical procedures: a review and synthesis. Clin Psychol. 2007;14:124–43.
31. Kain ZN, Caramico LA, Mayes LC, Genevro JL, Bornstein MH, Hofstadter MB. Preoperative preparation programs in children: a comparative examination. Anesth Analg. 1998;87:1249–55.
32. Nelson CC, Allen J. Reduction of healthy children's fears related to hospitalization and medical procedures: the effectiveness of multimedia computer instruction in pediatric psychology. Child Health Care. 1999;28:1–13.
33. Koetting O'Byrne K, Peterson L, Saldana L. Survey of pediatric hospitals' preparation programs: evidence of the impact of health psychology research. Health Psychol. 1997;16:147–54.
34. Klingman A, Melamed BG, Cuthberg MI, Hermecz DA. Effects of participant modeling on information acquisition and skill utilization. J Consult Clin Psychol. 1984;52:414–22.
35. Melamed BG, Yurcheson R, Fleece EL, Hutcherson S, Hawes R. Effects of film modeling on the reduction of anxiety-related behaviors in individuals varying in level of previous experience in the stress situation. J Consult Clin Psychol. 1978;46:1357–67.
36. Alger I, Linn S, Beardslee W. Puppetry as a therapeutic tool for hospitalized children. Hosp Community Psychiatry. 1985;36:129–30.
37. Atkins DM. Evaluation of pediatric preparation program for short-stay surgical patients. J Pediatr Psychol. 1987;12:285–90.
38. Morrison MIS, Herath K, Chase C. Puppets for prevention: "playing safe is playing smart". J Burn Care Res. 1988;9:650–1.
39. Shapiro DE. Puppet modeling technique for children undergoing stressful medical procedures: tips for clinicians. Int J Play Therapy. 1995;4:31–9.

40. Wanzer MB, Wojtaszczyk AM, Schimert J, et al. Enhancing the "informed" in informed consent: a pilot test of a multimedia presentation. Health Commun. 2010;25:365–74.
41. McDonagh JE, Minnaar G, Kelly K, O'Connor D, Shaw KL. Unmet education and training needs in adolescent health of health professionals in a UK children's hospital. Acta Paediatr. 2006;95:715–9.
42. Beale IL, Kato PM, Marin-Bowling VM, Guthrie N, Cole SW. Improvement in cancer-related knowledge following use of a psychoeducational video game for adolescents and young adults. J Adolesc Health. 2007;41:263–70.
43. Card JJ, Niego S, Mallari A, Farrell WS. The program archive on sexuality, health & adolescence: promising "prevention programs in a box". Fam Plann Perspect. 1996;28:210.
44. GetWellNetwork. (n.d.). Client community. http://www.getwellnetwork.com/company/about-us/client-community. Accessed 23 Feb 2013.

Chapter 9
Disparities in Adolescent Patient–Provider Communication Regarding Fertility Preservation Care

Amanda B. Fuchs and Robert E. Brannigan

Introduction

As survival rates of pediatric cancer now exceed 70 %, oncology providers have devoted increased attention to the future quality of life of young cancer survivors [1]. Cancer in the adolescent and young adult population represents a minority of all cancers diagnosed in the USA each year. Cancer in 15–30-year-olds is more than twice as common as in children under 15 years of age, yet these patients account for only 2 % of all invasive cancers in the USA [2]. As a result, improving the standard of care in the adolescent and young adult population has not been a primary focus for many oncology providers. The adolescent group in particular poses unique logistical and ethical challenges to oncologists; these patients are often cared for by pediatric providers, but possess widely varying levels of mature decision-making capacity. Often, parents are ultimately making long-term medical decisions for the patient, including decisions about fertility preservation.

In 2006, the American Society of Clinical Oncology (ASCO) published a set of recommendations suggesting that oncologists should not only inform patients of the possibility of infertility as a result of cancer treatment, but also discuss fertility preservation options with patients of childbearing age, including adolescents. Fertility preservation options for female and male oncology patients are overviewed in Table 9.1. At minimum, according to ASCO, "as long as the oncologist presents the options in enough detail for the patient to decide whether to seek a consultation,

A.B. Fuchs, B.A. (✉)
Feinberg School of Medicine, Northwestern University,
300 East Chicago Avenue, Chicago, IL 60611, USA
e-mail: amanda-fuchs@fsm.northwestern.edu

R.E. Brannigan, M.D.
Department of Urology, Feinberg School of Medicine,
Northwestern University, Chicago, IL, USA
e-mail: r-brannigan@northwestern.edu

T.K. Woodruff et al. (eds.), *Oncofertility Communication: Sharing Information and Building Relationships across Disciplines*, DOI 10.1007/978-1-4614-8235-2_9,

Table 9.1 Fertility preservation options for female and male oncology patients

Fertility preservation options for female oncology patients
Prepubertal
Ovarian shielding
Ovarian tissue cryopreservation (experimental)
Pubertal
Ovarian shielding
Ovarian tissue cryopreservation
Oocyte cryopreservation
Emergency IVF
Embryo cryopreservation
Fertility preservation options for male oncology patients
Prepubertal
Testicular tissue cryopreservation (experimental)
Pubertal
Testicular tissue cryopreservation
Ejaculated sperm cryopreservation

the detailed counseling could be done by an infertility specialist" [3]. These initial discussions with the oncologist can be a pivotal factor in a family's decision to seek fertility preservation for their adolescent child. Similarly, the ethics committee of the American Society for Reproductive Medicine (ASRM) states that "fertility programs should counsel cancer patients and survivors on the risks of cancer treatment on fertility and the options for and risks of preserving fertility and reproducing after cure or remission" [4]. However, it is apparent that fertility preservation counseling and services still have not reached a large proportion of the adolescent population who may benefit from these services [5, 6]. There are a number of barriers to discussing fertility preservation that are specific to the adolescent population. These barriers, as well as the disparities that currently exist in communicating the topic of fertility preservation to the adolescent population, will be discussed in this chapter.

Gender-Related Disparities in Fertility Preservation Care

Interviews with adult survivors of pediatric cancer have demonstrated that fertility is a significant concern for patients following potentially sterilizing oncologic treatment. While females are more likely than males to seek evaluation of fertility status following cancer treatment, there are numerous records of both males and females expressing regret for not having undergone fertility preservation prior to treatment [7]. In discussing fertility preservation with adolescent patients, providers are faced with a unique challenge; adolescents have varying levels of understanding of fertility, and therefore are unlikely to initiate fertility preservation discussion. However, it is clear that the majority of adolescents do articulate a desire to preserve future fertility. In one study, more than 90 % of female oncology patients between 10 and 21 years of age expressed a strong concern for their future. There was even a consensus among these patients and their parents about the value of pursuing "research treatment" in an effort to preserve fertility. It is important to note, however, that the majority of patients and parents agreed that they would not be willing to delay treatment 1 month or longer for the purpose of preserving fertility [8]. Some patients feel that the importance they placed on fertility changed once they understood the possibility of becoming infertile after cancer treatment. Unfortunately, for some, it is the realization that they are already infertile that introduced young patients to the issue of fertility; certain individuals discuss feeling "traumatized" after finding out that ovarian failure occurred following treatment. In focus groups with these patients and their families, parents expressed that their daughters' survival was their primary concern at the time of diagnosis, and late effects seemed secondary [9].

Some physicians have reflected on their experiences discussing fertility preservation with adolescents; these experiences have helped to illustrate that young male and female patients conceptualize the issue of fertility differently. The results of series of focused interviews with 24 pediatric oncologists in the state of Florida found that female patients were more receptive to a fertility preservation discussion than males of equal age [10]. In another study of male oncology patients between the ages of 13 and 21 who elected to preserve sperm, patients rated concerns about fertility low on a 10-point scale at the time of diagnosis. However, as in females, these male patients considered fertility to be more important once oncologic treatment had been successful [11]. In general, the parents of adolescent male cancer patients have had a positive initial response to the option of sperm cryopreservation prior to cancer treatment; in one study, 80.4 % of parents thought that sperm banking was a "great idea" [12]. Unfortunately, just as in females, many adult male survivors of pediatric cancer are surprised to learn that they are infertile, and they do not remember discussing the option of fertility preservation at the time of diagnosis [13]. In order to prevent regret on behalf of the patient in future years, it is important that physicians inform patients and their families about long-term effects of cancer treatments, and offer them the opportunity to consider fertility preservation options.

Barriers to Fertility Preservation Care

Though it is clear that fertility is important to both male and female adolescents, both genders face a considerable number of barriers to receiving fertility preservation care. Patients must sometimes delay the start of their treatment to undergo fertility preservation procedures. While male patients are limited only by their access to a fertility specialist or sperm bank, female patients must delay treatment for 3 weeks or more to allow for menstrual cycle synchronization, ovarian stimulation, and oocyte harvesting. Patients may face even longer delays in certain hospitals where there are a smaller number of providers who are familiar with fertility preservation procedures. Furthermore, if a patient has a particularly poor prognosis or is acutely ill at the time of diagnosis, the late effects of cancer treatment will be a secondary consideration to treatment and palliative care. Instead of delaying treatment, many families and physicians may choose to commence treatment as soon as possible, and consider fertility later, after the child has recovered.

In addition to the delay in treatment, families can incur a significant cost by choosing to preserve their child's fertility. For male patients, the typical cost of collecting three sperm samples is around $1,500, plus an additional $500 per year to cover the cost of storage. Because samples are generally stored for young patients for 10 years or more, the cumulative cost can be significant. The cost barrier is even higher for female patients; one cycle of oocyte retrieval costs $12,000, plus additional yearly storage fees. Insurance companies will rarely cover the cost of fertility preservation procedures in adolescent patients, and the families are responsible for the burden of these costs [14].

In addition to the barriers associated with the actual process of fertility preservation, there is a significant knowledge barrier that adolescent patients face in receiving fertility preservation care. Oncology providers can play a critical role in either overcoming knowledge-related barriers to fertility preservation care, yet as a group, pediatric oncology providers receive little or no formal education about fertility preservation methodology. Unfortunately, many providers are unaware of the options available to adolescent patients and the outcomes of these procedures. For this reason, as well as the sensitive nature of this topic in a vulnerable population, many providers feel uncomfortable discussing fertility preservation with their young patients. Because of the combination of personal discomfort and lack of familiarity with the subject, some providers many not stress the importance of consulting a fertility specialist or options for undergoing fertility preservation prior to treatment [15].

Gender-Based Barriers to Fertility Preservation Care

While the aforementioned barriers introduce a significant challenge to the delivery of health services to all adolescent patients, female patients are at a particular disadvantage in receiving appropriate fertility preservation care. Oocyte harvesting is not only more expensive and more time consuming than sperm banking by male patients, but is also a much more invasive procedure. Young girls will need to undergo a surgical procedure even before they start curative treatment for their cancer. Many parents express concern that prolonging the treatment course and performing elective procedures will add to the trauma of their daughter's experience. Lastly, cryopreserved sperm has been shown to be highly effective when used for in vitro fertilization (IVF), yielding pregnancies in up to 60 % of intracytoplasmic sperm injection (ICSI) procedures [16]. In contrast, there is considerable debate regarding the success rates in using frozen oocytes compared to frozen embryos for use in IVF. Historically, IVF was performed using only frozen embryos. However, in the last decade, some studies have shown that frozen oocytes can yield live births in up to 25 % of IVF attempts, which is the approximate success rate of

IVF with frozen embryos [17, 18]. These studies are limited by a small number of participants, as well as variability in existing protocols for IVF using frozen oocytes and embryos. Most specialists still recommend freezing whole embryos over individual oocytes, a practice that favors older patients who are in committed relationships. Between the cost, time commitment, and still experimental nature of oocyte cryopreservation, female adolescents face a more significant set of barriers in receiving fertility preservation care compared with male adolescents.

Practice patterns observed among physicians reflect the greater number of barriers that exist for the delivery of care to adolescent females. In one study, 80 % of pediatric oncologists agreed that threats to their young *male* patients' fertility are a major concern. In this same group of physicians, 87 % of pediatric oncologists agreed that threats to their young *female* patients' fertility are a major concern. However, while 66 % of these providers commonly refer male patients to a fertility specialist prior to treatment, only 23 % of providers commonly refer female patients to a fertility specialist prior to treatment [19]. These statistics indicate that male patients may be given greater access to fertility preservation consultation compared with female patients, adding to the disadvantage that young girls face when considering fertility preservation care. Special attention should be paid to the opportunity for discussing fertility preservation with adolescent female oncology patients, as there is much room for improvement in delivering care to this patient population.

Age-Related Disparities in Fertility Preservation Care

Discussing fertility preservation with adolescent oncology patients can be a particularly challenging task for pediatric providers, given their patients' young age and developmental stage. Reproductive function may be difficult to understand for patients who are physically mature, but who lack the intellectual maturity to consider fertility preservation within the context of their cancer care. These factors contribute to differences in the way that providers approach adult and adolescent fertility preservation care. A study from 1996 demonstrated that adolescent patients between the ages of 14 and 17 years with a variety of malignancies show hormone values, testicular volumes, and sperm concentrations that are comparable to those of adult patients with malignancies. Furthermore, semen parameters such as sperm motility and morphology were similar within the adolescent and adult groups [20]. Despite this, survey studies have shown that 24 % of adult male oncology patients bank sperm prior to treatment, compared to 18 % of adolescent male patients [13, 21]. These statistics demonstrate that while much can be done to extend access to fertility preservation to all oncology patients, there are additional age-related barriers to providing adequate fertility preservation care to the adolescent population in particular.

Young patients of both sexes who have not yet undergone puberty have a limited number of options for fertility preservation. For prepubescent females, the single option for fertility preservation is ovarian tissue cryopreservation, a surgical procedure in which part of one ovary is excised and stored for later use. Because there is no existing protocol to artificially advance the immature oocytes in these tissues to maturity, ovarian tissue cryopreservation is a purely experimental procedure that is available in a minority of academic medical centers. For prepubescent male patients, there is a similar procedure in which testicular tissue is surgically removed and frozen for future use; again, this procedure is experimental and has not yet produced any live births. Many physicians are unaware of these experimental procedures, and will simply not consider younger patients to be candidates for fertility preservation prior to cancer treatment.

Providing quality fertility preservation consultation can be complicated by a provider's inability to discern the developmental stage of the patient, either physically or intellectually. For example, it can be difficult to determine if a young male is prepubertal or postpubertal. Patient history, such as history of nocturnal emission, as well as Tanner stage, can help guide the practitioner, but these are not perfect predictors of sexual development or sperm maturation. In one prospective study of pediatric oncology providers in the UK over a 12-month period, researchers found that the effects of cancer treatment on fertility were discussed with 68 % of registered patients; the most commonly mentioned reason for not discussing the effects on fertility with a patient was young age. Within this study, physicians discussed fertility preservation with 83 % of postpubertal boys who were considered to be at high or medium risk of having compromised fertility following treatment. In comparison, this topic was discussed with only 39 % of male patients who were in early puberty. Individual providers determined their patients' pubertal status based on usual clinical practice [22]. This qualitative distinction of "early puberty" places limitations on access to fertility preservation care, as these patients may be able to produce viable sperm for cryopreservation via ejaculation or testicular sperm extraction. Given the evident disparity between physicians' approach to patients who are postpubertal compared to those in "early puberty," it is necessary to create a paradigm that more clearly defines which patients are candidates for fertility preservation; doing so would be a significant step toward addressing age-related disparities in fertility preservation care in this patient population.

When providers discuss fertility preservation with adolescent patients and their families, there is an implicit requirement that the patient has a certain level of understanding of sex and reproduction. Some providers might feel uncomfortable discussing these issues with pediatric patients, or struggle to address sex and reproduction in an age-sensitive way. In a survey-based study of 21 pediatric oncology nurses, a number of individuals expressed feeling uncomfortable and unprepared to discuss fertility with adolescent male patients. One respondent wrote that "The patient seemed very uncomfortable. I was uncomfortable talking about masturbation with his parents sitting there." Another respondent noted that she did not have adequate knowledge to answer patients' questions [23]. In a similar survey of pediatric oncologists in the state of Florida, some physicians noted they would feel more comfortable having fertility preservation discussions with their young male and female patients if there were more useful fertility-related educational materials for adolescents [24]. Because of the sensitive nature of fertility preservation discussions, physicians and nurses must be given every tool so that they are able to counsel and educate patients to the best of their ability.

In addition to physician factors that may affect the nature of fertility preservation discussions, patients' parents are extremely influential. Some parents may resist having conversations about fertility preservation based on cultural views of masturbation or sexual maturation. Other parents might be too overwhelmed with a new diagnosis of cancer to consider their child's future fertility. In the physician survey mentioned above, most oncologists noted that they would not pursue the issue fertility preservation if the patient's parents did not wish to discuss the topic [24]. Pediatric providers are in a unique position in which they must care for young patients while respecting the wishes of the patient's parents. Because infertility will likely compromise the patient's future quality of life, physicians have the challenge of balancing all of these interests while providing the highest quality of care.

Ethical Issues and Fertility Preservation Care in Adolescents

There are a number of ethical issues that are introduced when considering fertility preservation care in the adolescent population. Adolescents are not legally able to provide informed consent for fertility preservation procedures; they rely on the legal protection of their parents to do so. Parental consent must be provided for all aspects of fertility preservation care, including the use and storage of harvested gametes. Until the patient is of legal age, parents are the legal owners of sperm or oocytes. Historically, minors have not been able to provide informed consent because they are not considered legally competent to make medical decisions. Meisel and Lindz have included the following as tests in competency [25, 26]:

(a) Evidence of choice (expression of preference within the context of treatment alternative)
(b) "Reasonable outcome of choice" (option selection corresponds to a choice that a hypothetical reasonable person might take)
(c) "Rational" reasons (the treatment preference was derived from logical or rational reasoning)
(d) Understanding (comprehension of risks, benefits, and alternatives to treatment)

Based on these criteria, many older adolescents may, in fact, be competent to provide informed assent, if not legal consent. Assent would be possible for minors who are developmentally mature enough to consider their options and favor one course of treatment over alternatives [27]. In a study comparing the decision-making capacity of young patients to adults in a medical setting, Weithorn et al. determined that 14-year-old participants demonstrated a level of competency and informed decision making equal to those of adult participants. Furthermore, while 9-year-olds were found to be less competent in understanding medical information, they still satisfied the requirements of competence, specifically by demonstrating evidence of choice and reasonable outcome [28]. So while adolescent patients may not be able to give legal consent, it is important to acknowledge young patients' awareness of their illness and their ability to take an active role in their medical care. In an online focus group of survivors of pediatric cancer (diagnosed at 8–17 years of age), many young survivors expressed that they would have liked to be more involved in decision making and better informed during their treatment [29].

The dilemma between legal consent and informed assent in pediatric patients becomes even more complicated within the context of enrollment into experimental trials. In procedures such as ovarian or testicular tissue cryopreservation, there are few data on both short- and long-term outcomes for patients, and parents and physicians may be exposing minors to unjustified risk. Woodruff et al. discuss how research of this nature can also introduce an ethical problem by offering false hope of fertility to patients and their families; they concluded that documented accounts of regret related to infertility in adult survivors of pediatric cancer justifies presenting patients and their families with experimental opportunities [30]. In the majority of cases, patients and their parents will agree upon a given treatment course; however, if the situation does arise in which a patient and his or her parents are at odds in the decision-making process, the physician has the additional challenge of moderating a complicated family dynamic, an aspect of practice that is unique to pediatric providers. Input from a hospital Ethics Committee might be helpful in resolving disparate views and desires.

Conclusions

It is important for providers in the field of pediatric oncology to acknowledge the unique position of adolescents undergoing cancer treatment; while not legal adults, they can express preferences and consider adult issues such as fertility. With increasingly positive outcomes of pediatric cancer, the adolescent patient should be given the opportunity to maximize his or her future quality of life. The physician has the ability to advocate for adolescent patients who may be overlooked within the fields of pediatric and adult oncology care. By disseminating knowledge about fertility preservation options to relevant providers and producing targeted approaches to discussing fertility issues with adolescents, the medical field can assuage some of the existing disparities in the communication of, and access to, fertility preservation in this patient population.

Acknowledgments This work was supported by the Oncofertility Consortium NIH 5UL1DE019587.

References

1. Ries LAG, Melbert D, Krapcho M, et al., editors. SEER cancer statistics review, 1975–2004. Bethesda, MD: National Cancer Institute; 2006. http://seer.cancer.gov/csr/1975_2004/. Accessed 22 Feb 2013.
2. Bleyer A, O'Leary M, Barr R, Ries LAG, editors. Cancer epidemiology in older adolescents and young adults 15 to 29 years of age, including SEER incidence and survival: 1975–2000. Bethesda, MD: National Cancer Institute; 2006.

3. Lee SJ. American society of clinical oncology recommendations on fertility preservation in cancer patients. J Clin Oncol. 2006;24:2917–31.
4. Ethics Committee of the American Society for Reproductive Medicine. Fertility preservation and reproduction in cancer patients. Fertil Steril. 2005;83:1622–8.
5. Jeruss JS, Woodruff TK. Preservation of fertility in patients with cancer. N Engl J Med. 2009;360:2680–3.
6. Sheth KR, Sharma V, Helfand BT, et al. Improved fertility preservation care for male patients with cancer after establishment of formalized oncofertility program. J Urol. 2012;183:979–86.
7. Zeltzer LK. Cancer in adolescents and young adults psychosocial aspects. Long-term survivors. Cancer. 1993;71:3463–8.
8. Burns KC, Boudreau C, Panepinto JA. Attitudes regarding fertility preservation in female adolescent cancer patients. J Hematol Oncol. 2006;28:350–4.
9. Nieman CL, Kinahan KE, Yount SE, et al. Fertility preservation and adolescent cancer patients: lessons from adult survivors of childhood cancer and their parents. Cancer Treat Res. 2007;138:201–17.
10. Quinn GP, Vadaparampil ST. Fertility preservation and adolescent/young adult cancer patients: physician communication challenges. J Adolesc Health. 2009;44:394–400.
11. Edge B. Sperm banking in adolescent cancer patients. Arch Dis Child. 2005;91:149–52.
12. Ginsberg JP, Ogle SK, Tuchman LK, et al. Sperm banking for adolescent and young adult cancer patients: sperm quality, patient, and parent perspectives. Pediatr Blood Cancer. 2008;50:594–8.
13. Schover LR, Brey K, Lichtin A, et al. Knowledge and experience regarding cancer, infertility, and sperm banking in younger male survivors. J Clin Oncol. 2002;20:1880–9.
14. Fertile Hope. Pediatrics—information for parents. 2012. http://www.fertilehope.org/learn-more/cancer-and-fertility-info/pediatrics.cfm. Accessed 22 Feb 2013.
15. Schover LR, Rybicki LA, Martin BA, Bringelsen KA. Having children after cancer: a pilot survey of survivors' attitudes and experiences. Cancer. 1999;86:697–709.
16. Revel A, Haimovkochman R, Porat A, et al. In vitro fertilization-intracytoplasmic sperm injection success rates with cryopreserved sperm from patients with malignant disease. Fertil Steril. 2005;84:118–22.
17. Borini A, Bonu M, Coticchio G, Bianchi V, Cattoli M, Flamigni C. Pregnancies and births after oocyte cryopreservation. Fertil Steril. 2004;82:601–5.
18. Borini A, Lagalla C, Bonu MA, Bianchi V, Flamigni C, Coticchio G. Cumulative pregnancy rates resulting from the use of fresh and frozen oocytes: 7 years' experience. Reprod Biomed Online. 2006;12:481–6.
19. Köhler TS, Kondapalli LA, Shah A, Chan S, Woodruff TK, Brannigan RE. Results from the Survey for Preservation of Adolescent REproduction (SPARE) study: gender disparity in delivery of fertility preservation message to adolescents with cancer. J Assist Reprod Genet. 2010;28:269–77.
20. Kliesch S, Behre HM, Jürgens H, Nieschlag H. Cryopreservation of semen from adolescent patients with malignancies. Med Pediatr Oncol. 1996;26:20–7.
21. Neal M, Nagel K, Duckworth J, et al. Effectiveness of sperm banking in adolescents and young adults with cancer, a regional experience. Cancer. 2007;110:1125–9.
22. Anderson RA, Weddell A, Spoudeas HA, et al. Do doctors discuss fertility issues before they treat young patients with cancer? Hum Reprod. 2008;23:2246–51.
23. Nagel K, Neal M. Discussions regarding sperm banking with adolescent and young adult males who have cancer. J Pediatr Oncol Nurs. 2008;25:102–6.
24. Vadaparampil S, Quinn G, King L, Wilson C, Nieder M. Barriers to fertility preservation among pediatric oncologists. Patient Educ Couns. 2008;72:402–10.
25. Meisel A. The "exceptions" to the informed consent doctrine: striking a balance between competing values in medical decisionmaking. Wis Law Rev. 1979;2:413–88.
26. Meisel A, Roth LH, Lindz CW. Toward a model of the legal doctrine of informed consent. Am J Psychiatry. 1977;134:285–9.
27. Cohen CB. Ethical issues regarding fertility preservation in adolescents and children. Pediatr Blood Cancer. 2009;53:249–53.

28. Weithorn L, Campbell SB. The competency of children and adolescents to make informed treatment decisions. Child Dev. 1982;53:1589–98.
29. Zwaanswijk M, Tates K, Dulmen SV, Hoogerbrugge PM, Kamps WA, Bensing JM. Young patients', parents', and survivors' communication preferences in paediatric oncology: results of online focus groups. BMC Pediatr. 2007;7:35.
30. Zoloth L, Backhus L, Woodruff TK. Waiting to be born: the ethical implications of the generation of "NUBorn" and "NUAge" mice from pre-pubertal ovarian tissue. Am J Bioeth. 2008;8:21–9.

Chapter 10
Fertility Communication to Cancer Patients: A Hematologist–Oncologist's Perspective

Sara Barnato Giordano

As cancer treatments continue to advance, ~80 % of adolescents and young adults who receive a cancer diagnosis become long-term survivors. The increased survival has resulted in a focus in the long-term effects of therapy and a patient's quality of life. Oncologists must identify and address important quality of life issues that affect the well being of their patients. It is important both during treatment planning and in survivorship follow-up. Many studies have shown that young women with cancer have concerns related to sexual health, treatment-induced infertility, and menopause [1–3]. There is substantial room for improvement in communication and counseling of sexual health concerns, as well as the ability to provide resources and information for those women who demonstrate interest in fertility preservation.

Cancer treatments, including chemotherapy, radiation or surgical treatment may result in sexual dysfunction, cause menopausal symptoms, and/or impair fertility. Frequent complaints include loss of libido, vaginal dryness, dyspareunia, and decreased personal and partner satisfaction [4, 5]. Young women who experience amenorrhea as a result of their cancer treatment are likely to experience menopausal symptoms, including hot flashes, insomnia, and fatigue. Chemotherapy and radiation therapy may reduce the number of viable ovarian follicles in a drug- and dose-dependent manner, and surgical treatment may induce changes in a female's anatomy which can interfere with their ability to conceive after therapy is complete. Awareness and counseling by the physician is an integral part of patient care that is often overlooked or not discussed in premenopausal women with cancer.

The American Society of Clinical Oncology (ASCO) has recognized the need for improvement in counseling these women and for proper referrals to reproductive health care specialists. In 2006, ASCO published guidelines which suggested that oncologists "should address the possibility of infertility with patients treated during

S.B. Giordano, M.D. (✉)
Assistant Professor, Division of Hematology and Oncology, Medical University of South Carolina, 173 Ashley Avenue, BSB104, MSC 635, Charleston, SC 29425, USA
e-mail: sbarnato@gmail.com

T.K. Woodruff et al. (eds.), *Oncofertility Communication: Sharing Information and Building Relationships across Disciplines*, DOI 10.1007/978-1-4614-8235-2_10,

their reproductive years and be prepared to discuss possible fertility preservation options or refer appropriate and interested patients to a reproductive specialist" [6].

ASCO subsequently added two practice quality measures on fertility preservation to the Quality Oncology Practice Initiative (QOPI) program in 2007 to reflect the ASCO guidelines [7]. The QOPI program established age-based parameters to provide guidance on choosing appropriate patients for fertility discussions. Currently, conditions such as disease stage, disease prognosis, and curability do not exclude patients from the recommendations.

A survey conducted and published by Quinn and colleagues after the ASCO guidelines were created, demonstrated that less than half of oncologists are following these recommendations and that 25 % of oncologist reported routinely referring patients for fertility preservation, and only 38 % reported knowledge of the QOPI guidelines. Their reasons for lack of discussion or referral had to do with the lack of the oncologist's knowledge about referrals, their perception that patients could not delay treatment, and their perception that patients were not interested in discussing fertility preservation because it was not mentioned by the patient [8]. Data from the QOPI program also confirm many oncologists are not discussing infertility risk involved with chemotherapy and fertility preservation options. More research is needed to focus on the many barriers to the oncologist's ability to provide such discussions and resources and for the development of interventions to overcome such barriers.

Barriers to Fertility Preservation

With the release of ASCO guidelines in 2006, the role of the oncologist in discussing potential infertility due to cancer treatments and fertility preservation options has been delineated. Despite these guidelines, rates of discussion and referrals have been suboptimal. Several studies have identified significant barriers to this important communications process. Barriers exist within the health care system, by the physician, between the physician and patient, and by the patient.

Health Care System Barriers

While national guidelines exist regarding fertility discussion or referrals for fertility preservation, many hospital policies and practices do not correspond with the guidelines. The dissemination of guideline information is not instantaneous with physicians and nurses often unaware of practice guidelines. Even when parties are aware of the guidelines, there can be communication gaps within the health care system. Within an institution it is important to delegate which provider, the physician, pharmacist, mid-level, or nurse, will cover the discussion on the potential for infertility with the patient. In addition, it is critical for the provider to be aware of available sperm banks, reproductive urologists, and reproductive endocrinologists available at the institution or city [9].

Health insurance often poses a barrier to reproductive assisted technologies as insurance coverage is rarely available. The potential costs involved in most procedures are not only prohibitive for many cancer patients, but they also serve as a barrier for health care professionals to discuss these expensive options. No single state mandates coverage for fertility preservation for cancer patients prior to treatment. In addition, the legal definition of infertility does not apply to cancer patients who need fertility procedures in a timely manner. Infertility is defined as an inability to conceive despite attempts to become pregnant through unprotected intercourse for at least 1 year. For cancer patients who need to bank sperm or stimulate their ovaries for egg and/or embryo banking prior to their cancer therapy, they do not meet the state definition of infertility and may have difficulty obtaining reimbursement for the fertility preservation procedure [10]. LIVESTRONG's Sharing Hope program provides financial assistance to eligible patients undertaking fertility preservation at participating centers [9]. Access to the Sharing Hope program and the proposal of new health policies ultimately leading to insurance coverage can aide in solving one of the many issues young cancer patients face.

Physician Barriers

Even with national guideline recommendations in place, many physicians are reluctant to endorse fertility preservation. Studies looking at this specific topic have found physicians' knowledge about fertility and attitudes about discussing risks and preservation options as key barriers, as patients are strongly influenced by the messages they receive from their health care provider. A key obstacle is the concern among many oncologists that discussing the risk of infertility and fertility preservation is neither appropriate nor an immediate clinical priority. Also physicians often have perceptions that financial costs of fertility preservation may be too high for certain families. A study by Vadaparampil et al. considered barriers to fertility preservation among pediatric oncologists [11]. Interviews were conducted with pediatric hematologists/oncologists practicing in Florida. Responses were characterized by primary healthcare barriers, physician perceptions of desire for information, patient characteristics that may impact fertility preservation discussions, and issues unique to adolescent patients. Physician factors were related to lack of formal training in fertility preservation and lack of adequate referral information about fertility preservation. What was also noted in the survey was that the majority of pediatric oncologists expressed a desire for fertility preservation institutional guidelines.

A study by Kohler and colleagues surveyed pediatric oncologists' attitudes towards fertility preservation [12]. Results from the study suggest that while pediatric oncologists acknowledge the importance of addressing fertility preservation, less than half reported they refer male patients and only 12 % reported they refer female patients to a fertility specialist prior to treatment. In regard to the ASCO guidelines, 44 % noted they were familiar with them.

These studies are just a few of the many examples that demonstrate many providers often lack knowledge about fertility preservation, have the perception that the subject of fertility preservation adds more stress to the situation, and have general uncertainty about success of fertility preservation methods. In addition, many are unaware of current guidelines. Improved methods for information transmission are needed. Regardless of the uncertainty, there is general agreement that reproductive and sexual health of young cancer patients is important and the implementation of institutional guidelines for introducing, discussing, and providing fertility preservation services is warranted.

Communication Barriers

During a new patient consultation, patients are often flooded with new information regarding their diagnosis, therapeutic options, clinical trial availability, review of therapy-related toxicities, and discussion on prognosis. Each one of these issues requires attentive and delicate communication in a time efficient manner. With such patients, the delayed side effects of therapy, including infertility risk and fertility preservation are equally challenging and often times may seem inappropriate to both the physician and the patient. Some patient's feel discussing fertility at the time of diagnosis is futile as their focus is on saving their own life, vs. creating a new one. However multiple studies show patients experience regret once the shock of the initial diagnosis has lessened or once treatment is underway or complete [13].

Faulty timing of fertility preservation discussions and the way the information is provided to the patient is also a barrier to pursuing fertility preservation. The window is usually narrow for a woman to seek consultation for fertility preservation options and to undergo ovarian stimulation. Therefore the discussion is required during the initial hematology or oncology consultation. In addition, the delay in treatment initiation can also become a barrier. Some malignancies require immediate treatment, at which point fertility preservation should not be considered. Even so, the potential risk should still be discussed with the patient. The oncologist may also be concerned that a patient's choice to pursue fertility preservation could delay chemotherapy, possibly compromising treatment outcomes and impending the delivery of quality care. Studies looking at factors affecting decision-making about fertility preservation uniformly conclude with the suggested need for an early appointment with a fertility expert [14]. It is critical that the oncologist discuss these issues with the patient and not make a choice for the patient without the patient's consent.

Multiple studies and discussions with survivors suggest patients do not recall having a fertility preservation conversation with their doctor. What is not known is if these discussions did occur and were not remembered or if these conversations did not take place at all. What is known, however, is that the ability to have biological children in the future is extremely important to the vast majority of cancer patients. Feelings of decreased self-esteem, body image, and concern regarding intimate relationships are frequent among these patients. And even if having additional children may not be possible for a patient with incurable cancer, it is important for the patient to be aware of the risk and to be able to make the choice to pursue or forego fertility preservation independently on the basis of information provided by the oncologist.

Adolescent and Young Adult Barriers

Both males and females may experience emotional as well as physical barriers to using fertility preservation. Communication about sperm storage and ovarian stimulation may be uncomfortable for the young adult patient. In some cases, young men may be unprepared for the physical process of sperm banking and may need support from a team of experts. Also, the process of preservation is more complicated for women. Embryo and egg banking are both nonexperimental techniques for fertility preservation, however each with their own challenges. Egg cryopreservation is a less tested method, and depending on an institution's expertise, may not be an option for all female patients. Embryo cryopreservation poses a challenge if females do not have a sperm donor or if they are uneasy about using a sperm bank.

Parent Barriers

Parental communication barriers surrounding their teenager or young adult cancer diagnosis include lack of knowledge about emotional development and cognitive processes of the adolescent/young adult, and varying religious or culture values. Parents can lack information regarding the details about the cancer diagnosis, treatment plan, and side effects, all of which may provide an additional barrier to fertility preservation. There are times when the patient and the parents concerns are at odds. This is an area in which many physicians lack the training to effectively communicate with both parties.

Fertility Preservation in the Incurable Patient

On the basis of the ASCO guidelines [6], one of the QOPI measures assesses whether oncologists discuss infertility risk with their patients before they begin anticancer therapy. Discussing infertility risk and fertility preservation with patients not being treated with curative intent may be uncomfortable, and the topic should be handled carefully and sensitively. It is important for the oncologist to not withhold information from the patient regarding potential fertility loss and to assess each patient's wishes and concerns and facilitate access to information as needed. One suggestion is that after discussing the diagnosis with the patient and informing the cancer is not curable, the physician can acknowledge that often patients in similar situations still wonder about having children. At that point, recognizing the news is upsetting and referral to a fertility specialist should be offered.

Conclusion

Concerns about future fertility are common among patients with cancer and have a significant impact on quality of life. Ultimately the responsibility for conveying information about fertility and childbearing in relation to the cancer diagnosis and treatment lies in the hands of the medical professionals, specifically the treating oncologist. The ASCO guidelines recommend oncologists address these concerns with patients and their families. The QOPI measures are a useful mechanism for quality improvement efforts and assess whether discussion and referrals take. Also, stimulating greater communication and referral patterns between hematologist–oncologists and specialists in reproductive medicine will help ensure these patients are able to receive the specialty care they need. And with greater publicity surrounding this topic, patients and their families can become their own advocate and request information and services for fertility preservation and testing if their physician does not offer it.

Issues of fertility and reproduction are important to most patients with cancer of reproductive age. New methods of communication between all parties, physicians, patients, and parents, must be examined. Healthcare providers need training and guidelines on how to discuss fertility-related issues and concerns. Also, the ASCO guidelines and QOPI quality assessment measures regarding communication about infertility and fertility preservation options are appropriate additions to the overall effort to improve quality of care.

Acknowledgments This work was supported by the Oncofertility Consortium NIH 5UL1DE019587 and TL1CA133837.

References

1. Partridge AH, Gelber S, et al. Wed-based survey of fertility issues in young women with breast cancer. J Clin Oncol. 2004;22(20):4174–83.
2. Thewes B, Meiser B, et al. Fertility- and menopause-related information needs of younger women with a diagnosis of early breast cancer. J Clin Oncol. 2005;23(22):5155–65.
3. Nakayama K, Liu P, et al. Receiving information on fertility and menopause related treatment effects among women who undergo HSCT: changes in perceived importance over time. Biol Blood Marrow Transplant. 2009;11:1465–74.
4. Dizon D. Quality of life after breast cancer: survivorship and sexuality. Breast J. 2009; 15(5):500–4.
5. Schover LR. Premature ovarian failure and its consequences: vasomotor symptoms, sexuality, and fertility. J Clin Oncol. 2008;26:753–8.

6. Lee S, Schover LR, et al. American Society of Clinical Oncology recommendations on fertility preservation in cancer patients. J Clin Oncol. 2006;24(18):2917–31.
7. American Society of Clinical Oncology: QOPI Methodology. http://qopi.asco.org/Methodology
8. Quinn GP, Vadaparampil ST, et al. Physician referral for fertility preservation in oncology patients: a national study of practice behaviors. J Clin Oncol. 2009;27(35):5952–7.
9. Kelvin JF, Reinecke J. Institutional approaches to implementing fertility preservation for cancer patients. Adv Exp Med Biol. 2012;732:165–73.
10. Knapp CA, Quinn GP, et al. Patient provider communication and reproductive health. Adv Exp Med Biol. 2012;732:175–85.
11. Quinn GP, Vadaparampil ST. Fertility preservation and adolescent young adult cancer patients: physician communication challenges. J Adolesc Health. 2009;44(4):394–400.
12. Kohler TS, Kondapalli LA, et al. Results from the survey for preservation of adolescent reproduction (SPARE) study: gender disparity in delivery of fertility preservation message to adolescents with cancer. J Assist Reprod Genet. 2011;28(3):269–77.
13. Crawshaw MA, Glaser AW, et al. Male and female experiences of having fertility matters raised alongside a cancer diagnosis during the teenage and young adult years. Eur J Cancer Care. 2009;18(4):381–90.
14. Peddie VL, Porter MA, et al. Factors affecting decision making about fertility preservation after cancer diagnosis: a qualitative study. BJOG. 2012;119:1049–57.

Part II
Communicating with Healthcare Professionals, Stakeholders and the Public

Chapter 11
An Interprofessional Approach to Shared Decision Making: What it Means and Where Next

France Légaré and Dawn Stacey

Introduction

Given the emphasis on integrated healthcare services and engagement of patients as partners in their care, finding effective ways to involve patients in shared decision making is critical [1–3]. An interprofessional healthcare team approach is a process by which two or more professionals collaborate to provide integrated and cohesive patient care to address the needs of their population [4]. Professionals include any healthcare workers involved in patient care across the spectrum from prevention to treatment and/or rehabilitation. An interprofessional approach to shared decision making enables interprofessional teams to support patients facing decisions, meet their decisional needs, and reach healthcare choices that are agreed upon by the patient and the interprofessional team together [5, 6]. To date, shared decision making models are limited to the patient–physician dyad, yet care is increasingly planned and delivered through interprofessional teams [4, 7–12]. An interprofessional approach to shared decision making has the potential to link multiple professionals (e.g., physicians, nurses, physical therapists, psychologists) and healthcare levels with patients and their families, thereby bridging gaps and minimizing the silos that

---

F. Légaré (✉)
Centre Hospitalier Universitaire de Quebec Research Centre, Hôpital St-François D'Assise, 10 rue Espinay, Québec, QC, Canada G1L 3L5

Department of Family Medicine and Emergency Medicine, Université Laval, Québec, QC, Canada G1K 7P4
e-mail: france.legare@mfa.ulaval.ca

D. Stacey
Faculty of Health Sciences, School of Nursing, University of Ottawa, 451 Smyth Road, Ottawa, ON, Canada K1H 8M5

Clinical Epidemiology Program, Ottawa Hospital Research Institute, Ottawa, ON, Canada

T.K. Woodruff et al. (eds.), *Oncofertility Communication: Sharing Information and Building Relationships across Disciplines*, DOI 10.1007/978-1-4614-8235-2_11,

exist within the healthcare system. In other words, an interprofessional approach to shared decision making could improve the quality of decisions made by patients and their healthcare teams by fostering integrated healthcare services and continuity across health sectors and throughout the continuum of care [13]. This in turn could increase quality of care, reduce practice variations, and improve the fit between what patients want and what they receive throughout the life cycle [14].

Oncofertility care exemplifies the necessity and potential for interprofessional shared decision making. Oncologists, reproductive endocrinologists, nurses, and psychologists must work together in order to provide quality oncofertility care. Even if a patient does not want to engage in fertility preservation, the oncologist and his or her staff must be familiar with the topic of cancer-related infertility in order to broach the topic and provide appropriate information and referrals. In addition, several institutions have found success using midlevel providers as oncofertility "point persons" to ensure that patients receive information in a timely manner.

This chapter reviews the state of knowledge regarding an interprofessional approach to shared decision making in healthcare. It also summarizes the lessons learned from current initiatives and provides suggestions for future research and development in this area.

Do Patients Want to Be Engaged in Decision Making, and Are They?

In a systematic review of optimal matches of patient preferences about information, decision making, and interpersonal behavior, findings from 14 studies, a majority of which were conducted among cancer patients, showed that a substantial proportion of patients (26–95 %, with a median of 52 %) was dissatisfied with the information given, and preferred to have an active role in decisions concerning their health, especially when they understood the expectations around this role [15]. The same review showed that the better the match between the information desired and the information received, the better the patient outcomes [15]. Patient participation in making decisions with their health providers is also linked to favorable patient outcomes [16–18]. However, in a recently published systematic review of 33 studies which took place in nine countries and assessed the extent to which healthcare providers involve patients in decision making from a third-party perspective, the mean OPTION score was 23 ± 14 % (0 = no involvement at all to 100 % = maximum involvement) [19]. The most prevalent clinical topic was cancer screening and/or treatment. Patients across the world are thus not being actively engaged in decision making pertaining to their health, and oncology clinical settings are no exception.

What Interventions are Effective for Engaging Patients in Decision Making?

A Cochrane systematic review of 86 studies of patients making treatment or screening decisions showed that patient decision aids improve patient engagement in decision making. Of these 86 studies, 18 were focused on cancer screening, 11 on cancer surgery, 9 cancer genetic testing, and 2 chemotherapy. Furthermore, patient decision aids were found to enhance decision quality by reducing uncertainty and among patients, improving the decision process measures of feeling informed and being clear about values [20]. These programs have been found to improve the clinical decision-making process by reducing overuse of options not clearly associated with benefits for all [21] and by enhancing use of options clearly associated with benefits for the majority [22]. In other words, patient decision aids foster a shared understanding among providers and patients, which in turn is positively associated with resolution of problems and symptoms [23, 24], satisfaction with the provider [25] and the clinical encounter [26], trust in and endorsement of the provider's recommendations [27], adherence to the chosen option [28], and self-efficacy when faced with a chronic disease [29]. However, these studies are limited to the patient's perspective and that of one health provider, without consideration of family members or of an interprofessional team.

We published two systematic reviews on interventions to improve the adoption of shared decision making by healthcare providers: a Cochrane review with outcomes evaluated from a third-party perspective, and another review with outcomes reported by the patient [30, 31]. We recently updated these reviews and found 20 new eligible studies. Overall, out of the 40 identified studies, 13 showed increased use of shared decision making in clinical practice. Effective interventions included patient-mediated interventions such as patient decision aids often provided together with training of providers. Only three focused on an interprofessional approach by training two professions in shared decision making: physicians and nurses regarding end-of-life treatment care [32], diabetes management [33], and colorectal cancer screening [34]. Interestingly, these three studies were found to be positive. In summary, engaging an interprofessional team in shared decision making may make better use of the particular contributions of each professional involved, allowing them to work to the full scope of their practice, and thus making implementation of shared decision making both more effective and more sustainable.

An Interprofessional Healthcare Team Approach to Shared Decision Making

When two or more healthcare professionals collaborate with the patient to reach an agreed upon decision, interprofessional shared decision making has been achieved. Interprofessionality involves continuous interaction, open communication and knowledge sharing, understanding of professional roles and common health goals [8, 35]. Interprofessionality also involves exploring a variety of education and care issues, all the while seeking to optimize the patient's participation. Interprofessional collaborations build on the strengths of each profession's approach to care delivery such that professionals practice within their full scope of practice and without intentional duplication of services. Theories about decision making suggest that people do not have stable and preexisting beliefs about self-interest but construct them in the process of eliciting information [36]. Therefore, the way healthcare providers as a team give information is crucial in assisting patients to construct preferences and then decide on a course of action. In others words, an interprofessional approach to shared decision making is about improving the decision-making process among healthcare teams and their patients so that decisions can lead to a choice that is not only informed by the best evidence but also in line with what patients value most.

However, constraining factors on the optimization of interprofessional collaboration in the health sector are numerous and well documented. Mainly they relate to differences in professional perspectives that arise from differing core values [37] and levels of responsibility among professions, as well as from hierarchical relations between professions [38, 39]. Moreover, in a systematic review addressing barriers and facilitators perceived by health professionals from 18 countries for implementing shared decision making in clinical practice, the vast majority of participants ($n=3{,}231$) were physicians (89 %), i.e. there was little interprofessional perspective [40].

In oncofertility clinical practice, there are additional barriers at the organizational level that interfere with achieving an interprofessional approach. These include the different schedules of oncology (often crisis-based) and reproductive endocrinology clinics mainly consumer demand-driven [41]. Oncologists often do not have standing relationships with reproductive endocrinologists, and patients are left to themselves to find fertility-related information and care concurrent with cancer treatment planning [42, 43]. Some have called for a specific specialty of oncofertility care [44], although this would not obviate the need for interprofessional collaboration.

A Model for an Interprofessional Approach to Shared Decision Making

Since 2007, guided by the *Knowledge to Action* (KTA) framework [45], and with the overarching goal of implementing shared decision making using an interprofessional approach, an interdisciplinary and international group have devised a conceptual model to support applied research in this field [5, 6]. This model was based on an extensive review of the literature combined with theory analysis [46]. Briefly, the interprofessional shared decision making model has two main axes: a vertical axis representing the shared decision making process and a horizontal axis representing individuals involved in the process (Fig. 11.1). Elements at the micro level are

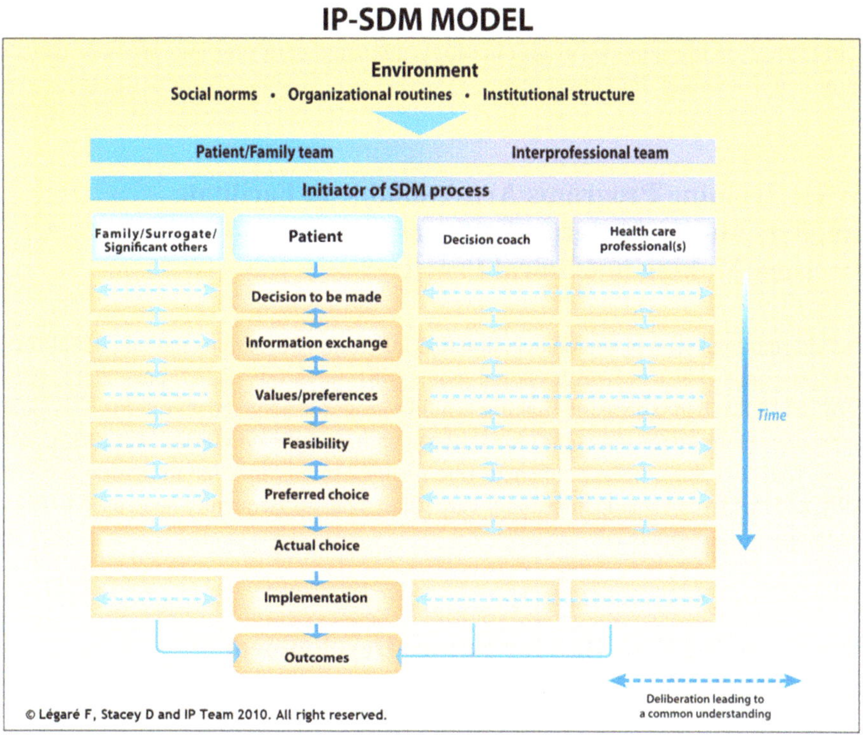

Fig. 11.1 Interprofessional shared decision making model

embedded within family and interprofessional team systems; both are situated within broader environmental influences. There are four key assumptions underlying the model. First, involving patients in the shared decision making process is essential for achieving patient-centered care and reaching decisions that are informed and based on individual patient values. Second, achieving a common understanding of the essential elements of the shared decision making process among the interprofessional team and recognizing the influence of the various individuals on this process will improve success in reaching a shared decision. Third, achieving an interprofessional approach to shared decision making may occur synchronously in the example of family conferences in the intensive care unit, but more often occurs asynchronously and therefore requires a shared framework with this common understanding. Fourth, family or significant others are important stakeholders involved or implicated by the decision and their values and preferences may not be the same as those of the patient.

We recently completed a pilot study of an interprofessional approach to shared decision making with an interprofessional home care team in Quebec City and another, in Edmonton [47]. We developed a toolkit (i.e. a training program, educations tools, and a video) to facilitate the implementation of an interprofessional approach to shared decision making and overcome barriers to implementation (See Appendix). We found that most providers had a high intention to engage in interprofessional shared decision making but depending on their profession, the barriers varied.

This model has also been applied in research projects focused on decisions about withdrawal of life support in an oncology intensive care unit and prostate cancer treatment for newly diagnosed men.

What Training Programs Are Available to Facilitate Implementing an Interprofessional Approach to Shared Decision Making in Clinical Practice?

An international scan of shared decision making training programs indicated that very few programs target interprofessional teams [48]. In fact as of February 2013, only four out of 80 shared decision making training programs targeted an interprofessional approach (http://decision.chaire.fmed.ulaval.ca/index.php?id=180&L=2#c406). Of these four, two have been published: one from Germany in a rehabilitation context [49], and one from Canada in primary care [6] that has subsequently been used to train oncology professionals.

What Are the Priorities for Future Development and Research?

More can be done to refine the preliminary work in conceptual models underlying an interprofessional approach to shared decision making. More specifically, existing models can be validated across clinical settings and cultural contexts. Very little has been achieved in the area of measurement of interprofessional approaches to shared decision making. In a recent review, we were not able to find any existing instruments to measure such an approach. Also, implementation challenges to achieving an interprofessional approach to shared decision making will need to be overcome given that different factors influence different professions. Finally, rigorous studies to evaluate the implementation of an interprofessional approach to shared decision making are required, but these types of studies will involve large numbers of a diverse range of health professionals. Furthermore both the costs and the outcome measures for such studies may be quite different from those for traditional health services research.

Conclusion

The current healthcare context in many countries reinforces the need for interprofessional teams to address the emerging challenges in providing more patient-centered healthcare. An interprofessional approach to shared decision making is needed now because the number of patients facing difficult treatment decisions and needing patient-centered decision support is growing rapidly and clinical decision-making processes need to be improved to better involve patients and recognize their preferences. The interprofessional approach to shared decision making model provides a framework that can guide healthcare teams in making decisions with their patients. However, more research is required to determine effective ways to implement such an interprofessional approach in clinical practice. Oncology, particularly with respect to oncofertility, is no exception. Importantly, an interprofessional approach to shared decision making may prove instrumental in allowing oncofertility patients to become partners in their own care without having to search for their own speciali sts and coordinate their own care. Medical care, and cancer care in particular, is increasingly interdisciplinary. Models of shared decision making should take account of this fact and determine how to best engage patients while promoting interprofessional dialogue.

Acknowledgments This work was supported by the Canadian Institutes of Health Research.

References

1. Flynn D, Knoedler MA, Hess EP, Murad MH, Erwin PJ, Montori VM, et al. Engaging patients in health care decisions in the emergency department through shared decision-making: a systematic review. Acad Emerg Med. 2012;19(8):959–67.
2. Ricciardi L, Mostashari F, Murphy J, Daniel JG, Siminerio EP. A national action plan to support consumer engagement via e-health. Health Aff (Millwood). 2013;32(2):376–84.
3. Dentzer S. Rx for the 'blockbuster drug' of patient engagement. Health Aff (Millwood). 2013;32(2):202.
4. D'Amour D, Ferrada-Videla M, San Martin Rodriguez L, Beaulieu MD. The conceptual basis for interprofessional collaboration: core concepts and theoretical frameworks. J Interprof Care. 2005;19 Suppl 1:116–31.
5. Legare F, Stacey D, Pouliot S, Gauvin FP, Desroches S, Kryworuchko J, et al. Interprofessionalism and shared decision-making in primary care: a stepwise approach towards a new model. J Interprof Care. 2011;25(1):18–25.
6. Legare F, Stacey D, Gagnon S, Dunn S, Pluye P, Frosch D, et al. Validating a conceptual model for an inter-professional approach to shared decision making: a mixed methods study. J Eval Clin Pract. 2011;17(4):554–64.
7. Coulter A. Paternalism or partnership? Patients have grown up-and there's no going back [editorial; comment] [see comments]. BMJ. 1999;319(7212):719–20.
8. D'Amour D, Oandasan I. Interprofessionality as the field of interprofessional practice and interprofessional education: an emerging concept. J Interprof Care. 2005;19 Suppl 1:8–20.
9. Oandasan I. Teamwork and healthy workplaces: strengthening the links for deliberation and action through research and policy. Healthc Pap. 2007;7 Spec No. 98–103; discussion 9–19.
10. Oandasan I, Reeves S. Key elements of interprofessional education. Part 2: Factors, processes and outcomes. J Interprof Care. 2005;19 Suppl 1:39–48.
11. Oandasan I, Reeves S. Key elements for interprofessional education. Part 1: The learner, the educator and the learning context. J Interprof Care. 2005;19 Suppl 1:21–38.
12. Health Professions Network Nursing and Midwifery Office Within the Department of Human Resources for Health. Framework for action on interprofessional education & collaborative practice. Geneva: World Health Organization; 2010.

13. Haggerty JL, Reid RJ, Freeman GK, Starfield BH, Adair CE, McKendry R. Continuity of care: a multidisciplinary review. BMJ. 2003;327(7425):1219–21.
14. Bisognano M, Goodman E. Engaging patients and their loved ones in the ultimate conversation. Health Aff (Millwood). 2013;32(2):203–6.
15. Kiesler DJ, Auerbach SM. Optimal matches of patient preferences for information, decision-making and interpersonal behavior: evidence, models and interventions. Patient Educ Couns. 2006;61(3):319–41.
16. Carlsen B, Aakvik A. Patient involvement in clinical decision making: the effect of GP attitude on patient satisfaction. Health Expect. 2006;9(2):148–57.
17. Hack TF, Degner LF, Watson P, Sinha L. Do patients benefit from participating in medical decision making? Longitudinal follow-up of women with breast cancer. Psychooncology. 2006;15(1):9–19.
18. Hibbard JH, Greene J. What the evidence shows about patient activation: better health outcomes and care experiences; fewer data on costs. Health Aff (Millwood). 2013;32(2):207–14.
19. Couët N, Desroches S, Robitaille H, Vaillancourt H, Leblanc A, et al. Assessments of the extent to which healthcare providers involve patients in decision making: a systematic review of studies using the OPTION instrument. Health Expect. 2013 Mar 4.
20. Stacey D, Bennett CL, Barry MJ, Col NF, Eden KB, Holmes-Rovner M, et al. Decision aids for people facing health treatment or screening decisions. Cochrane Database Syst Rev. 2011(10):CD001431.
21. Evans R, Edwards A, Brett J, Bradburn M, Watson E, Austoker J, et al. Reduction in uptake of PSA tests following decision aids: systematic review of current aids and their evaluations. Patient Educ Couns. 2005;58(1):13–26.
22. O'Connor AM, Bennett C, Stacey D, Barry MJ, Col NF, Eden KB, et al. Do patient decision aids meet effectiveness criteria of the international patient decision aid standards collaboration? A systematic review and meta-analysis. Med Decis Making. 2007;27(5):554–74.
23. Starfield B, Wray C, Hess K, Gross R, Birk PS, D'Lugoff BC. The influence of patient-practitioner agreement on outcome of care. Am J Public Health. 1981;71(2):127–31.
24. Bass MJ, Buck C, Turner L, Dickie G, Pratt G, Robinson HC. The physician's actions and the outcome of illness in family practice. J Fam Pract. 1986;23(1):43–7.
25. Krupat E, Rosenkranz SL, Yeager CM, Barnard K, Putnam SM, Inui TS. The practice orientations of physicians and patients: the effect of doctor-patient congruence on satisfaction. Patient Educ Couns. 2000;39(1):49–59.
26. Fagerberg CR, Kragstrup J, Stovring H, Rasmussen NK. How well do patient and general practitioner agree about the content of consultations? Scand J Prim Health Care. 1999; 17(3):149–52.
27. Krupat E, Bell RA, Kravitz RL, Thom D, Azari R. When physicians and patients think alike: patient-centered beliefs and their impact on satisfaction and trust. J Fam Pract. 2001;50(12): 1057–62.
28. Sewitch MJ, Abrahamowicz M, Barkun A, Bitton A, Wild GE, Cohen A, et al. Patient nonadherence to medication in inflammatory bowel disease. Am J Gastroenterol. 2003;98(7): 1535–44.
29. Heisler M, Vijan S, Anderson RM, Ubel PA, Bernstein SJ, Hofer TP. When do patients and their physicians agree on diabetes treatment goals and strategies, and what difference does it make? J Gen Intern Med. 2003;18(11):893–902.
30. Legare F, Ratte S, Stacey D, Kryworuchko J, Gravel K, Graham ID, et al. Interventions for improving the adoption of shared decision making by healthcare professionals. Cochrane Database Syst Rev. 2010(5):CD006732.
31. Legare F, Turcotte S, Stacey D, Ratte S, Kryworuchko J, Graham ID. Patients' perceptions of sharing in decisions: a systematic review of interventions to enhance shared decision making in routine clinical practice. Patient. 2012;5(1):1–19.
32. Murray MA, Stacey D, Wilson KG, O'Connor AM. Skills training to support patients considering place of end-of-life care: a randomized control trial. J Palliat Care. 2010;26(2):112–21.

33. Mullan RJ, Montori VM, Shah ND, Christianson TJ, Bryant SC, Guyatt GH, et al. The diabetes mellitus medication choice decision aid: a randomized trial. Arch Intern Med. 2009; 169(17):1560–8.
34. Schroy III PC, Emmons K, Peters E, Glick JT, Robinson PA, Lydotes MA, et al. The impact of a novel computer-based decision aid on shared decision making for colorectal cancer screening: a randomized trial. Med Decis Making. 2011;31(1):93–107.
35. Xyrichis A, Ream E. Teamwork: a concept analysis. J Adv Nurs. 2008;61(2):232–41.
36. Tversky A, Kahneman D. The framing of decisions and the psychology of choice. Science. 1981;211:453–8.
37. Oddi L, Cassidy V. The message of SUPPORT: study to understand prognosis and preferences for outcomes and risks of treatment. Change is long overdue. J Prof Nurs. 1998;14(4):165–74.
38. Emanuel L. Structured deliberation to improve decision-making for the seriously ill. Hastings Cent Rep. 1995;25(6):S14–8.
39. Sundin-Huard D, Fahy K. Moral distress, advocacy and burnout: theorizing the relationships. Int J Nurs Pract. 1999;5(1):8–13.
40. Legare F, Ratte S, Gravel K, Graham ID. Barriers and facilitators to implementing shared decision-making in clinical practice: update of a systematic review of health professionals' perceptions. Patient Educ Couns. 2008;73(3):526–35.
41. Knapp CA, Quinn GP. Healthcare provider perspectives on fertility preservation for cancer patients. Cancer Treat Res. 2010;156:391–401.
42. Loren AW, Brazauskas R, Chow EJ, Gilleece M, Halter J, Jacobsohn DA, et al. Physician perceptions and practice patterns regarding fertility preservation in hematopoietic cell transplant recipients. Bone Marrow Transplant. 2013 July 17.
43. Vadaparampil S, Quinn G, King L, Wilson C, Nieder M. Barriers to fertility preservation among pediatric oncologists. Patient Educ Couns. 2008;72(3):402–10.
44. Kondapalli LA. Oncofertility: a new medical discipline and the emerging scholar. Cancer Treat Res. 2007;138:221–34.
45. Graham ID, Logan J, Harrison MB, Straus SE, Tetroe J, Caswell W, et al. Lost in knowledge translation: time for a map? J Contin Educ Health Prof. 2006;26(1):13–24.
46. Stacey D, Legare F, Pouliot S, Kryworuchko J, Dunn S. Shared decision making models to inform an interprofessional perspective on decision making: a theory analysis. Patient Educ Couns. 2010;80(2):164–72.
47. Legare F, Stacey D, Briere N, Fraser K, Desroches S, Dumont S, et al. Healthcare providers' intentions to engage in an interprofessional approach to shared decision-making in home care programs: a mixed methods study. J Interprof Care. 2013;27(3):214–22.
48. Legare F, Politi MC, Drolet R, Desroches S, Stacey D, Bekker H. Training health professionals in shared decision-making: an international environmental scan. Patient Educ Couns. 2012 Feb 1.
49. Korner M, Ehrhardt H, Steger AK, Bengel J. Interprofessional SDM train-the-trainer program "Fit for SDM": provider satisfaction and impact on participation. Patient Educ Couns. 2012 May 28.

Chapter 12
Oncofertility Communication Tools for Professionals and the Public

Stefani Foster LaBrecque, Harlan Wallach, and Kate E. Waimey

Introduction

Oncofertility clinicians, researchers, and support staff—who are working to address the reproductive needs of young cancer patients—face the challenge of disseminating information about an interdisciplinary topic to a wide target audience. Oncofertility clinicians must communicate with their partners in reproductive medicine, as well as with oncologists who may have very different academic and clinical backgrounds. Clinicians must also impart their knowledge—specifically, the reproductive impact of cancer treatment on fertility and the available fertility preservation options—to patients, their partners, and parents, often in the chaotic period of time just after a cancer diagnosis. In addition, researchers and other oncofertility support staff must distill complex topics in fertility preservation science for both professional and public audiences. For the past 5 years, the Oncofertility Consortium has developed a diverse set of communication tools that can help oncofertility professionals present authoritative, expert, and accessible information to a wide audience.

These tools range from the traditional, such as publishing primary and review articles in the academic literature, to next-generation tools like social media and other Internet-based programs. Each communication method has its own

S.F. LaBrecque, B.S. (✉)
Northwestern University Advanced Media Production Studio,
1970 Campus Drive, 2-EAST, Evanston, IL 60208, USA
e-mail: stefanifoster@gmail.com

H. Wallach, B.F.A., M.F.A.
NUIT—Northwestern University Information Technologies, Chicago, IL, USA
e-mail: Wallach@northwestern.edu

K.E. Waimey, Ph.D.
Department of Obstetrics and Gynecology, Feinberg School of Medicine,
Northwestern University, Chicago, IL, USA
e-mail: ktimmerman@northwestern.edu

T.K. Woodruff et al. (eds.), *Oncofertility Communication: Sharing Information and Building Relationships across Disciplines*, DOI 10.1007/978-1-4614-8235-2_12,

advantages and disadvantages. For example, academic publications have credibility with funding sources and in scholarly environments; however, they often reach a relatively small group of already engaged stakeholders. In contrast, social media has the ability to communicate to very large audience, but is considered to be a much less credible source due to the lack of a peer review process [1]. Thus, though the Oncofertility Consortium has created many communication tools, it is important that oncofertility professionals appreciate how to select and use the most effective tools to tell the oncofertility story in an engaging way to their peers as well as the broader public.

Tools to Educate Scientific and Medical Professionals

Most oncofertility professionals are familiar with the traditional route used to communicate biomedical topics via academic publications; however, emerging tools, such as Web sites, virtual meetings, and mobile tools, have the advantage of rapid dissemination of oncofertility information to a larger professional audience, beyond the academic journals' readership. Academic publication often takes months or years from initial submission to final publication and may ultimately be read by only a handful of experts already within the field. While the peer review system of academic publication ensures that the highest quality data are presented, it may not be the best vehicle to propagate research findings to a wider audience.

Medical education programs designed to disseminate emerging research to various clinical communities have been extensively studied to determine the most effective education methods. Continuing medical education is presented to clinicians at professional conferences, with printed clinical materials, and in train-the-trainer programs [1]. Yet, traditional in-person education programs can be expensive to implement and connect with limited numbers of clinicians over restricted geographic regions [2, 3]. While print education for clinicians, such as brochures and booklets, transcend the regional restrictions of in-person events, they can quickly become outdated in rapidly advancing interdisciplinary fields such as oncofertility.

Even within a single field, individual professionals may prefer certain modes of education. For example, clinicians are twice as likely as researchers, public health experts, and academics to prefer education through print media, such as journal articles, and annual society meetings [4]. Familiarity with technology must also be taken into account when developing educational programs, as medical professionals comprise early, middle, and late technology adopters who utilize technology to different degrees and for different reasons [4, 5]. In addition, professionals may be more or less comfortable with certain types of information presented online. In a recent survey, providers were asked what tools they would most like to see from an online authoritative resource; the respondents indicated that they would like to see information about screening and treatment options [5, 6].

To combat the limitations of print and in-person education, and to better tailor scientific education to different audiences, researchers have investigated the effectiveness of online and mobile education, which can reach an unlimited audience size and geographic locations [7, 8]. These studies indicate that learning achieved from Internet-based education programs is equivalent to that from traditional printed materials [9, 10]. The capacity for frequent content updates makes online education programs ideal for communicating research breakthroughs to the clinical community in rapidly advancing interdisciplinary fields, such as oncofertility. Interactive Internet-based education can also improve learning outcomes with practice exercises and repetition of information that is not possible with print products [11].

Two strategies that were recently integrated into the Oncofertility Consortium communication effort are social media and mobile-based presentations, with the goal of expanding the reach of educational programs and resources beyond computer-based browsers. During the first 5 years of the Consortium, mobile devices were quickly being adopted as a common basis of online interaction. In response, the Consortium developed standalone mobile apps, started direct sharing of all content items to social media platforms, and began using HTML5 Web standards for all Web presentations. The goal was to maximize the accessibility of the content by using the greatest number of available platforms; this has been possible with the widespread adoption of HTML5 Web standards.

Professional Web sites

In response to the shift in education to Web-based and mobile platforms, the oncofertility community has developed Web-based print materials and programs in order to reach a larger community of reproductive health and oncology researchers and clinicians in a timely and credible manner. These Web-based tools have been utilized to disseminate information to researchers and clinicians, and promote continuing professional education.

The 5-year history of oncofertility communication is characterized by a continuous evolution of technology tools developed to meet the needs of the Oncofertility Consortium. The goal of these efforts was and continues to be the reinforcement of connections between clinicians and the emerging science, using a common language for both internal coordination and external outreach. This process has involved a deep and ongoing introspection of how to align the technology to the changing needs of the Oncofertility Consortium goals, ideas, and audiences.

The original documentation, communication, and outreach plans for online oncofertility communication focused on utilization of the World Wide Web, in an environment in which online media was primarily consumed via standard-sized display/browser windows, without the need to be responsive to the variety of portable devices that are now commonplace. This initial effort was accomplished primarily through the development of the main Oncofertility Consortium Web site (http://oncofertility.northwestern.edu/) for internal communication, and a public-facing Web site, MyOncofertility (http://myoncofertility.org/) for direct outreach (Fig. 12.1). Both of these sites were initially developed in platforms that quickly

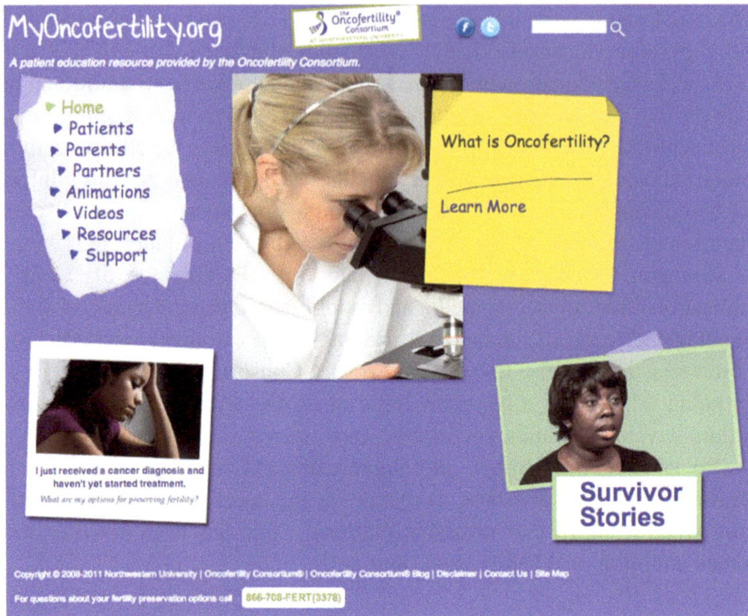

Fig. 12.1 The original professional and public-facing oncofertility Web sites, Oncofertility. Northwestern.edu and MyOncofertility.org

proved to be insufficient to reach a wide target audience. Within 18 months of the project launch, both sites were migrated from their original platforms to newer systems to better leverage more contemporary network communication. This immediately moved the online communication of oncofertility into a modern dynamic content system that directly supported and sustained reader interest and engagement.

A core component to successfully implementing these features was the use of human-readable URLs and Web permalinks, thus enabling dramatic gains in search engine optimization (SEO). All of these features were the first deep integration of contemporary online communication methods that recognize the interconnected nature of publishing online data. It was not enough to merely publish; the data needed to be presented in ways that allowed it to be found by clinicians and patients, as the common ways of searching, communicating, and staying current had evolved in the short time since the launch of the consortium.

Archived data included on professional Web sites can serve as a valuable resource. The Oncofertility Consortium utilizes its Web site for professionals (http://oncofertility.northwestern.edu/) for this purpose, posting all publications funded through the Consortium and recordings of lectures as enduring educational materials. These include videos and slide decks of presentations from the annual conferences and past virtual grand rounds. Finally, this portal provides a method for the Oncofertility Consortium to disseminate new evidence-based tools that providers can use, such as brochures and decision tools. Due to the broad array of content available, this single Web site receives more than 22,000 visits annually from around the globe.

The professional Oncofertility Consortium Web site also assists oncologists and other specialists in finding information on fertility preservation. A map of reproductive specialist Oncofertility Consortium members helps physicians identify fertility preservation experts in their region. The Web site also promotes the national fertility hotline, FERTline, which is staffed by a fertility preservation patient navigator who can refer physicians to reproductive specialists in their region who have experience in fertility preservation.

The evolving, broad-based communication approach taken by the Oncofertility Consortium can be appreciated in the responsive design and implementation of its latest online resource, the Fertility Preservation Patient Navigator Web site (http://preservefertility.northwestern.edu/). All content on the site is presentable and useable on any mobile device. Efforts to make the availability of oncofertility science and outreach as widespread as possible is reflected in the continual improvement of all Consortium online publishing platforms; as communication technologies change, the tools are adapted to remain relevant and accessible.

Virtual Meetings

Established and next-generation communication tools can be used to develop and maintain team unity across diverse disciplines, which is essential to the field of oncofertility. The Oncofertility Consortium developed tools to both educate professionals and to support team-building to advance the pace of interdisciplinary research and adoption of fertility preservation into clinical practice. For interdisciplinary fields such as oncofertility, virtual meetings can provide researchers and clinicians an opportunity to communicate across long distances and in real time.

The Oncofertility Consortium developed two types of virtual meetings to foster such communication. Researchers within the Consortium utilize Virtual Lab Meetings to share emerging data. As with in-person lab meetings, these provide an opportunity for trainees to present their initial findings and discuss research problems with peers and established academics. The virtual nature of these meetings allows researchers from multiple perspectives to participate in discussions across the research pipeline. For example, when scientists discuss improving the media used to culture mouse follicles, clinical researchers can provide input about how those changes may affect human ovarian tissue culture. Having these discussions as researchers are developing a method can save time and money when that method is later translated into clinical care. The technology used for these meetings is the Vidyo videoconferencing system, which allows for face-to-face audio, video, and data sharing between Oncofertility Consortium members. Investigators and their teams can join from any computer or mobile device in the world, accessing the meeting from their institution's conference room or from their mobile device.

The Oncofertility Consortium also hosts virtual grand rounds to engage the larger oncofertility community, including researchers, clinicians, advocates, and grant officers from around the country. Virtual grand rounds allow experts in the oncofertility field to communicate current research findings and clinical care updates with cancer and fertility researchers and clinicians using Adobe Connect (San Jose, CA). With this technology, a single presenter broadcasts video and data slides and viewers ask text-based questions that can be answered in real time. The Consortium has utilized this software to host external presentations from experts in the field. Recordings of the data slides and video are then posted on Oncofertility Consortium Web site, expanding viewership of the Rounds. Typically, approximately 40 people attend the live virtual grand rounds from across the United States and an additional 400 watch recordings of the archived videos over the following year.

> Feedback on the oncofertility virtual grand rounds:
> I think the virtual grand rounds meetings have really bridged the gap between clinical work and basic science research and really allowed a conversation to happen between those two realms which often don't have an opportunity to talk. So I can say, 'We see these patients, they are going through IVF, they don't respond well, or there are issues. What is the best way to stimulate these patients, how can we get the eggs out, how should we prepare the tissue?' And then they can go back and look at different things in the laboratory, you know, in the primate model and in the mouse and say, 'Well we're finding, this is true.' I think it's really helping to inform the basic science and even the basic science is helping to inform the clinical practice.
>
> — Interview with Clarisa R. Gracia, MD, MSCE, June 30, 2011, Philadelphia, PA

> ...we could say that all the virtual doors are open 24 hours a day, 7 days a week. You can expect an email, or a Skype, or a virtual lab meeting at almost any time, any day. And it may involve not only just the members of the Consortium, but consultants that we bring in from around the country, around the world. And we all recognize, we support the confidentiality of what we present, but within the Consortium itself, it's basically one big brain trust.
>
> — Interview with Richard L. Stouffer, Ph.D., June, 28, 2011, Beaverton, OR

Though virtual communication tools help to build and maintain interdisciplinary teams across long distances and educate researchers and clinicians, there is no replacement for in-person communication. Within the Oncofertility Consortium, an annual conference provides an opportunity for researchers, clinicians, and others to learn about cutting-edge advances in fertility preservation and discuss how these can be incorporated into clinical practice. Attendees include professionals from across the research pipeline, including principal investigators, trainees, and research staff. In addition, professionals from the health care, advocacy, and bioethics join the annual oncofertility conference to foster interdisciplinary collaborations through formal networking sessions and informal sessions, such as dinners and poster presentations.

While the person-to-person interaction of the Oncofertility Consortium conferences provides an opportunity for team building, professionals who are unable to travel can also watch the educational content through live streaming of conference presentations through Adobe Connect. This next-generation technology allows individuals to participate in the conference despite demanding clinical schedules. Recordings of presentations are then posted online using Mediasite lecture capture (Madison, WI), which allow viewers to view searchable data slides and presenter videos simultaneously. Continuing medical education credits can also be given for viewing online oncofertility lectures. These virtual meetings and tools to broadcast in-person activities allow transient events to reach the global oncofertility community.

Mobile Tools

Next generation technologies, such as mobile handheld technology, can facilitate clinical education and communicate advances in healthcare. Mobile handheld technologies, which can be viewed on PDAs, tablet PCs, and smartphones, can increase access to information for physicians [12, 13]. In a recent study, 72 % of clinicians reported using such devices in a medical setting for indirect patient care (such as for preparation for cases) [14]. Interestingly, that same study indicated that few clinicians use mobile handheld technology for direct patient consultation, such as answering clinical questions in the exam room.

In the relatively short period that the oncofertility field has been in existence, the opportunities to communicate through mobile technologies have expanded rapidly. A simple example of this evolution is that neither iPhone nor Android smart phones had been released when the Oncofertility Consortium was founded and funded by the National Institutes of Health Roadmap Grant, and today, the need to communicate through these technological platforms (smartphones) is key to reaching contemporary audiences.

The Oncofertility Consortium embraced this opportunity by developing a mobile application compatible with the iPhone to disseminate oncofertility education to providers. This app, iSaveFertility, offers providers the ability to view educational pocket guides about fertility preservation for women, men, and children on their smart phones (Fig. 12.2). A companion Web site (http://www.savemyfertility.org/) was launched in parallel to make the content available to other mobile and desktop platforms beyond iOS devices. Users of the app, which has been downloaded more than 1,000 times, spend almost 10 min reviewing the material, providing some of the first evidence that clinicians may learn new health information through mobile devices. Despite the presence of the app, clinicians also frequently request print copies of the pocket guides, indicating that individual preferences for print materials also come into play when educating healthcare providers.

Tools to Disseminate Oncofertility Information to the Public

While reproductive scientists and oncologists and other disease specialists are the gatekeepers to clinical discussions with patients, anecdotal evidence and research studies indicate that many patients do not currently receive timely information

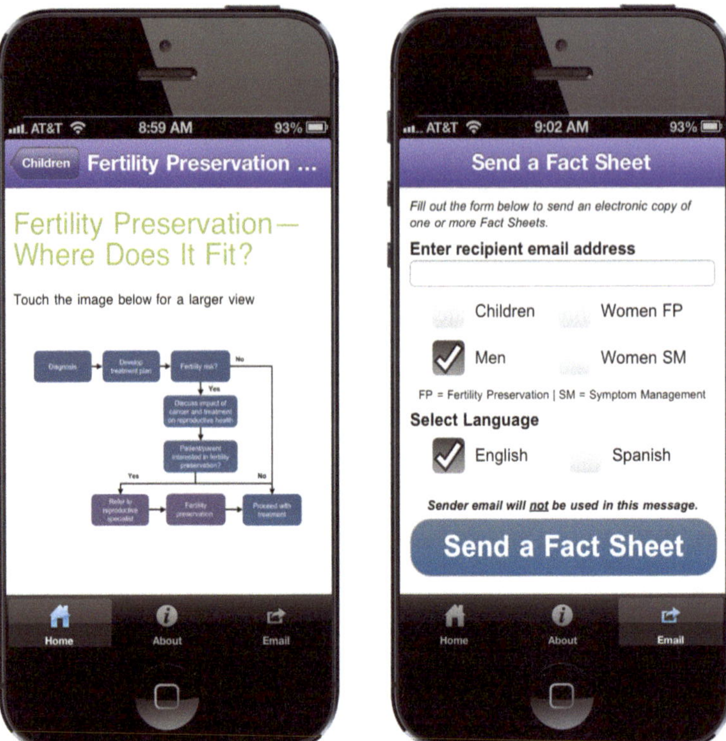

Fig. 12.2 Screen shots of the iSaveFertility iPhone App, which provides clinical education for healthcare providers and the ability to directly e-mail oncofertility fact sheets to patients

regarding fertility preservation prior to the onset of cancer treatment. As such, professional groups have developed patient-oriented, authoritative materials that are appropriate for the general public and patient audiences. Print materials have been developed to facilitate provider discussions with patients and increase access to specialists, but studies show that these are currently of limited use [15–17]. A combination of physician–patient discussion and printed material distribution is one of the most effective ways to provide health care education to patients [18]. While oncologists are in the best position to provide such dual education, only 13 % of oncologists report frequent distribution of fertility preservation materials and these materials may not be distributed in an appropriate manner [15–17]. Furthermore, only a quarter of those who provide materials to patients believe they are relevant to the patient [16]. Thus, there is a significant need for oncofertility materials to be developed and distributed based on feedback from oncology clinicians and patients, and disseminated to patients in a manner that is appropriate to their knowledge level and comfort with the topic.

Younger cancer patients, who may be particularly interested in a reproductive future, are the ideal audience for oncofertility communication using online tools, such as Web sites, social media, and mobile applications, as they may be more likely to seek out health care information online than the general population. The Oncofertility Consortium has leveraged the technical savvy of young survivors to develop a series of tailored tools and raise awareness and education about fertility in cancer patients. These tools include Web sites such as MyOncofertility, SaveMyFertility, and the Fertility Preservation Patient Navigator, each of which has specific public-facing content. The creation of relevant media with clear messaging and relatable information is critical to the success of the oncofertility mission. Smart engagement with the target audience, specifically young patients, using creative storytelling, polished esthetics, and a demonstration of modern media savvy will help propel the message into the communities that most need to receive it, increasing the likelihood that awareness will be passed along to the general public.

Adolescent and young adult cancer patients make up approximately 10 % of the cancer population and have unique needs that don't fall into the realm of the typical cancer patient. This underserved community lacks resources and information regarding their future reproductive options after cancer treatment, a gap that is being addressed by the Oncofertility Consortium and other groups. One goal of patient-directed oncofertility communication is to reduce the feeling of isolation faced by many young people with cancer and give a sense of hope after a cancer diagnosis. As these patients are bombarded with information from the moment they are diagnosed, it is critical that the oncofertility community ensures the availability of consistent, credible information and connection with key resources.

> ...if they wouldn't have mentioned [fertility preservation] as an option, as something we should consider, I don't know if we would have even known to do it. Without the doctor recommending it, we never would have done it, I don't think. We would have just accepted the fact [that children weren't in our future]...
>
> — David Majors, from an interview with David and Tiffany Majors, July 26, 2011, Chicago, IL

Because some cancer treatments, as well as some fertility preservation procedures, are extremely time-sensitive, fast and accurate access to information can be critical for certain patients. Spouses or family members might discourage the patient from taking time to consider and pursue fertility-preservation options because they are more concerned with the immediate goal of saving the life of their loved one rather than future concerns about fertility.

For some patients, access to a wide range of information, such as ethical and legal issues surrounding oncofertility, is extremely important, and can heavily influence their decision to pursue fertility preservation options. Communication tools are not only an important source of information, but also necessary to counter misinformation. For newly diagnosed patients and family members, the Internet is a huge source of information with varying degrees of reliability, and this information will often be sought without discretion in times of great concern and stress. It is critical to ensure that this audience is getting the correct and relevant information in the most straightforward and timely manner possible.

Public-Facing Web sites

The MyOncofertility Web site was the first oncofertility Web site developed to aid patients, their parents, and partners in making fertility preservation decisions during the high-stress time after a cancer diagnosis. The Web site houses short videos of patients, scientists, and health care providers, and animations of fertility preservation techniques. This visual approach can be particularly useful for children, individuals with poor literacy, and those struggling with the oncofertility decision-making process. The site also employs a question-and-answer model that mimics a dialogue between provider and patient, creating an interactive learning experience. The MyOncofertility Web site aims to provide the information that patients require to make informed oncofertility decisions, help mitigate stress, empower users, and help them identify with other patients in similar situations [19]. The Web site was initially built in English but has since been developed into a Spanish-language site (http://es.myoncofertility.org/), to provide oncofertility information to the more than 34 million people worldwide who speak Spanish as their primary language. Research has shown that minority cancer patients (African American, Asian, Hispanic, Multiracial, Native Hawaiian/Other Pacific Islander, Native American/Native Alaskan) are more distressed by loss of fertility due to cancer treatment and more likely to want fertility preservation information than Caucasians, but are less likely to receive information from clinicians who do not speak Spanish at their primary language [20]. The Spanish-language site now receives greater than 10 % of the total MyOncofertility Web site traffic, with more than 20,000 visits per year.

In the years since the MyOncofertility Web site launch in 2007, user feedback highlighted the need to provide more concise information to patients, which the Consortium adopted in two new Web sites. One simplified site, the Fertility Preservation Patient Navigator site (http://fertilitypreservation.northwestern.edu), provides information to patients regarding fertility preservation but does so using an interactive patient decision tool, stories of patients who underwent fertility preservation prior to cancer treatment, and animated tutorials about fertility preservation procedures. The decision tool, called "What are My Options," guides patients through the key factors that are considered when making decisions about fertility preservation, such as sex, pubertal status, and progress of the cancer treatment plan. It also directs patients to a fertility preservation patient navigator. In addition to the decision tool, six patient stories are communicated in 1–2 min videos, rather than the short videos found on the My Oncofertility Web site. These extended videos allow viewers time to identify with and develop relationships with the patients on the screen, which can help patients, partners, and parents feel more comfortable with the fertility preservation decision-making process.

The SaveMyFertility microsite (http://www.savemyfertility.org/) was developed by the Oncofertility Consortium and Hormone Health Network to provide patients fact sheets on fertility and endocrine health. The information is tailored to women, men, and parents of children with cancer and is viewable on the Web and available as downloadable PDFs. The Web site also includes oncofertility information geared to medical professionals interested in learning clinical information about reproductive health after cancer and the fertility preservation process. The SaveMyFertility Web site was built in conjunction with the iSaveFertility mobile application discussed previously, as it provides information to both the clinical and patient communities.

Social Media

While the patient-facing oncofertility Web sites described here provide enduring online materials to the public, they also require significant development costs, time, and marketing to drive traffic to the sites. To complement the information on the Web, the Oncofertility Consortium also uses social media to disseminate medical and research information. The interactivity and continuous contact possible with online social media can keep emerging topics and information in the consciousness of patients and the public. Social media tools include blogs, Facebook, Twitter, You Tube, Pinterest, and the seemingly endless number of new tools that are emerging every day. The adoption of social media allows professionals in science and medicine, including researchers and clinicians, to engage and communicate information to the larger community.

The Oncofertility Consortium uses Facebook, Twitter, and You Tube to communicate to the public and advocacy communities, and to engage patients during and after the treatment process. With these tools, it is possible to keep a large community informed of upcoming events, existing didactic tools of the consortium, and other information. In contrast to traditional media such as publications, or even Web sites, social media tools take little time to establish but may require updates on a weekly, daily, or hourly basis, in order to achieve the goals of the program. Furthermore, there is a need to tailor messaging and language for each social media audience.

The term blog is derived from Web log, a common form of Web publishing that allows individuals or organizations to post entries in a reverse chronological manner. This allows readers to quickly identify the most recent blogs, making it an ideal way to disseminate timely information. Blog hosting sites, such as Wordpress and Blogger, simplify blog development and maintenance for non-computer programmers. The Oncofertility Consortium utilizes its blog (http://blog.oncofertility.northwestern.edu), to post a variety of educational and community-oriented information. These include summaries of recent publications, descriptions of new research studies, and updates for the oncofertility community. The Oncofertility Consortium blog contains RSS networked feeds in order to grow and maximize its reader base, and allows for direct subscription via e-mail as an option for communicating to the community.

Future Directions in Oncofertility Communication

The field of oncofertility poses unique communication challenges and opportunities for clinicians, researchers, and others wishing to disseminate information at the intersection of cancer and reproductive health. The continued expansion of communication technologies provides content experts with new ways to target information to distinct audiences. The Oncofertility Consortium has principally utilized these technologies to educate clinicians, researchers, and the public. One example of an emerging tool being developed by the Oncofertility Consortium to advance research is called iExperiment. This technology integrates traditional videoconferencing and microscopic imaging to allow researchers to share live microscope images and discuss them in real time. These discussions can occur between researchers across the globe, allowing them to provide input on experiments in progress. While developed for oncofertility researchers, technologies like iExperiment have the ability to be translated to a broad array of fields to transform the pace of scientific research. In addition to the adoption of new technologies, advances in interpersonal understanding will also guide communication within this interdisciplinary field.

On the public-facing side, survivors must continue to work together with clinicians and professionals, sharing their personal stories and opinions on how the fertility-preservation process did or didn't work for them. Discussing past experiences is critical to creating a better path for future patients to follow. Survivors can connect with new patients and provide the perspective of someone who has gone through the process. They can provide encouragement and share options for handling treatment and its side effects that the new patient might not have considered or known about, and help patients take the long view to what life after cancer might look like. Organizations that have collaborated with the Oncofertility Consortium, such as Imerman Angels and Stupid Cancer, are examples of how the survivor-patient connection fits into the broader view of public outreach, turning survivors into communication and outreach professionals.

> I don't think that people realize that just calling and making the appointment for the family, not giving them a phone number, makes all the difference. Asking them, 'What time will work for you?' and getting them that appointment time. It's just simple, it's simple things, but it just makes it happen. [Newly diagnosed patients and their families] don't have the wherewithal at that point in their world to be able to do that kind of thing. So just taking control of that for them and saying, 'Just show up.'...It works.
>
> — Interview with Jill P. Ginsberg, MD, June 30, 2011, Philadelphia, PA

> Many oncology clinicians have set practice patterns when dealing with young cancer patients, patterns that they learned from mentors as students, and those historically have not included discussions about fertility. It is important to change their skill set to include offering information about oncofertility and have the ability to talk about it with patients in a natural and confident manner such that the patient and their family believe in what you're offering and the safety and the rationale for that.
>
> — Interview with Jacqueline S. Jeruss, MD, PhD, July 28, 2011, Chicago, IL

Acknowledgments This work was supported by the Oncofertility Consortium NIH 5UL1DE019587.

References

1. Yarbro CH. International nursing and breast cancer. Breast. 2003;9 Suppl 2:S98–100.
2. Rosenberg M. E-learning: strategies for delivering knowledge in the digital age. Columbus, OH: McGraw-Hill; 2001.

3. Bates T. Technology, e-learning and distance education. New York, NY: Routledge; 2005.
4. Blakely JT, Sinkowitz-Cochran RL, Jarvis WR. Infectious diseases physicians' preferences for continuing medical education on antimicrobial resistance and other general topics. Infect Control Hosp Epidemiol. 2006;27:873–5.
5. Galvin JE, Meuser TM, Boise L, Connell CM. Internet-based dementia resources: physician attitudes and practices. J Appl Gerontol. 2011;30:513–23.
6. Quinn GP, Vadaparampil ST, Gwede CK, Miree C, King LM, Clayton HB, Wilson C, Munster P. Discussion of fertility preservation with newly diagnosed patients: oncologists' views. J Cancer Surviv. 2007;1:146–55.
7. Sinusas K. Internet point of care learning at a community hospital. J Contin Educ Health Prof. 2009;29:39–43.
8. Kuo GM, Ma JD, Lee KC, Halpert JR, Bourne PE, Ganiats TG, Taylor P. Institutional profile: University of California San Diego Pharmacogenomics Education Program (PharmGenEd): bridging the gap between science and practice. Pharmacogenomics. 2011;12:149–53.
9. Cook DA, Levinson AJ, Garside S, Dupras DM, Erwin PJ, Montori VM. Internet-based learning in the health professions: a meta-analysis. JAMA. 2008;300:1181–96.
10. Ruiz JG, Mintzer MJ, Leipzig RM. The impact of E-learning in medical education. Acad Med. 2006;81:207–12.
11. Cook DA, Levinson AJ, Garside S, Dupras DM, Erwin PJ, Montori VM. Instructional design variations in internet-based learning for health professions education: a systematic review and meta-analysis. Acad Med. 2010;85:909–22.
12. Prgomet M, Georgiou A, Westbrook JI. The impact of mobile handheld technology on hospital physicians' work practices and patient care: a systematic review. J Am Med Inform Assoc. 2009;16:792–801.
13. Kho A, Henderson LE, Dressler DD, Kripalani S. Use of handheld computers in medical education. A systematic review. J Gen Intern Med. 2006;21:531–7.
14. Shurtz S, von Isenburg M. Exploring e-readers to support clinical medical education: two case studies. J Med Libr Assoc. 2011;99:110–7.
15. Clayman ML, Harper M, Quinn GP, Shah S, Reinecke J. The status of oncofertility resources at NCI-designated comprehensive cancer centers. J Clin Oncol. 2011;29 Suppl 15:Abstract 9123.
16. Quinn GP, Vadaparampil ST, Malo T, Reinecke J, Bower B, Albrecht T, Clayman ML. Oncologists' use of patient educational materials about cancer and fertility preservation. Psychooncology. 2011;21:1244–9.
17. Schover LR, Brey K, Lichtin A, Lipshultz LI, Jeha S. Oncologists' attitudes and practices regarding banking sperm before cancer treatment. J Clin Oncol. 2002;20:1890–7.
18. Rudd RE, Moeykens BA, Colton TC. Health and literacy: a review of medical and public health literature. In: Comings J, Garners B, Smith C, editors. Health and literacy. New York, NY: Jossey-Bass; 1999.
19. Jona K, Gerber A. MyOncofertility.org: a web-based patient education resource supporting decision making under severe emotional and cognitive overload. Cancer Treat Res. 2010; 156:345–61.
20. Loscalzo MJ, Clark KL. The psychosocial context of cancer-related infertility. Cancer Treat Res. 2007;138:180–90.

Chapter 13
Educating Providers on Evidence-Based Medical Guidelines

Lauren N.C. Johnson and Clarisa R. Gracia

Introduction

Fertility preservation is a relatively new field, and as such, few standardized guidelines are available to guide clinicians in the care of patients. Furthermore, this field presents unique challenges to the implementation of clinical research. Young patients who are interested in preserving fertility are generally a heterogeneous population. These patients range in age from newborns to individuals in their late reproductive years, and they come from a variety of socioeconomic backgrounds. They may have a wide range of malignant and non-malignant disorders that are treated with various gonadotoxic therapies. Furthermore, these patients often have only a short period of time between diagnosis and the start of radiation or chemotherapy—often a few days to weeks at most—to pursue fertility-sparing treatments, making participation in clinical trials difficult and evidence-based guidance scarce. Despite these challenges, the number of studies published in the area of fertility preservation is increasing exponentially. Therefore, it is of critical importance that clinicians caring for this population stay up to date on the current literature, which requires mastery of the concept of evidence-based medicine.

The Old Paradigm

For centuries, the practice of medicine and medical decision making relied heavily on individual clinical experience and on an understanding of pathophysiology [1, 2]. Based on this foundation and the nature of their training, physicians were

L.N.C. Johnson, M.D. (✉) • C.R. Gracia, M.D., M.S.C.E.
Department of Reproductive Endocrinology and Infertility, University of Pennsylvania, 3701 Market Street, Suite 800, Philadelphia, PA 19104, USA
e-mail: lauren.johnson2@uphs.upenn.edu; cgracia@obgyn.upenn.edu

T.K. Woodruff et al. (eds.), *Oncofertility Communication: Sharing Information and Building Relationships across Disciplines*, DOI 10.1007/978-1-4614-8235-2_13,

considered to be well equipped to judge the efficacy of new tests or procedures. When faced with a clinical question to which he/she did not know the answer, the clinician would reflect on his knowledge of pathophysiology, refer to a textbook, or consult a more senior colleague. As a result, patient care decisions were often made based on individual biases instead of scientific methods or objective data.

Evidence-based medicine emerged during the late twentieth century and is generally considered to be a paradigm shift in the way that clinicians make decisions about patient care [1]. This new paradigm highlights the critical importance of utilizing objective data to guide medical decisions [1–3]. Three principles are emphasized. First, by relying on systematically recorded and reproducible data, physicians can minimize bias and increase their confidence in the certainty of a diagnosis or test result. In the absence of systematically collected data, physicians must rely on clinical judgment, recognizing that their individual experiences may be misleading. Second, while understanding pathophysiology of disease is necessary for the practice of medicine, it is not sufficient for clinical decision making. Third, the correct interpretation of systematic observations requires knowledge of the rules of evidence.

What Is Evidence-Based Medicine?

Broadly speaking, Evidence-Based Medicine (EBM) is a tool for solving clinical questions. When evidence-based medicine was first introduced in the 1990s, it was defined as "the conscientious, explicit, and judicious use of current best evidence in making decisions about the care of individual patients" [4]. This definition was later refined to include the critical role of the patient in his or her health care decisions. Evidence-based medicine is now defined as a systematic approach to clinical problem solving that allows "the integration of the best available research evidence with clinical expertise and patient values" [5]. This concept can be understood more completely by considering the EBM triad (Fig. 13.1). This diagram emphasizes the concept that EBM occurs at the intersection of individual clinical expertise, the best external evidence, and patient values and expectations. Each of these components is essential for making good clinical decisions in patient care.

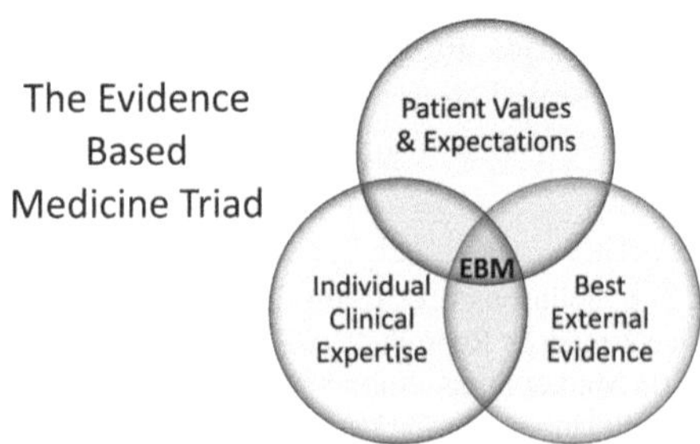

Fig. 13.1 The evidence based medicine triad

Some have the perception that EBM is only possible when excellent evidence exists, i.e., randomized trials and meta-analyses. Because fertility preservation is a young discipline with very limited randomized trial data, some would argue that EBM is not possible for this field. However, it is important to understand that while randomized trials and meta-analyses are the gold standard of evidence, EBM involves utilizing the best *available* evidence in clinical decision making. Thus, the lack of randomized trials should not be a barrier to use of the medical literature and EBM.

Asking Clinical Questions: The PICO Model

One of the fundamental tools used in EBM is the generation of an important clinical question that is targeted to address a specific clinical situation. A literature search is then performed to assess the quality of the evidence on this topic. Physicians make two critical mistakes when searching the literature. The first is performing a search with broad terms, which yields hundreds of results. On the other hand, some perform searches that are so specific that the search yields no results. For this reason, generating an appropriate clinical question is paramount in order to efficiently identify the most relevant literature.

"PICO" is a commonly used mnemonic to facilitate generation of a robust clinical question [3, 5, 6].

"P" stands for Patient, Problem, or Population. Who are the patients that you are interested in learning about? What is the particular medical problem or population that your clinical query addresses?

"I" stands for Intervention, which includes the treatment, exposure, diagnostic test, or prognostic factor that you are interested in studying.

"C" stands for Comparison. Are you interested in comparing two treatment regimens or two different diagnostic tests? What is the main alternative to intervention that you are interested in exploring? In some cases, there will not be a comparison group.

"O" stands for Outcome. What is the result that you are interested in? What is the outcome of the exposure? Generally, patient-centered outcomes are preferred if data are available.

Let's consider the following clinical scenario: A 28-year-old nulligravid female presents for a fertility preservation consultation. She was recently diagnosed with breast cancer and desires to pursue controlled ovarian hyperstimulation and oocyte cryopreservation. However, she is concerned that in vitro fertilization will increase her chance of recurrence. What do you tell her? Our PICO components are:

*P*atient: Young women with breast cancer
*I*nvention: Fertility preservation via controlled ovarian hyperstimulation
*C*omparison: No fertility preservation
*O*utcome: Breast cancer recurrence

Using the PICO format, we can generate the following clinical question: "In young women with breast cancer, does fertility preservation via controlled ovarian hyperstimulation increase the risk of breast cancer recurrence compared to no fertility preservation?" We can then use this clinical question to search the literature for related citations. Most clinicians turn to PubMed for their search; however, there are several EBM databases that may facilitate identification of high-quality, evidence-based data, including the Cochrane Library, the United States Preventive Services Task Force (USPSTF), InfoPOEMS, and others.

Grading the Evidence

Once the literature search on a specific medical question is complete, the body of evidence must be systematically and objectively evaluated. Several rating scales have been developed to help medical professionals evaluate the quality of the evidence for a particular study or practice guideline. The best known rating scale was first described by the USPSTF in 1989 [7]. Under this system, the evidence is assigned a score of I to III based on the design of the studies that contributed to the recommendation. The highest level of evidence is scored as I and includes at least one properly designed randomized controlled trial. Controlled trials without randomization, cohort studies, and case–control studies are described as level II. Evidence from expert opinions or cases reports is deemed to be the lowest level of evidence and is given a score of III (Table 13.1). Recommendations that are made after review of the evidence are assigned a letter grade of A, B, or C based on the highest level of evidence used to generate the recommendation.

In 2007, the USPSTF updated their evaluation system. Under the new system, the quality of evidence is graded on a three-point scale, in which evidence is

Table 13.1 Evaluation system of the United States Preventative Services Task Force prior to May 2007

Quality of evidence
I Evidence obtained from at least one properly designed randomized controlled trial
II-1 Evidence obtained from well-designed controlled trials without randomization
II-2 Evidence obtained from well-designed cohort or case–control analytic studies, preferably from more than one center or research group
II-3 Evidence obtained from multiple time series with or without the intervention. Dramatic results in uncontrolled experiments also could be regarded as this type of evidence
III Opinions of respected authorities, based on clinical experience, descriptive studies, or reports of expert committees
Strength of recommendations[a]
Level A—Recommendations are based on good and consistent scientific evidence
Level B—Recommendations are based on limited or inconsistent scientific evidence
Level C—Recommendations are based primarily on consensus and expert opinion

[a]Recommendations are graded based on the highest level of evidence found in the data

Table 13.2 Evaluation system of the United States Preventative Services Task Force after May 2007

Quality of evidence	
Good	Evidence includes consistent results from well-designed, well-conducted studies in representative populations that directly assess effects on health outcomes
Fair	Evidence is sufficient to determine effects on health outcomes, but the strength of the evidence is limited by the number, quality, or consistency of the individual studies, generalizability to routine practice, or indirect nature of the evidence on health outcomes
Poor	Evidence is insufficient to assess the effects on health outcomes because of limited number or power of studies, important flaws in their design or conduct, gaps in the chain of evidence, or lack of information on important health outcomes

Strength of recommendation and suggestions for practice

Grade	Definition	Suggestions for practice
A	The USPSTF recommends the service. There is high certainty that the net benefit is substantial	Offer or provide this service
B	The USPSTF recommends the service. There is high certainty that the net benefit is moderate or there is moderate certainty that the net benefit is moderate to substantial	Offer or provide this service
C	Clinicians may provide this service to selected patients depending on individual circumstances. However, for most individuals without signs or symptoms there is likely to be only a small benefit from this service	Offer or provide this service only if other considerations support the offering or providing the service in an individual patient
D	The USPSTF recommends against the service. There is moderate or high certainty that the service has no net benefit or that the harms outweigh the benefits	Discourage the use of this service
I	The USPSTF concludes that the current evidence is insufficient to assess the balance of benefits and harms of the service. Evidence is lacking, of poor quality, or conflicting, and the balance of benefits and harms cannot be determined	Read the clinical considerations section of USPSTF Recommendation Statement. If the service is offered, patients should understand the uncertainty about the balance of benefits and harms

described as "good, fair, or poor" (Table 13.2) [8]. Unlike the previous system, this updated grading system is more accessible, as medical professionals can understand it quickly even if they do not have a detailed knowledge of study design. With this revision, the USPSTF also provides an updated grading system for recommendations as well as suggestions for practice for each recommendation.

Many additional systems for grading the evidence have been developed to better meet the needs of clinicians. For example, in 2004, editors from several primary care journals developed the Strength-of-Recommendation Taxonomy (SORT) system [9]. This system focuses primarily on patient-centered outcomes, such as mortality, quality of life, and symptom improvement, instead of disease-centered outcomes, defined primarily as surrogate markers. This system is widely used across family practice journals and is easy to understand and incorporate into practice (Table 13.3).

Table 13.3 Strength-of-recommendation taxonomy (SORT)

Code	Definition
A	Consistent, good-quality patient-oriented evidence[a]
B	Inconsistent or limited-quality patient-oriented evidence[a]
C	Consensus, disease-oriented evidence[a], usual practice, expert opinion, or case series for studies of diagnosis, treatment, prevention, or screening

[a]Patient-oriented evidence measures outcomes that matter to patients: morbidity, mortality, symptom improvement, cost reduction, and quality of life. Disease-oriented evidence measures immediate, physiologic, or surrogate end points that may or may not reflect improvements in patient outcomes (e.g., blood pressure, blood chemistry, physiologic function, pathologic findings)

Other frequently used systems include the Oxford Centre for Evidence-Based Medicine and Grading of Recommendations Assessment, Development and Evaluation (GRADE) [10]. While the original USPSTF system is the most widely used, clinicians should be aware that other systems are equally valid and can be very helpful when evaluating data.

The State of Evidence-Based Medicine in Fertility Preservation and Oncofertility

Until recently, few researchers were interested in the impact of cancer therapies on fertility, mainly due to the low rate of long-term survival. However, with vast improvements in cancer treatments and survival rate over the past decade, patients and health care providers have started to focus more attention on the long-term medical issues that cancer survivors face, including infertility. Moreover, improvements in reproductive technologies have expanded the options available for fertility preservation in reproductive-age individuals who face gonadotoxic treatments for malignant or non-malignant conditions. As oncofertility has gained attention, there has been more research conducted in this area, and there has been a steady rise the number of articles with the keyword "fertility preservation" published in the last 10 years (Fig. 13.2).

While the data in some areas of fertility preservation are limited, the literature in other areas of oncofertility research has evolved rapidly, moving from Level III evidence to Level I evidence. For example, in 1986, a case report published in *Lancet* described the first human birth from a cryopreserved oocyte (Level III evidence) [11]. During the next 2 decades, observational data were reported for a variety of clinical questions, including clinical outcomes with cryopreserved oocytes vs. fresh oocytes [12, 13], pregnancy rates with cryopreserved oocytes based on maternal age [14], and rates of birth defects in children conceived using cryopreserved oocytes (Level II evidence) [15]. Finally, between 2008 and 2011, four randomized controlled trials were published that compared implantation rates

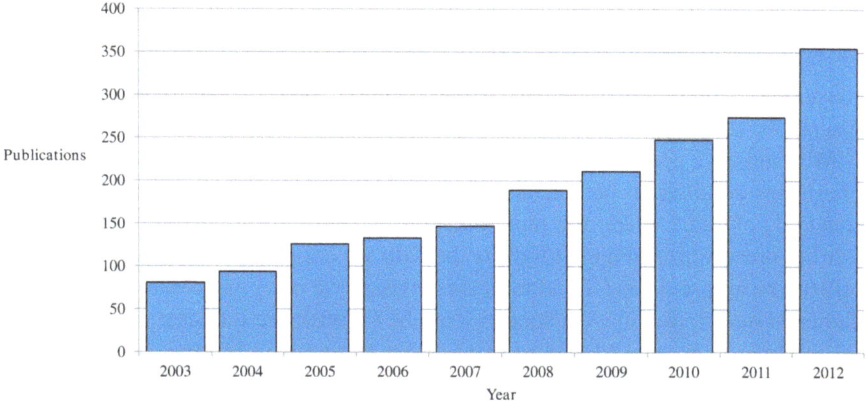

Fig. 13.2 Number of articles retrieved by year in PubMed with keyword "Fertility preservation." Accessed January 3, 2013

and clinical pregnancy rates in cycles utilizing vitrified oocytes vs. fresh oocytes (Level I evidence) [16–19]. Based on the quality of the current data (Grade A), the American Society for Reproductive Medicine (ASRM) recently reclassified oocyte cryopreservation, moving it from an experimental procedure to an established technique [20]. This example illustrates how EBM has been used to inform clinical decision-making in fertility preservation.

On the other hand, ovarian tissue cryopreservation is still in early stages of development, and the data available today are limited to case reports of live births from this technique (Level III evidence). While these reports are encouraging, the number of women attempting pregnancy via ovarian tissue cryopreservation is unknown at this point. While there may never be randomized controlled trials for this procedure, large, prospective observational studies comparing pregnancy rates among those who used transplanted tissue vs. those who did not will undoubtedly be conducted and will provide valuable information to inform clinical decisions using EBM.

As the field of fertility preservation evolves, there are three critical factors that must be in place to ensure that clinical decisions are based on strong evidence. First, high-quality research must be conducted and published. Given the heterogeneous nature of the fertility preservation population, it is likely that successful completion of high-quality research with patient-based outcomes will require collaboration between institutions to enroll sufficient participants. Second, substantial funding must be available to conduct these high-quality studies in an environment where fertility preservation research is a high priority. Finally, it is critical that clinicians possess strong EBM skills so that they can easily access emerging data, interpret the data correctly, and use the data when making clinical decisions with their patients.

Evidence-Based Medicine and Physician Education

Because fertility preservation is a rapidly evolving field, it is of critical importance that physicians caring for this patient population pursue continuing medical education (CME) and have access to the most up-to-date information. How do we ensure that physicians continue to be educated and are informed of the latest data regarding standards of care? Given the multidisciplinary nature of the patient care team in fertility preservation and oncofertility, how do we ensure that educational tools are utilized by all providers? To address these issues, we must first consider some fundamental questions. How do doctors learn best? What are the most effective tools for teaching physicians? Do physicians prefer lecture-based formats or case-based instruction?

The question of how to deliver effective CME to physicians has been explored extensively. In 1995, Davis et al. conducted a systematic review summarizing the impact of educational strategies or interventions on physician performance or health care outcomes [21]. The authors identified 99 randomized controlled trials containing 160 physician interventions. Of those trials focused on physician performance, 70 % of interventions resulted in an improvement in physician performance in at least one major area. However, for trials focused on health care outcomes, only 48 % of interventions resulted in major changes in outcomes. The magnitude of the effect was small to moderate in most cases. Additionally, the authors found that attendance at conferences, one of the most widely utilized CME delivery systems, was ineffective in improving physician performance. This analysis clearly demonstrated that CME strategies employed at the time were not as successful as hoped.

In 2009, this analysis was updated, and the authors issued recommendations regarding the delivery of CME activities based on their findings [22, 23]. First, the authors recommended that the goal of CME activities should be to improve physician performance and clinical outcomes. Second, the authors concluded that instructional media utilizing multiple platforms was effective in improving physician performance and clinical outcomes. Their data also suggested that physician performance may be improved through use of live media alone and that exclusive use of print media is not effective. Finally, the authors suggested that effective CME interventions should utilize multiple instructional techniques and include multiple exposures.

Other authors have attempted to determine which CME techniques are the most effective in terms of altering physician behavior and improving patient outcomes [24]. A systematic review of meta-analyses investigated the effectiveness of eight commonly utilized CME tools (Table 13.4). The author concluded that interactive techniques, including physician reminders, audit/feedback, and academic detailing/outreach, were the most effective at both improving clinical outcomes and amending physician practice patterns. The least effective techniques were use of opinion leaders and clinical practice guidelines. The most commonly used CME techniques—use of printed materials and didactic presentations—offered little to no benefit. Despite these findings, use of less of effective techniques continues to dominate the landscape of CME offerings.

Table 13.4 Education methods tested by BS Bloom in "Effects of continuing medical education on improving physician clinical care and patient health: A review of systematic reviews." *Int J Technol Assess Health Care*. 2005; 21(3): 380–385

Educational method	Description
Didactic programs	Predominantly lectures and presentations that may include question and answer periods
Information only	Distribution of printed materials alone or as part of lecture sessions
Opinion leaders	Those persons recognized locally or nationally as experts who set norms for appropriate clinical practice behavior
Clinical practice guidelines	Structured clinical diagnostic and treatment strategies based on synthesis of best available evidence, preferably from randomized controlled trials and meta-analyses
Interactive education	Interactive sessions of participants and presenter or leader. Interactive techniques may include role playing, case discussion, and honing newly acquired practice skills
Audit and feedback	A review of current practitioner clinical practice behavior, usually for a specified diagnosis, and recommendations for new clinical behavior if warranted
Academic (counter-) detailing/outreach	Utilizes a personal visit by a trained professional to a physician to provide best available information on health and medical care interventions
Reminders	Prompts to the practitioner to provide a specific clinical intervention under defined clinical circumstances

Educational Activities Within Oncofertility

A variety of resources—some of which provide CME credit—are available to help physicians learn about topics within oncofertility. The Oncofertility Consortium hosts an annual conference with didactic sessions as well as hands-on, small-group training courses. Additionally, the group conducts a Web-based "virtual grand rounds" each month where leaders in the field present recent data and discuss advances. These sessions are archived on the Oncofertility Consortium Web site and are accessible free-of-charge. Furthermore, the Web site enables clinicians to obtain CME credits by accessing the online materials and answering questions from the material [25].

Fertile Hope, an advocacy and support group dedicated to providing cancer patients with information about reproductive options, offers risk assessment calculators and summary tables to estimate the likelihood that a woman will experience amenorrhea after her cancer treatment [26]. The Web site also offers other clinical tools, including a detailed summary of fertility preservation options and algorithms for management. Finally, there are links to published research studies in a variety of areas, links to ongoing clinical trials, and access to printed materials.

Practice guidelines for fertility preservation in cancer patients have been published by several professional societies, including the American Society for Clinical Oncology (ASCO), ASRM, and the British Fertility Society [27–29]. In addition,

ASCO offers online training modules focused on female and male fertility preservation, with CME credit available [30]. Similarly, ASRM provides online CME courses focused on mature oocyte cryopreservation as well as fertility preservation strategies for men [31]. Finally, through The Endocrine Society, physicians can access online educational materials and prerecorded lectures detailing fertility preservation options and the use of assisted reproductive technologies in adolescents and young adults [32].

Conclusions

Oncofertility is an exciting and rapidly evolving field with the potential to improve quality of life for many cancer survivors. Fertility preservation options are being extended to reproductive age patients with a range of malignant and non-malignant conditions that will be treated with gonadotoxic therapies. However, appropriate physician education is critical for improving patient outcomes. Knowledge of the principles of EBM, combined with access to high-quality, patient-oriented literature, will allow physicians to deliver excellent care to patients seeking fertility preservation services. Ultimately, the utilization of EBM offers providers the best chance to optimize the reproductive health and fertility preservation options for individuals facing gonadotoxic therapies.

Online resources for physician education

http://oncofertility.northwestern.edu
www.fertilehope.org
http://university.asco.org/fertility-preservation-issues-aya-females
http://university.asco.org/fertility-preservation-issues-aya-males
https://www.asrm.org/eLearnCatalog
http://www.endosessions.org/portal

Acknowledgments This work was supported by the Oncofertility Consortium NIH 5UL1DE019587 and the Specialized Cooperative Centers Program in Reproduction and Infertility Research NIH U54HD076188.

References

1. Evidence-Based Medicine Working Group. Evidence-based medicine: a new approach to the teaching of medicine. JAMA. 1992;268:2420–5.
2. Grimes DA. Introducing evidence-based medicine into a department of obstetrics and gynecology. Obstet Gynecol. 1995;86:451–7.
3. Guyatt G, Rennie D, Meade M, Cook D. Users' guides to the medical literature: a manual for evidence-based clinical practice. 2nd ed. New York: McGraw-Hill; 2008.
4. Sackett D, Rosenberg W, Gray J, Haynes R, Richardson W. Evidence based medicine: what it is and what it isn't. BMJ. 1996;312:71–2.

5. Sackett DL, Strauss SE, Richardson WS, Sackett DL, Rosenberg W, Haynes RB. Evidence-based medicine: how to practice and teach EBM, vol. 2. Edinburgh: Churchill-Livingstone; 2000.
6. Richardson W. The well-built clinical question: a key to evidence based decisions. ACP J Club. 1995;123:A12–3.
7. US Preventive Services Task Force. Grade definitions page. Available at: http://www.uspreventiveservicestaskforce.org/uspstf/grades.htm. Accessed 18 Dec 2012.
8. US Preventive Services Task Force. Guide to clinical preventive services. 2nd ed. Washington, DC: US Department of Health and Human Services; 1996.
9. Ebell MH, Siwek J, Weiss BD, Woolf SH, Susman J, Ewigman E, et al. Strength of recommendation taxonomy (SORT): a patient-centered approach to grading evidence in the medical literature. Am Fam Physician. 2004;69:548–56.
10. Guyatt G, Oxman AD, Akl E, Kunz R, Vist G, Brozek J, et al. GRADE guidelines 1. Introduction-GRADE evidence profiles and summary of findings tables. J Clin Epidemiol. 2011;64:383–94.
11. Chen C. Pregnancy after human oocyte cryopreservation. Lancet. 1986;1:884–6.
12. Borini A, Levi Setti PE, Anserini P, De Luca R, De Santis L, Porcu E, et al. Multicenter observational study on slow-cooling oocyte cryopreservation: clinical outcome. Fertil Steril. 2010;94:1662–8.
13. Scaravelli G, Vigiliano V, Mayorga JM, Bolli S, De Luca R, D'Aloja P. Analysis of oocyte cryopreservation in assisted reproduction: the Italian National Register data from 2005 to 2007. Reprod Biomed Online. 2010;21:496–500.
14. Rienzi L, Cobo A, Paffoni A, Scarduelli C, Capalbo A, Vajta G, et al. Consistent and predictable delivery rates after oocyte vitrification: an observational longitudinal cohort multicentric study. Hum Reprod. 2012;27:1606–12.
15. Noyes N, Porcu E, Borini A. Over 900 oocyte cryopreservation babies born with no apparent increase in congenital anomalies. Reprod Biomed Online. 2009;18:769–76.
16. Cobo A, Kuwayama M, Perez S, Ruiz A, Pellicer A, Remohi J. Comparison of concomitant outcome achieved with fresh and cryopreserved donor oocytes vitrified by the Cryotop method. Fertil Steril. 2008;89:1657–64.
17. Cobo A, Meseguer M, Remohi J, Pellicer A. Use of cryo-banked oocytes in an ovum donation programme: a prospective, randomized, controlled, clinical trial. Hum Reprod. 2010; 25:2239–46.
18. Rienzi L, Romano S, Albricci L, Maggiulli R, Capalbo A, Baroni E, et al. Embryo development of fresh 'versus' vitrified metaphase II oocytes after ICSI: a prospective randomized sibling oocyte study. Hum Reprod. 2010;25:66–73.
19. Parmegiani L, Cognigni GE, Bernardi S, Cuomo S, Ciampaglia W, Infante FE, et al. Efficiency of aseptic open vitrification and hermetical cryostorage of human oocytes. Reprod Biomed Online. 2011;23:505–12.
20. The Practice Committees of the American Society for Reproductive Medicine and the Society for Assisted Reproductive Technology. Mature oocyte cryopreservation: a guideline. Fertil Steril. 2013;99:37–43.
21. Davis DA, Thomson MA, Oxman AD, Haynes B. Changing physician performance: a systematic review of the effect of continuing medical education strategies. JAMA. 1995;274:700–5.
22. Mazmanian PE, Davis DA, Galbraith R. Continuing medical education effect on clinical outcomes. Effectiveness of continuing medical education: American College of Chest Physicians evidence-based educational guidelines. Chest. 2009;135:49S–55.
23. Davis DA, Galbraith R. Continuing medical education effect on practice performance. Effectiveness of continuing medical education: American College of Chest Physicians evidence-based educational guidelines. Chest. 2009;135:42S–8.
24. Bloom BS. Effects of continuing medical education on improving physician clinical care and patient health: a review of systematic reviews. Int J Technol Assess Health Care. 2005;21:380–5.
25. The Oncofertility Consortium at Northwestern University. Health professionals page. Available at: http://oncofertility.northwestern.edu. Accessed 4 Jan 2013.

26. Fertile Hope. Healthcare professionals page. Available at: http://www.fertilehope.org. Accessed 4 Jan 2013.
27. Lee SJ, Schover LR, Partridge AH, Patrizio P, Wallace WH, Hagerty K, et al. American Society of Clinical Oncology recommendations on fertility preservation in cancer patients. J Clin Oncol. 2006;24:2917–31.
28. Ethics Committee of the American Society for Reproductive Medicine. Fertility preservation and reproduction in cancer patients. Fertil Steril. 2005;83:1622–8.
29. Multidisciplinary Working Group Convened by the British Fertility Society. A strategy for fertility services for survivors of childhood cancer. Hum Fertil (Camb). 2003;6:A1–39.
30. American Society of Clinical Oncology. The ASCO University focus under forty page. Available at: http://university.asco.org/focus-under-forty. Accessed 4 Jan 2013.
31. American Society for Reproductive Medicine. eLearning catalog page. Available at: https://www.asrm.org/eLearnCatalog. Accessed 18 Jan 2013.
32. The Endocrine Society. EndoSessions page. Available at: http://www.endosessions.org/portal. Accessed 18 Jan 2013.

Chapter 14
Incorporating Insurance Education into the Fertility Preservation Process

Laxmi A. Kondapalli and Alice Crisci

Overview

Over the last several decades, cancer survival rates have tremendously increased, largely due to enhanced early detection and improved therapeutics. What was once considered a "death sentence," now allows survivors to imagine a life after cancer with expectations beyond survival [1]. These medical achievements should be tempered by the resultant gonadotoxic effects. As such, survivorship issues are of increasing importance. Fertility loss is of particular concern for the approximately 135,000 pediatric, adolescent, and young adults (AYA) diagnosed each year [2]. Infertility caused by cancer treatment is *iatrogenic*, meaning any adverse condition induced by medical interventions including reactions from prescribed drugs or from medical and surgical procedures. Iatrogenic infertility is typically caused by cancer treatments such as chemotherapy, radiation, or surgical removal of reproductive organs. While the focus of this chapter will be specific to cancer patients, fertility may be compromised by treatments for other conditions such as autoimmune disorders.

While cancer screening, diagnosis and treatment are commonly covered under most insurance plans, fertility preservation (FP) is not, despite growing evidence of reproductive dysfunction resulting from treatments [3–5]. Further, many insurance

L.A. Kondapalli, M.D., M.S.C.E. (✉)
Division of Reproductive Endocrinology and Infertility,
Department of Obstetrics and Gynecology, University of Colorado
Denver Anschutz Medical Campus, 12700 East 19th Avenue,
Mail Stop 8613, Research Complex II, Room 3006, Aurora, CO, USA
e-mail: laxmi.kondapalli@ucdenver.edu

A. Crisci, B.S.
Fertile Action, P.O. Box 3526, Manhattan Beach, CA 90266, USA
e-mail: alice@fertileaction.org

T.K. Woodruff et al. (eds.), *Oncofertility Communication: Sharing Information and Building Relationships across Disciplines*, DOI 10.1007/978-1-4614-8235-2_14,

companies will cover treatment for other iatrogenic conditions cause by cancer treatment [6], such as breast reconstruction after mastectomy for breast cancer. Patients at risk for iatrogenic infertility are different from patients treated for infertility. Infertility is defined as the inability to conceive after 12 months. Cancer patients may not have infertility at the time of diagnosis, but they need to undergo fertility preservation services prior to initiation of cancer treatments, which may impart risk of becoming infertile in the future. For example, a young woman with newly diagnosed lymphoma may choose to cryopreserve oocytes before starting treatment. Although she may have normal reproductive function at the time, her ability to have biological children in the future may be impaired. Therefore, she may choose to preserve oocytes to secure her fertility wishes. Even when traditional insurance has provisions for infertility treatments, cancer patients are often denied coverage because they do not meet the strict criteria of infertility, which limits coverage to those who have been trying to conceive for at least 6–12 months. This definition excludes most cancer patients attempting to access fertility preservation treatment.

While there is ongoing discussion and debate about insurance coverage for fertility preservation at a local and national level, the following sections outline strategies that may facilitate assess to fertility preservation services for patients.

Preauthorization for Oncofertility Consultation and Treatment

Most insurance companies have provisions covering consultations with specialists. An important component to ensure this coverage is the referral to an oncofertility specialist. It is critical for patients and office staff to understand the process to receive pre-authorization coverage for consultations with a reproductive endocrinologist. These patients benefit from understanding the full endocrine impact from their specific cancer treatment and all the potential associated side effects including menstrual irregularities, sub-fertility and infertility, sexual dysfunction, metabolic disturbances, cardiovascular and bone health. See Appendix 1 for a sample oncofertility referral form.

While there may be differences in specific procedures for pre-authorization across insurance companies, most will have guidelines about the process that are accessible via phone or online. Many insurance companies have specific pre-authorization forms that are available on their Web site that can be faxed to your office. Another important component to achieving insurance coverage is the use of appropriate diagnosis codes for the visits. The International Classification of Diseases (ICD) is the classification system used to code and classify disease states and mortality data and was designed to promote international comparability of these statistics [7]. Health care providers use the ICD system to code diagnoses associated with particular hospital and office visits, and are used by insurance companies to justify coverage for the visit.

Table 14.1 Supplemental V codes for fertility preservation

V codes for fertility preservation	
V 26.42	• Encounter for fertility preservation counseling • Encounter for fertility preservation counseling prior to cancer therapy • Encounter for fertility preservation counseling prior to surgical removal of gonads
V 26.82	• Encounter for fertility preservation procedure • Encounter for fertility preservation procedure prior to cancer therapy • Encounter for fertility preservation procedure prior to surgical removal of gonads

Providers can add these codes to the primary cancer diagnosis when submitting insurance bills. Note that these codes can be added to any primary diagnosis, not only cancer, such as rheumatologic and hematologic disease, and not gender-specific

For oncofertility patients, it is essential to use the cancer diagnosis as the primary diagnosis code for the consultation. In addition, there is a supplementary classification of factors, known as V codes, which influence the patient's health status and contact with health services. In fact, special V codes for fertility preservation have been developed and are billable medical codes that can be used on reimbursement claims. These V codes should be used for preauthorization and all subsequent visits (Table 14.1). If a patient wishes to proceed with FP treatment, it will be helpful to submit a separate pre-authorization form for the specific FP procedure. Often, this is coupled with a Letter of Medical Necessity.

Communication About Medical Necessity for Fertility Preservation Procedures

Insurance companies often use medical necessity to review benefits coverage and/or provider payment for services, tests or procedures that are medically appropriate and cost-effective for its members.

For example, one insurance company, Cigna Healthcare®, states that the medical necessity process is based on health care services that a Physician, exercising prudent clinical judgment, would provide to a patient, and that are:

- In accordance with the generally accepted standards of medical practice;
- Clinically appropriate, in terms of type, frequency, extent, site, and duration, and considered effective for the patient's illness, injury, or disease; and
- Not primarily for the convenience of the patient or Physician, or other Physician, and not more costly than an alternative service or sequence of services at least as likely to produce equivalent therapeutic or diagnostic results as to the diagnosis or treatment of that patient's illness, injury, or disease [8].

Oncofertility specialists can submit a comprehensive letter that establishes medical necessity, which includes the following topics:

- Patient name and date of birth
- Insurance carrier name and patient identification number
- Clinical diagnosis and ICD code
- Cancer treatment plan
- Side effects of the treatment plan associated with reproductive health
- Proposed ICD-10 codes and associated V-codes that you are requesting coverage
- Case for coverage (see below)
- Physician signature
- Your contact details

Case for Insurance Coverage for Oncofertility Services

There are a number of factors that can be included in the letter of medical necessity to support insurance coverage for patients. These include [9]:

- *Guidelines from professional organizations*: The American Society of Clinical Oncology (ASCO) and American Society of Reproductive Medicine (ASRM) promote discussion of fertility impact of treatment at the time of diagnosis and have published guidelines discussing the incorporation of oncofertility in cancer care.
- *Iatrogenic Condition*: Cancer patients often undergo gonadotoxic treatments that are medically necessary to overcome malignancy, but that may impart iatrogenic infertility. Cancer benefits typically include insurance coverage for the remedy of iatrogenic conditions. This includes procedures that are otherwise considered elective, such as surgical scar revision.
- *Right to Parity*: This concept is related to *non-maleficence* meaning to "do no harm" and argues that insurance practice should mitigate iatrogenic effects caused by cancer treatment.
- *Benefit Already Exists*: Some patients may have infertility coverage in their insurance plans. Although they may not meet the strict criteria for infertility, an argument can be made that they are at significant risk of permanent infertility as a consequence of cancer treatment. Fertility may be so impaired that assisted reproduction will be ineffectual in the future; therefore they will not be able to take advantage of this covered benefit.
- *Low Usage, Low Cost, and Positive Returns*: The at-risk population is small and the proportion of insured members that will utilize the service is also small. Further, the cost per member per month is low with potential for significant positive cost offsets in the future. Patients who are unable to pursue FP prior to cancer therapy may become subfertile and utilize more assisted reproductive resources in the future.

- *Avoids Risk of Adverse Selection*: The narrow window of time between cancer diagnosis and initiation of treatments discourages patients from switching insurance policies to take advantage of a FP benefit.

In addition to diagnostic codes, some insurance companies require a list of procedures associated with FP that a patient is seeking insurance coverage. The Current Procedural Terminology (CPT) is a universal coding system in which numbers are assigned to every medical service a medical practitioner may provide to a patient including medical, surgical and diagnostic services. Insurance companies use these codes to determine which procedures are covered and the amount of reimbursement. Table 14.2 outlines CPT codes for standard fertility preservation treatments that are useful in writing letters of medical necessity (Table 14.2) [10].

Table 14.2 Standard ICD codes to use for fertility preservation procedures

CPT code	Code description
Fertility preservation methods	
77334	Shielding of gonads during radiation therapy
58825	Transposition of the ovary(s)
57531	Radical trachelectomy
89259	Sperm cryopreservation
89258	Embryo cryopreservation
0059T	Oocyte cryopreservation
0058T	Ovarian tissue cryopreservation
89335	Cryopreservation, reproductive tissue, testicular/ovarian
89240	Experimental/investigational fertility preservation treatments
Monitoring and laboratory services	
76830	Complete pelvic ultrasound with image documentation
76857	Limited pelvic ultrasound for follicular monitoring
36415	Venipuncture
83001	Follicle stimulating hormone
83002	Luteinizing hormone
82670	Estradiol
84144	Progesterone
99211	Nursing visit
98960	Injection teaching
Oocyte retrieval and embryology lab procedures	
00840	Anesthesia for intraperitoneal procedure
58970	Follicle puncture for oocyte retrieval
76948	Ultrasonic guidance for aspiration of oocytes
89254	Oocyte identification from follicular fluid
89250	Culture of oocytes
89251	Culture of oocytes/embryos, < 4 days, with coculture of oocytes/embryos
89320	Semen analysis

(continued)

Table 14.2 (continued)

CPT code	Code description
89259	Insemination of oocytes
89280	Intracytoplasmic sperm injection (ICSI), when necessary
89281	Assisted oocyte fertilization, microtechnique; >10 oocytes
89272	Extended culture of oocytes/embryos, when necessary
Gamete storage	
89342	Storage per year, embryo(s)
89343	Storage per year, sperm/semen
89344	Storage per year, reproductive tissue, testicular/ovarian
89345	Storage per year, oocyte(s)

The following codes are typically excluded, but may be possible in other aspects of an insurance plan:

- Assisted reproductive technologies for future conception
  - Intrauterine insemination (58321, 58322, 58323)
  - Thawing of cryopreserved embryos (89352)
  - Thawing of cryopreserved sperm (89354)
  - Preparation of embryo for transfer (89255)
  - Embryo transfer (58974, 58976)
- Preimplantation genetic diagnosis (PGD) and other genetic testing (89290, 89291)
- Assisted embryo hatching procedures (89253)
- Donor egg, sperm or embryos (S4023, S4025, S4026)

A Letter of Medical Necessity is a critical aspect of insurance advocacy for patients and a letter template is provided in Appendix 2. Although it does not guarantee coverage for fertility preservation consultations or treatment, it may be the only opportunity a patient has to successfully appeal.

Appeal Process

The Affordable Care Act ensures a patient's right to appeal health insurance decisions, including asking insurers to reconsider its decision to deny payment for a service or treatment. Plans created after March 23, 2010 specifically spell out how insurers must handle the appeal process. The law even permits its members to have an independent review organization decide whether to uphold or overturn the plan's decision. The Letter of Medical Necessity and physician referral form are assets required for this process.

Insurers are required to let its members know:

- The reason the claim was denied.
- The insured's right to file an internal appeal.

- The insured's right to request an external review if the internal appeal was unsuccessful.
- The availability of a Consumer Assistance Program (when their state has one).

The law further protects your patients by requiring insurers:

- To give their decision within 72 h after receiving a request for an appeal regarding the denial of a claim for urgent care. (If the appeal concerns urgent care, you may be able to have the internal appeal and external review take place at the same time.)
- 30 Days for denials of nonurgent care not yet received.
- 60 Days for denials of services already received.

Many insurance companies facilitate the appeals process online for its members and is historically something your patient must work through independently with the support of your Letter of Medical Necessity, summary notes and physician referral. Patients can also submit a letter of appeal for fertility preservation on their own behalf (Appendix 3), in addition to letters of support from patient advocacy groups.

Insurance Reform: State Laws Related to Insurance Coverage for Infertility Treatment

Over the past 30 years, 15 states—Arkansas, California, Connecticut, Hawaii, Illinois, Louisiana, Maryland, Massachusetts, Montana, New Jersey, New York, Ohio, Rhode Island, Texas, and West Virginia—have passed laws that require insurers to either cover or offer coverage for infertility diagnosis and treatment. While most these states require inclusion of coverage for in vitro fertilization (IVF), California, Louisiana, and New York have laws that specifically exclude coverage for IVF. These mandates, which are not specific to cancer treatments, are illustrated in Table 14.3 [11]. In contrast, states across the nation currently do not require insurance coverage for infertility treatments for people who may become infertile as a result of cancer or medical treatments.

To date, three states have introduced legislation proposed to expand existing coverage of infertility caused by cancer treatments. However, none of these measures have become law. In 2011, California Assembly member Anthony Portantino was the first legislator to author a fertility preservation bill. California Assembly Bill 428 required health plans and policies to cover "medically necessary expenses for standard fertility preservation services when a necessary medical treatment may directly or indirectly cause iatrogenic infertility to an enrollee [12, 13]" The California Health Benefits Review Program analyzed the fiscal impact of this bill and estimated an increase premium of $0.03 per member per month. This bill was not approved by the state appropriations committee and will be reintroduced at a later time.

Table 14.3 Mandated coverage for infertility treatments available in 15 states

State	Coverage
Arkansas	Requires health insurance companies to cover in vitro fertilization (IVF) by a licensed facility that conforms to guidelines and minimum standards of the American College of Obstetricians and Gynecologists and the American Society for Reproductive Medicine
California	Requires health care service plan for group contracts and insurers to offer coverage for the treatment of infertility, except IVF
Connecticut	Requires health insurance organizations to provide coverage for medically necessary expenses in the diagnosis and treatment of infertility, including IVF procedures
Hawaii	Requires all accident and health insurance policies that provide pregnancy-related benefits to include a one-time only benefit for outpatient expenses arising from IVF procedures
Illinois	Requires certain insurance policies that provide pregnancy-related benefits to provide coverage for the diagnosis and treatment of infertility. Coverage includes a variety of procedures including IVF and four completed oocyte retrievals
Louisiana	Prohibits the exclusion of coverage for the diagnosis and treatment of a medical condition otherwise covered by the policy solely because the condition results in infertility. The law does not require insurers to cover fertility drugs, IVF or other assisted reproductive techniques
Maryland	Prohibits certain health insurers that provide pregnancy-related benefits from excluding benefits for all outpatient expenses arising from IVF procedures performed
Massachusetts	Requires general insurance policies, nonprofit hospital service corporations, medical service corporations and health maintenance organizations that provide pregnancy related benefits to also provide coverage for the diagnosis and treatment of infertility, including IVF
Montana	Requires health maintenance organizations to cover infertility services as part of basic health services on a prepaid basis
New Jersey	Requires health insurers to provide coverage for medically necessary expenses incurred in diagnosis and treatment of infertility. Coverage includes medications, surgery, IVF and four completed egg retrievals per lifetime of the covered person
New York	Requires certain insurers to cover infertility treatment for women between 21 and 44. Coverage includes hospital, surgical and medical care for diagnosis and treatment of "correctable medical conditions otherwise covered by the policy solely because the medical condition results in infertility." However, coverage does not include IVF
Ohio	Requires health maintenance organizations to provide basic health care services, including infertility services when medically necessary
Rhode Island	Requires insurers to provide coverage of medically necessary expenses for the diagnosis and treatment of infertility
Texas	Requires all health insurers to offer and make available coverage for services and benefits for expenses incurred or prepaid for outpatient expenses that may arise from IVF procedures, provided the couple has a history of infertility for at least 5 years or have specified medical conditions resulting in infertility
West Virginia	Requires health maintenance organizations to cover infertility services

According to the National Conference of State Legislatures, 15 states have laws requiring private insurers to cover or offer coverage for a variety of infertility diagnoses and treatments

In 2012, two states attempted to pass legislation for fertility preservation. A bill introduced in New Jersey aimed to require insurers to cover medically necessary expenses for preventing infertility in *women* undergoing chemotherapy or radiation therapy for the treatment of cancer through *oocyte cryopreservation*. This differs from Hawaii House Bill 2105, which provides coverage for established preservation procedures to both men and women who are: (1) of reproductive age, and (2) diagnosed with a cancer or undergo cancer treatments that may adversely affect fertility. However, the bill identifies only two specific fertility preservation methods—*sperm and embryo cryopreservation* [14].

Finally, Senator Claire McCaskill (D-MO) introduced a provision in the National Defense Bill which would provide "additional coverage of fertility treatments for military members who may require such treatments due to chemotherapy, radiation or surgery in order to ensure military service members who face loss of fertility due to medical treatments have a chance to preserve their ability to have children."

As the national conversation for expanded insurance coverage to include fertility preservation evolves, a number of advocacy groups are actively collaborating with key legislators to address this issue. For instance, the Livestrong Foundation and the Cancer Legal Resource Center joined together to develop a position statement outlining standards for health insurance coverage to address the fertility needs at the time of a cancer diagnosis. Key points include statements regarding insurance coverage for standard fertility preservation services for iatrogenic infertility should be dependent on a diagnosis of a medical condition requiring treatment that may cause infertility, not a diagnosis of infertility; and that all coverage language should be written so that when experimental fertility preservation treatments become standard practice as determined by appropriate professional societies, they become a covered benefit [15].

Acknowledgement This work was supported by the Oncofertility Consortium NIH 5UL1DE019587 and NIH K12-HD001271-13 (LAK).

Appendix 1

Oncofertility Referral Form

Patient Name: ____________ MRN: ______ DOB: ______ Age: ______

Attending Physician: ____________ UPI # ______
Ordering Healthcare Provider: ____________ Pager# ______

REFERRING TO:
Department: OBGYN > ReproMed > Oncofertility Clinic
Specialist:

Appointment for:

- ☐ Fertility Preservation Consultation
- ☐ Evaluation and Treatment
- ☐ Surgical
- ☐ Second Opinion

Is the Patient:

- ☐ Inpatient
- ☐ Outpatient
- ☐ Children's Patient?

Room Number? ______

Reason for Visit (Include Patient Diagnosis):

ICD9 Code for DX: ______

Priority

- ☐ Urgent
- ☐ ASAP
- ☐ Routine

Treatment Prescribed to Treat Condition Above:

- ☐ Surgery Date______
- ☐ Chemotherapy Date______
- ☐ Radiation Date______
- ☐ BMT Date______
- ☐ Other Date______

Form completed by: ____________ Title ______ Date ______

Approved By ____________

Phone Number: ____________

Appendix 2

[Center Letterhead]
[Date]
[Insurance Name] Review Unit
By fax: (999) 999-9999
Attn: Appeals
RE: Doe, Jane
D.O.B: 9-30-1984
Blue Cross Blue Shield ID #: 9999999999
Group #: 99999
To Whom It May Concern:

Ms. Jane Doe is a 35-year-old with Stage 4 colon cancer diagnosed in January 2009. The patient's plan of care for this diagnosis includes chemotherapy and likely subsequent radiation. Many of these therapies that so effectively help increase survival have side effects that may cause the loss of fertility. The patient is not currently infertile but may be rendered sterile by the cancer treatment (a covered benefit under her plan).

In preparation for these treatments, the patient saw me in consultation to review fertility preservation options as per American Society of Clinical Oncology (ASCO) and American Society for Reproductive Medicine Guidelines (Attached). After discussing the probable impact of the proposed cancer treatment on her fertility, we reviewed the range of options available.

(Select the appropriate paragraph and delete the others.)

After discussing the spectrum of options, based on cancer treatment, age, diagnosis and the window of time available to the start of cancer treatment the decision was made to bank [oocytes / embryos / ovarian tissue cryopreservation] [Oocyte / embryo] banking is the standard of care for fertility preservation for someone in her circumstances.

After discussing the spectrum of options, based on the cancer treatment, age, diagnosis and window of time available to the start of cancer treatment the decision was made to perform a fertility sparing unilateral salpingo-oophorectomy and ovarian cryopreservation prior to beginning her treatment. Surgical intervention is the standard of care for obtaining ovarian tissue for cryopreservation.

Note on Male Patients: This can be customized to include a description of the male diagnosis if the male is the patient. Use of sperm banking, donor sperm and/or assisted reproductive technologies to treat couples where the man has been rendered infertile by cancer treatment is NOT the same as infertility from other causes and often covered.

Therefore, we request that this treatment as well as related procedures and testing, which have been previously denied, be reconsidered for coverage for this patient. As noted, the patient did not present with infertility but this fertility preservation treatment is essential to preserving fertility prior to beginning cancer treatment.

If you have any questions or need further information, please do not hesitate to contact me.

Sincerely,

John Smith, MD

Lead Physician

Center for Advanced Reproductive Services

Attachments:

1. American Society of Clinical Oncology Recommendations on Fertility Preservation in Cancer Patients. Journal of Clinical Oncology 24: 917–2931, 2006.
2. Fertility preservation and reproduction in cancer patients. Fertility and Sterility, Vol. 83, No. 6, June 2005.

Appendix 3

Jane Doe

22 Fair Avenue

Chicago, IL

[date]

[Insurance Company Name] Review Unit

By fax: (999) 999-9999

Attn: Appeals

RE: Doe, Jane

D.O.B: 9-30-1984

Blue Cross Blue Shield ID #: 9999999999

Group #: 99999

To Whom It May Concern:

I am a 35-year-old with stage 4 colon cancer diagnosed in January 2009. My plan of care for this diagnosis includes chemotherapy and likely subsequent radiation. Many of the therapies that so effectively help increase survival have side effects that may cause the loss of fertility. I am not currently infertile but may be rendered sterile by the cancer treatment (a covered benefit under their plan). In preparation for these treatments, I met with Dr. John Smith in consultation to review the possible impact of my cancer treatment on my fertility and my options for fertility preservation options as per American Society of Clinical Oncology (ASCO) and American Society for Reproductive Medicine Guidelines (see below).

(Select the appropriate paragraph and delete the others.)

After discussing the range of options available, based on my cancer treatment, age, diagnosis and time available to the start of my cancer treatment the decision was made to bank embryos. Embryo banking is the standard of care for fertility preservation for someone in my circumstance.

After discussing the range of options available, based on my cancer treatment, age, diagnosis and time available to the start of my cancer treatment the decision was made to bank eggs. Egg banking is the standard of care for fertility preservation for someone in my circumstance.

After discussing the range of options available, based on my cancer treatment, age, diagnosis and time available to the start of my cancer treatment the decision was made to perform a fertility sparing unilateral salpingo-oophorectomy and ovarian cryopreservation prior to beginning her treatment. Surgical intervention is the standard of care for obtaining ovarian tissue for cryopreservation.

Note on Male Patients: This can be customized to include a description of the male diagnosis if the male is the patient. Use of sperm banking, donor sperm, and/or assisted reproductive technologies to treat couples where the man has been rendered infertile by cancer treatment is NOT the same as infertility from other causes and often covered.

Therefore, we request that this procedure as well as related procedures and testing previously denied for coverage be reconsidered. As noted, I do not have infertility but this treatment was essential to preserving my fertility before my cancer treatment could begin.

If you have any questions or need further information, please do not hesitate to contact Dr. Smith at [Practice Name] or me.

Sincerely,

Jane Doe

References:

1. American Society of Clinical Oncology Recommendations on Fertility Preservation in Cancer Patients. Journal of Clinical Oncology 24: 917–2931, 2006.
2. Fertility preservation and reproduction in cancer patients. Fertility and Sterility, Vol. 83, No. 6, June 2005.

References

1. ACS. American Cancer Society Cancer Facts and Figures 2012. Atlanta: American Cancer Society; 2012.
2. SEER. Surveillance, Epidemiology, and End Results (SEER) Program Populations (1969–2009) (http://www.seer.cancer.gov/popdata), National Cancer Institute, DCCPS, Surveillance Research Program, Cancer Statistics Branch, released January 2011; 2011.
3. Bath LE, et al. Depletion of ovarian reserve in young women after treatment for cancer in childhood: detection by anti-Mullerian hormone, inhibin B an d ovarian ultrasound. Hum Reprod. 2003;18(11):2368–74.
4. Chemaitilly W, et al. Acute ovarian failure in the childhood cancer survivor study. J Clin Endocrinol Metab. 2006;91(5):1723–8.
5. Letourneau JM, et al. Acute ovarian failure underestimates age-specific reproductive impairment for young women undergoing chemotherapy for cancer. Cancer. 2012;118(7):1933–9.
6. Campo-Engelstein L. Consistency in insurance coverage for iatrogenic conditions resulting from cancer treatment including fertility preservation. J Clin Oncol. 2010;28(8):1284–6.
7. Prevention, C.f.D.C.a. International Classification of Diseases, Tenth Revision (ICD-10). 2011 [cited 2013 01/18/2013]; Available from: http://www.cdc.gov/nchs/icd/icd10.htm.
8. Cigna. Medical Necessity Definitions. 2013 [cited 2013 01/18/2013]; Available from: http://www.cigna.com/healthcareprofessionals/resources-for-health-care-professionals/clinical-payment-and-reimbursement-policies/medical-necessity-definitions.html.
9. Livestrong. Position Statement: Insurance Coverage for Iatrogenic Infertility. 2011 [01/18/2013]; Available from: http://www.livestrong.org/What-We-Do/Our-Approach/Platforms-Priorities/Health-Insurance-Coverage-for-Iatrogenic-Infertility.
10. Policy NM. Fertility preservation in cancer patients. 2012 [cited 2013 01/18/2013]; Available from: https://http://www.healthnet.com/.
11. NCSL. Mandated Health Insurance Benefits and State Laws. 2012 [01/15/2013]; Available from: http://www.ncsl.org/issues-research/health/mandated-health-insurance-benefits-and-state-laws.aspx.
12. HEALTH, A.C.O. Assembly Bill 428. 2011 [01/15/2011]; Available from: http://www.leginfo.ca.gov/pub/11-12/bill/asm/ab_0401-0450/ 428_cfa_20110501_122908_asm_comm.html.
13. (CHBRP), C.H.B.R.P. Analysis of Assembly Bill 428: Fertility Preservation, in Report to California State Legislature 2011, Oakland, CA.
14. Auditor O.o.t. Mandatory health insurance coverage for fertility preservation procedures for people of reproductive age diagnosed with cancer. A report to the Governor and the Legislature of the State of Hawai'i, 2012;12(09).
15. CLRC, L.F.H. Position Statement: Health Insurance Coverage for Iatrogenci Infertility; 2011

Chapter 15
Research Recruitment and Dissemination in Young Adults with Cancer

H. Irene Su and Kathleen Lin

Oncofertility is a survivorship issue that affects primarily young cancer patients. In the USA, there are more than 550,000 adolescent and young adult (AYA) cancer survivors who are between 15 and 39 years old [1]. While several age ranges have been used to describe the AYA population, we use this definition, consistent with the AYA Oncology Progress Review Group recommendations, to encompass patients of reproductive age [2].

Due to improvements in cancer treatments, the AYA cancer survivor population is growing, and research on late effects, including loss of fertility, is needed to address and prevent untoward health problems that stem from cancer treatment. Oncofertility research efforts, including epidemiologic studies on reproductive outcomes and clinical trials on fertility preservation strategies, all require the recruitment and participation of young cancer patients. The objective of this chapter is to discuss challenges and approaches in research recruitment and dissemination in AYA cancer patients.

Challenges in Research Recruitment

There are a myriad of challenges in recruiting AYAs with cancer, including lower disease incidence, limited prior research focus on the population, and immense psychosocial changes that occur over young adult life. AYA is a low incidence

H.I. Su, M.D., M.S.C.E. (✉)
Division of Reproductive Endocrinology and Infertility, Department of Reproductive Medicine, University of California, San Diego, 3855 Health Sciences Drive, Dept 0901, La Jolla, CA 92093-0901, USA
e-mail: hisu@ucsd.edu

K. Lin, M.D., M.S.C.E.
Reproductive Endocrinology and Infertility, Seattle, WA, USA
e-mail: kathleenlinmd@gmail.com

T.K. Woodruff et al. (eds.), *Oncofertility Communication: Sharing Information and Building Relationships across Disciplines*, DOI 10.1007/978-1-4614-8235-2_15,

cancer population. AYA patients constitute 4–5 % of the cancer survivor population [1]. Therefore, while there is a significant overall AYA population, the number of young patients at individual medical institutions is limited and a barrier to single institution research studies.

AYA patients have had less access to clinical trials due to oncology cooperative group structures and practice patterns in adult medical oncology. Oncology cooperative groups, first developed in the 1950s to 1970s, are credited with improvements in survival because of improved quality-of-care, attention while on trial from a broader group of specialized professionals, and the ability to conduct appropriately powered studies across centers [3]. Cooperative groups are traditionally divided between pediatric and adult patients, and AYA patients fall in the gap between these two groups. Consequently, AYA patients have been under-represented in trials from both groups. For example, greater than 90 % of children younger than age 15 diagnosed with cancer are treated at institutions with clinical trials programs sponsored by the National Cancer Institute, with 40–70 % enrolled in clinical trials [4]. In contrast, it is estimated that 10 % of patients aged 15–19 and 1–2 % of patients aged 20–39 are enrolled in clinical trials in the USA [4]. In addition, while most pediatric patients are treated in academic centers, older AYA patients are frequently treated by adult oncologists in a myriad of settings. Most adult oncologists practice in the community rather than in academic centers, and as such, access to clinical trials is more limited.

The AYA population comprises the largest and fastest growing group of underinsured Americans [5]. Nearly one-third of 18–24-year-old Americans are uninsured or underinsured. Until recently, parental insurance policies rarely cover young patients after age 23, and Medicaid and Child Health Insurance Programs stop coverage at age 19. Many jobs filled by young people offer limited or no health insurance benefits. With enactment of the Affordable Care Act, some subgroups of AYAs may benefit, such as those younger than age 26 who may now remain on their parents' private insurance. Indeed, for the first year after initiation of the Affordable Care Act, a significant gain in private insurance coverage for the 19–24-year-old group has been demonstrated [6]. However, no increase in insurance coverage was demonstrated for young adults older than 26, nor for those without individual or family access to private insurance. To date, utilization data are lacking. Without appropriate insurance coverage, AYA cancer patients face challenges in accessing quality healthcare and continuity of care. As many research studies utilize clinic-based recruitment, young patients who lack this interface with medical care would not be recruited.

Young adult years are a time of high mobility because of education, employment opportunities, marriage, shifts in residence, and other personal life changes. This mobility renders young adult cancer survivors difficult to follow longitudinally, thus limiting traditional, regionally based recruitment strategies. It is also possible that increased insurance coverage for certain subgroups under the Affordable Care Act may not necessarily mean increased utilization as mobile AYAs have limited access to regional in-network providers [7].

Psychosocial factors: The AYA years are a critical time for maturation and development of skills to increase autonomy, capacity for self-awareness, ability to comprehend complex and abstract information, and evolving personal relationships, social roles, identities, and responsibilities [8]. Elements of this psychosocial context will affect a patient's inclination and ability to participate in research studies. Most studies on psychosocial functioning report encouraging outcomes. However, approximately 25 % of pediatric cancer survivors demonstrate difficulties, including neurocognitive deficits (especially in subjects treated with cranial irradiation and/or central nervous system chemotherapy), academic problems, interpersonal difficulties, low self-esteem, anxiety, and features of depression or posttraumatic stress [9]. Previous studies have also suggested that the cultural complexities of the doctor–parent–patient communications surrounding sex and fertility may make it difficult for an adolescent, young adult or their parent/legal guardians to engage in discussions, including those on oncofertility research, directly with a healthcare provider [10].

Of note, until age 18, parental consent is needed in addition to adolescent assent to research studies. Preparation for recruitment would need to account for procedures to obtain appropriate assent and consent for adolescent patients.

Approaches to Research Recruitment

Research recruitment strategies range from clinic- to population-based. Different approaches provide unique challenges and opportunities. Traditionally, recruitment efforts have focused on individual clinics or research cooperatives composed of several clinics or research centers. On a broader basis, national cancer registries facilitate access to subjects from many regions that could potentially improve generalizability of results. The advent of the Internet and social media offers the advantage of a wide audience, but at the potential cost of bias, since these users represent a self-selected group of patients. How best to harness the power of the Internet for study recruitment is still an important unanswered question.

Clinic-Based Recruitment

Single site, clinic-based recruitment is a common approach to study accrual. Medical oncology, surgical oncology, and long-term survivorship clinics are all sources of young adult patients. There are multiple advantages to clinic-based recruitment. It is possible for direct study involvement by potential participants' healthcare providers. Providers can inform the study team of whether a protocol is appropriate, as well as help introduce and/or recruit for the study. It is also possible to screen and approach all eligible patients presenting to the clinic, limiting selection bias. Medical records for treatment summaries can be readily accessed.

As well, face-to-face contact with patients can facilitate piloting different recruitment approaches and materials and soliciting feedback. This approach requires resources for a single site. The primary disadvantage to clinic-based recruitment is limited sample size and generalizability of data to the type of population seen at the clinic. Secondary disadvantages are limitations in the number of concurrent studies any individual patient may participate in, thus further diluting the pool of potential participants for any given study.

Cooperative Group

Cancer cooperative groups afford multicenter recruitment, aiding in achieving larger sample sizes. Cooperative group infrastructure partly alleviates substantial resources otherwise needed to fund accrual at multiple sites. Rather than devote all resources at one site, cooperative group studies take advantage of the ability to recruit from dozens to hundreds of clinic sites. The efficiency gained is in centralized coordinating centers for study conduct and data management.

As cooperative group studies are based in oncology practices, there are similar benefits to clinic-based recruitment in terms of provider participation and access to medical records. The primary limitations to cooperative groups are an emphasis on studies on survival and large investigator teams. Because of focus on trials to treat cancer and improve survival, other research areas such as oncofertility may not be prioritized. Large investigator groups also result in competition to initiate studies through this mechanism. Potential differences in patient care patterns across centers can result in heterogeneity in the data set. An example of a multi-institutional study of fertility in cancer survivorship is the Childhood Cancer Survivor Study (CCSS) [11]. Through the combined efforts of 27 participating centers, the CCSS is a retrospective cohort study that has recruited 40–45 % of 5-year survivors of childhood cancer diagnosed prior to age 21 between 1970 and 1986 in the USA. In total, the CCSS successfully recruited 57 % of eligible female patients [12].

Cancer Registries

Nearly all newly diagnosed cancer cases in the USA are reported to national cancer registries, making these databases an important source for population-based recruitment of young cancer patients. Registries such as the Surveillance, Epidemiology, and End Results (SEER) Program of the National Cancer Institute in the USA collect population-based information on cancer incidence, patient demographics, primary tumor location, tumor characteristics and stage at diagnosis, first course of treatment, and survival [13]. Currently, 18 SEER registries cover approximately 28 % of the US population. Together with the CDC's National Program of Cancer Registries (NPCR), these two registries ensure that 98 % of newly diagnosed cancer cases and 100 % of mortality data are collected in the USA each year. Research studies may be conducted in collaboration with these registries where potential eligible patients are identified and contacted by registry personnel to introduce research studies, followed by recruitment efforts by the research team.

The strength of cancer registries is comprehensive coverage of cancer cases in a population. The sample should reasonably represent AYA cases in the general population, minimizing selection bias. Because cancer registries cover large areas, achieving sufficiently large sample sizes is feasible. There are several challenges in conducting research through cancer registries. Recruiting newly diagnosed patients is difficult because of lag time between diagnosis and required reporting by medical facilities to the registry. Locating patients who are further out from diagnosis can be difficult in mobile populations as contact information is collected at diagnosis. Indeed, lost to follow-up is a major hurdle in the AYA population characterizing nearly two-thirds of potential subjects whose contact information is no longer accurate [12, 14]. However, a variety of tracing procedures may be undertaken to locate potential participants, from contacting healthcare providers and family members to accessing public records such as Voter Registration [14]. But these tracing procedures may be resource intensive. Passing research protocols through institutional review boards of multiple cancer registries also can be lengthy. In addition, some studies require clinicians' active consent prior to contacting patients.

Recruitment of AYA participants via cancer registries has met variable success (7.8–43 %) [14–16]. From these studies, it is evident that response rates differ by cancer type, sex, and race. For example, in one study assessing various posttreatment quality of life and healthcare delivery issues demonstrated a 38 % response rate for acute lymphocytic leukemia and sarcoma compared to 51 % for Hodgkin's lymphoma. Males, non-Hispanic blacks, and Hispanic patients are significantly less likely to participate. Hispanic patients are also more than twice as likely than any other ethnic group to be lost to follow-up (32 % vs. 12 % non-Hispanic white and 14 % non-Hispanic black).

Advocacy Groups

A number of cancer advocacy groups provide outreach to AYA cancer patients. These include large, well-established groups such as the American Cancer Society and Livestrong, disease-specific organizations such as the Young Survival Coalition, and young adult focused groups such as Stupid Cancer and Planet Cancer. In the AYA population, these organizations provide an invaluable forum for information and peer support. However, advocacy and cancer support group participants may not be representative of all cancer patients [17]. For example, cancer support group participants tend to be of higher socioeconomic background and are more anxious and distressed [18]. Depending on the study objectives, results from participants derived from advocacy sources may not be generalizable across all AYA cancer patients.

A variety of cancer advocacy groups have supported research recruitment. Organizations including the American Cancer Society and Livestrong have recruited and followed cancer patients for the organizations' ongoing cohort studies. There are also opportunities to partner with these groups for investigator-initiated studies. Advocacy groups can help to disseminate study information and encourage participation in studies of interest to their constituents via mailings, e-mail, Web site postings, and social media outreach [19]. Studies have reported recruitment at cancer advocacy venues such as the Susan G. Komen Race for the Cure and the American Cancer Society Relays for Life [20].

The advantages to recruitment with the support of advocacy organizations include targeting specific cancer populations (by disease or age group), outreach to young patients who may not interface with the medical community or are lost to follow-up by cancer registries, and peer-to-peer dissemination of study information. Dependent on the study design, it is possible to have a single establishment's institutional review board protocol to approve national recruitment, in contrast to cooperative groups and cancer registry studies.

The use of social media for AYA recruitment is a new and powerful method for accruing large samples in a time and cost-efficient manner. Eighty-three percent of young adults ages 18–29 use a social networking site of some kind [21], supporting the potential power of social media outreach in facilitating research. For example, at the time of this writing, there are over 57,000 "likes" directed at the StupidCancer.org Web site, where an icon specifically links to ongoing clinical trials [22]. Implicit endorsement of the study may encourage followers to learn more about study participation. For example, under the "Clinical Trials" tab of the YSC.org (Young Survival Coalition) Web site, an introduction states: "Participating in clinical trials is one of the most meaningful actions we, as members of this community of young women, can take to help each other. Working together with medical researchers, we have the power to ensure good data that's relevant to us all—while answering those questions that continue to confound young women and doctors alike" [23]. The increased exposure and advocacy for research offered by social media Web sites is a powerful tool to improve study recruitment.

Our recent experience with recruitment for a cohort study on reproductive outcomes demonstrates responses to Facebook posts by Stupid Cancer (Fig. 15.1). This study asks participants to complete annual Web-based questionnaires and provide access to their medical records. Over five bimonthly posts, the number of responders interested in participation grew; as well, increasing numbers of individuals liked or shared the post, which in turn exposes more Facebook users to the study. Participants are highly motivated and almost all agreed to contact for future studies.

The primary limitation is participant self-selection with implications on study generalizability. For example, in our study on reproductive outcomes, our study population skews toward higher educational levels, and recruitment of black and Hispanic AYA survivors has been more challenging. Moreover, in contrast to registry studies where it is possible to compare responders from nonresponders, there is not an established method to identify nonresponders in recruitment via social media.

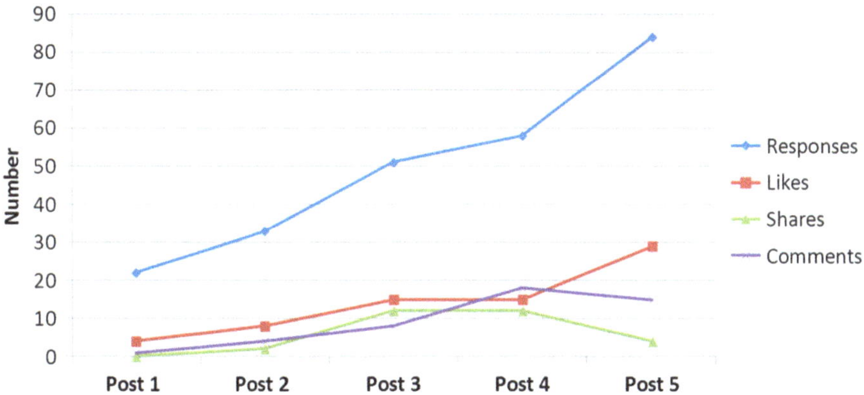

Fig. 15.1 Responses to Facebook recruitment posts by adolescent and young adult (AYA) advocacy group

Research Dissemination

Similarly, research results can be disseminated on social media Web sites with the ability to reach a wide network. Since study participants may have learned of a particular study through a Web site, it also makes sense that they would turn to the same source for information on research results.

However, this powerful ability for information exchange must be carefully used. How best to integrate scientists and physicians to ensure accurate and understandable content is still being evaluated with real-time activity ahead of best practices recommendations [24]. Scientific findings are usually not presented in their primary format for the Internet user to interpret. Rather, Web sites are more likely to take positions based on their interpretation of relevant research results, which could have a significant impact on the public's response to a finding. Until specific standards for the reporting of research news are devised with cross-references to credible agencies, there does remain a risk of misinterpretation and hype.

Conclusion

One of the challenges facing oncofertility research in AYA cancer patients is successful recruitment. Recruitment strategies in this population require an understanding of barriers to research participation, careful consideration of pros and cons of various approaches, and, in many instances, harnessing multiple approaches to optimize participation. Beyond traditional methods, social media and advocacy groups in young adults with cancer may play a significant role in research recruitment and dissemination, but more studies are needed to delineate efficacy and optimize these novel approaches.

Acknowledgment This work was supported by the Oncofertility Consortium NIH 5UL1DE019587, PL1CA133835, NIH HD058799, and ACS MRSG-08-110-01-CCE.

References

1. SEER Cancer Statistics Review, 1975–2008 [http://seer.cancer.gov/csr/1975_2008/, based on Nov 2010 SEER data submission, posted to the SEER web site, 2011].
2. Closing the gap: research and care imperatives for adolescents and young adults with cancer. A report of the Adolescent and Young Adult Oncology Progress Review Group. Department of Health and Human Services, National Institutes of Health, National Cancer Institute and the LiveStrong Young Adult Alliance. National Cancer Institute; 2006.
3. Ferrari A, Bleyer A. Participation of adolescents with cancer in clinical trials. Cancer Treat Rev. 2007;33(7):603–8.
4. Burke ME, Albritton K, Marina N. Challenges in the recruitment of adolescents and young adults to cancer clinical trials. Cancer. 2007;110(11):2385–93.
5. DeNavas-Walt C, Proctor BD, Lee CH. Income, poverty, and health insurance coverage in the United States: 2005. In: Bureau USC, editor. Current population reports. Washington, DC: U.S. Government Printing Office; 2006. p. 60–229. http://www.census.gov/prod/2008pubs/p60-235.pdf
6. Sommers BD, Buchmueller T, Decker SL, Carey C, Kronick R. The Affordable Care Act has led to significant gains in health insurance and access to care for young adults. Health Aff (Millwood). 2013;32(1):165–74.
7. Andrews M. Young and doubly insured: a modern health dilemma. In: National Public Radio; 2013. http://www.npr.org/blogs/health/2013/01/08/168863301/young-and-doubly-insured-a-modern-health-dilemma
8. Freyer DR. Transition of care for young adult survivors of childhood and adolescent cancer: rationale and approaches. J Clin Oncol. 2010;28(32):4810–8.
9. Patenaude AF, Kupst MJ. Psychosocial functioning in pediatric cancer. J Pediatr Psychol. 2005;30(1):9–27.
10. Quinn GP, Vadaparampil ST. Fertility preservation and adolescent/young adult cancer patients: physician communication challenges. J Adolesc Health. 2009;44(4):394–400.
11. Leisenring WM, Mertens AC, Armstrong GT, Stovall MA, Neglia JP, Lanctot JQ, Boice Jr JD, Whitton JA, Yasui Y. Pediatric cancer survivorship research: experience of the Childhood Cancer Survivor Study. J Clin Oncol. 2009;27(14):2319–27.
12. Green DM, Kawashima T, Stovall M, Leisenring W, Sklar CA, Mertens AC, Donaldson SS, Byrne J, Robison LL. Fertility of female survivors of childhood cancer: a report from the childhood cancer survivor study. J Clin Oncol. 2009;27(16):2677–85.
13. http://seer.cancer.gov/about/
14. Harlan LC, Lynch CF, Keegan TH, Hamilton AS, Wu XC, Kato I, West MM, Cress RD, Schwartz SM, Smith AW, et al. Recruitment and follow-up of adolescent and young adult cancer survivors: the AYA HOPE Study. J Cancer Surviv. 2011;5(3):305–14.
15. Clinton-McHarg T, Carey M, Sanson-Fisher R, Tracey E. Recruitment of representative samples for low incidence cancer populations: do registries deliver? BMC Med Res Methodol. 2011;11(1):5.
16. Letourneau JM, Ebbel EE, Katz PP, Katz A, Ai WZ, Chien AJ, Melisko ME, Cedars MI, Rosen MP. Pretreatment fertility counseling and fertility preservation improve quality of life in reproductive age women with cancer. Cancer. 2012;118(6):1710–7.
17. Napoles-Springer AM, Ortiz C, O'Brien H, Diaz-Mendez M, Perez-Stable EJ. Use of cancer support groups among Latina breast cancer survivors. J Cancer Surviv. 2007;1(3):193–204.
18. Grande GE, Myers LB, Sutton SR. How do patients who participate in cancer support groups differ from those who do not? Psychooncology. 2006;15(4):321–34.

19. Cantrell MA, Conte T, Hudson M, Shad A, Ruble K, Herth K, Canino A, Kemmy S. Recruitment and retention of older adolescent and young adult female survivors of childhood cancer in longitudinal research. Oncol Nurs Forum. 2012;39(5):483–90.
20. Bondurant KL, Harvey S, Klimberg S, Kadlubar S, Phillips MM. Establishment of a southern breast cancer cohort. Breast J. 2011;17(3):281–8.
21. 65 % of online adults use social network sites. http://pewinternet.org/Reports/2011/Social-Networking-Sites.aspx
22. http://stupidcancer.com/index.shtml
23. http://www.youngsurvival.org/breast-cancer-in-young-women/living-with-breast-cancer/clinical-trials/
24. Fordis M, Street Jr RL, Volk RJ, Smith Q. The prospects for web 2.0 technologies for engagement, communication, and dissemination in the era of patient-centered outcomes research: selected articles developed from the Eisenberg conference series 2010 meeting. J Health Commun. 2010;2011(16 Suppl 1):3–9.

Chapter 16
Improving Legislation with the Help of Objective Scientific Advice

Gregory Dolin

Introduction

Otto von Bismarck is rumored to have quipped that "legislation is like sausage: it's better not to watch it being made" [1, 2].[1] It may well have been sound advice when the laws were made in service of a monarchy without much consideration of the views or the desires of the populace. Americans however "have ignored this advice and have widely subscribed to the view that a truly democratic people must have access to governmental decision-making …." [3]. In reality, despite an expectation of public participation, the public is often shut off from the legislative process. Furthermore, when Congress legislates in areas that deal with science and technology, it tends to prove Bismarck right, because it legislates in the dark, without understanding the underlying issues or the full impact that legislation is likely to have on the progress of science [4].[2] In those instances, it truly is better to avoid seeing the legislative process. The solution, however, is not to avert our gaze, but to improve the process so that the result is as worthy as sausages are tasty.

Congress enacts, on a nearly continuous basis, a variety of laws that affect scientific research and progress. Some of these laws have an unquestionably positive effect. For instance, Congress' creation of the National Institutes of Health [5], the National Academy of Sciences [6], NASA [7], various appropriations to fund groundbreaking research [8], and multitude of other laws have incalculably advanced human

[1] The quote is likely apocryphal, but it is oft-quoted by lawyers and judges alike, despite there being no definitive proof that Bismarck actually uttered these words.

[2] "[A]ccording to the Congressional Research Service, the technically trained among the 435 members of the House include one physicist, 22 people with medical training (including 2 psychologists and a veterinarian), a chemist, a microbiologist and 6 engineers."

G. Dolin, M.D. (✉)
Center for Medicine and Law, University of Baltimore School of Law, The Johns Hopkins University School of Medicine, 1415 Maryland Avenue, Baltimore, MD 21201, USA
e-mail: gdolin@ubalt.edu

T.K. Woodruff et al. (eds.), *Oncofertility Communication: Sharing Information and Building Relationships across Disciplines*, DOI 10.1007/978-1-4614-8235-2_16,

knowledge, and it is to Congress' great credit that these laws have been and are continuing to be enacted. However, not all laws that affect the progress of science are an unalloyed good. Quite the opposite, often the laws aim to, and in fact do, slow the progress of scientific research [9].[3] The question then is whether the benefit from those laws outweighs the costs imposed on scientific progress. At one extreme, one may consider the Nuclear Test Ban Treaty [10]. The treaty certainly had the effect of limiting the study of nuclear physics [11, 12].[4] Yet, there is some value in banning nuclear tests, and Congress has attempted to strike a balance between the two [10, 11, 13].[5] The problem is that too many laws are enacted without any serious consideration of these costs and benefits, because these laws are considered without the full understanding of the impact that they will have on scientific research [14].[6]

In Part I, I discuss what the general public is often taught and told about the lawmaking process versus the actual reality of the process. According to the civics textbooks, the lawmaking begins in a committee where the proposal is carefully studied, debated, amended, and voted on, and then the process is repeated on the floor of the house, and then again, from scratch, in the other house. The reality, of course, is much different. First, bills often skip the committee process, and amendments are often added last minute without a chance for a meaningful debate. But even where the process is followed as described, it is often hard to describe the committee hearings as a true deliberative process. Instead, they are often described as a "Kabuki theater" [15–19],[7] where the Chair and the Ranking Member designate the witnesses they wish to call to support the preformulated position [20].[8] Interested

[3] "To give example of legal restrictions on technology is to survey much of modern American law .... Food and drug law has become recognized as a discrete area of study that includes cases where new products have been delayed in reaching the market or prevented from doing so altogether. In other areas, ranging from communications to computers, regulation is a fact of modern life. At the state level, statutes and judicial decisions, concerning, for example, malpractice, products liability, and exposure to radioactive materials, have subjected technology to extraordinarily close scrutiny."

[4] "[T]he nuclear weapons problem is one that deeply implicates science and technology. A relevant role from modern international law is to come to grips with the possibilities and limitations of science and technology in order to provide the goal guidance that is both relevant and steeped in realism."

[5] For example, the United States ratified the 1963 Nuclear Test Ban Treaty [10], but balked at ratifying the new Comprehensive Nuclear Test Ban Treaty [13]. One of the reasons for the opposition to the Treaty was the stated effect on scientific testing [11].

[6] "Scientists argue that risks of experimentation in biotechnology cannot be discussed rationally unless participants understand the subject matter. ... According to many scientists, rapidly-moving research simply is not amenable to safety regulations by nonscientific decision makers. ... Public participants in scientific discussions tend to be intimidated by scientists, and are hesitant to raise technical issues for fear of embarrassment."

[7] While most criticisms focus on nomination, especially judicial nomination hearings, legislative hearings are little different.

[8] "Because of the unique control that committee chairs have over the design and content of hearings—including who testifies and on what—testimony at hearings may be viewed simply as an additional forum for interest group influence in the form of witnesses. It is up to the chair to decide the extent to which individuals will be heard by the committee or to which their written views will

parties cannot provide testimony unless asked to do so by the relevant committee [21, 22].[9] Thus, oftentimes the people with the deepest knowledge, but few political skills, are cut out of the process [20].[10] The end result is that Congress votes on legislation without fully understanding the implications thereof [14]. The voters are also injured in that it is hard to hold Congress accountable if one cannot point out that it ignored the views of the scientific communities [23, 24].[11]

In Part II, I discuss a specific example of uninformed legislating and its effect on scientific progress. The Dickey-Wicker Amendment (DWA) was enacted in 1996 as part of the annual appropriation process [25]. The Amendment bars federal funding for any research on a human embryo, which is in turn defined as any organism "derived by fertilization, parthenogenesis, or any other means from one or more human gametes" [25]. This rider was enacted without any separate vote on the issue and was attached to "must-pass" legislation [26]. It has been reenacted every year since 1996 [27]. The problem is that in enacting this legislation, no one considered whether differences between fertilization, cloning, and parthenogenesis exist, and if so whether they are of sufficient magnitude to treat each process differently [28].[12] As it turns out, such differences do exist [29], yet they were not taken into account, precisely because no one asked the right question, and there was no one in the room to answer it. The DWA has stymied research in areas such as fertility, assisted reproductive technology, and stem cells, all because of Congress' basic lack of understanding of the underlying scientific principles [29].

Part III of this chapter proposes a solution to the problem. I argue that bills that affect the progress of science ought to be evaluated by an independent body similar to the Congressional Budget Office (CBO) [30].[13] Like the CBO, this body would not have any authority to block a bill, but it would be able to "score" it, i.e., provide information on the effect the bill will have on research [30]. In order to accomplish its task, this newly created body would be required to provide notice of pending legislation and then seek comments from the interested parties, much like what is

---

be placed in the committee record.... In general, the committee chair retains power to set the agenda and format of any hearings and determine all witnesses in consultation with the ranking member of the minority party on the committee."

[9] "[T]he information Congress receives ... is limited by the set of parties invited to participate." [21].

Reference [22] describes a hearing on adult industry where only scientists opposed to pornography were invited to participate, but those holding contrary views or who questioned the basis of the studies presented to the committee were not.

[10] "[W]itnesses reflecting minority viewpoints are often heard from last and end up speaking to few Members and empty hearing rooms."

[11] Stating that for electoral accountability, "citizens must have access to information about what their government is doing and how decisions have been reached." [23].

"Broad availability of information is an essential element of a strong democracy—quality collective decision-making and electoral accountability both depend upon an informed polity." [24].

[12] As discussed below, the bill was written, considered, passed, and signed within 48 h, leaving essentially no time to debate the merits of any of its provisions.

[13] Reference [30] gives a history and the description of the functions of the Congressional Budget Office.

done in the administrative rule-making process [31].[14] The comments would then be collected and analyzed with the final report presented to Congress before it votes. Congress will continue to be able to vote as it pleases, but with this process in place, it will be forced to do so with its eyes wide open. By understanding the full scope and the implications for scientific progress of the bills it wishes to enact, Congress will produce better legislation that is less detrimental to scientific progress.

The Legislative Process: Myths and Realities

Millions of Americans think of the legislative process by reference to Schoolhouse Rock's *I'm Just a Bill* [32] and Jimmy Stewart's *Mr. Smith Goes to Washington* [33]. The process that is imprinted in the public's mind is one with exhaustive debates in the committees and on the floor where the views of people most likely to be affected by the legislation and most knowledgeable in the subject matter provide input to Congress before it reaches its decision [32]. This view is bolstered by Congressional Webpages that list committees and their areas of jurisdiction, Congressional mailings touting a particular member's membership on certain committees that are supposedly relevant to the specific concerns of the Congressman's district, and even C-SPAN programming that shows committee hearings where Congressmen and Senators hear testimony and question proponents and opponents of proposed bills. With such media presentations, the public can be forgiven for thinking that each bill undergoes serious scrutiny and debate before being voted on and enacted into law. The reality, however, is quite different.

In the last few years, Congressional hearings have often been called "kabuki theater"[15] [16, 17] or a "dog and pony show" [18, 19].[16] While the moniker is most often applied to the judicial confirmation hearings [16, 17] the same is true about all other hearings [19]. The hearings are no longer designed to elicit unbiased expert testimony to aid the deliberative process, but rather to provide support for preexisting political viewpoints [20–22]. The appearance of witnesses in the Congressional hearings is not a matter of right for the public, but a matter of prerogative for committee chairs and the ranking members [20–22]. The chairman is a particularly powerful figure in the committee, with the authority to decide not only which proposals are considered and in what order (or for that matter whether they are considered at all) but also which witnesses will be called and what will be testified to [34, 35].[17]

[14] Reference [31] describes the notice-and-comment process in the administrative agencies.

[15] Reference [16] describes confirmation hearings as "kabuki" and reference [17] quotes then-Senator Joe Biden describing the hearings as a "Kabuki dance."

[16] "I find this for me more helpful than a congressional hearing and what some would call a dog and pony show, which is what a lot of the hearings turn out to be."—quoting Rep. Brad Ellsworth.

[17] "Power is particularly concentrated in the hands of committee chairs, who hold sway over the committees' agendas and the bills reported to the floor." [34].

Reference [35] notes that committee chairs control the agenda and that "[t]he rules for setting the agenda become a powerful means for manipulating a divided legislature to converge on those outcomes favored by the agenda setters."

The exercise of this power was on display when the late Senator Jesse Helms, the then-Chairman of the Senate Foreign Relations Committee, refused to hold hearings on the nomination of William Weld to be the US Ambassador to Mexico [36]. When even Helms' Republican colleagues rebelled against this approach, Helms was forced to hold a hearing [37]. However, at that hearing, it was not Governor Weld who testified in support of his nomination [37]. Rather, Helms engaged in a soliloquy about the Senate traditions of allowing the committee chairmen to refuse to bring up matters for hearings or votes, and then adjourned the hearing when he was done [38]. Ultimately, Weld was never brought up for a vote and his nomination was withdrawn [39]. A committee chairman also has the authority to draft a bill on his own and have that bill form the basis of discussions, rather than anything that may have been debated in a subcommittee, or during the initial hearings in the full committee [40].[18] Thus, the chairman has a near-complete control of the scope and substance of discussion that takes place in the committee [34, 35].

The modern absurdity of committee hearings is perhaps best illustrated by the appearance of the comedian Stephen Colbert in front of the House Judiciary Committee in July of 2010 [41]. Mr. Colbert used the opportunity to mock Congress and the process of considering bills [42].[19] Mr. Colbert, however, did not just "show up" at the hearing room. He was invited by the panel's chairwoman and Committee Chair, the long-serving Representative Zoe Lofgren [43]. Instead of a real debate on the merits of the Farm Bill, the committee (and by extension, the public) was treated to a mocking performance of a satirist [43].

What's more, committee hearings are rarely fully attended by the committee members [44].[20] In some ways, this is not surprising given that each member of Congress serves on a number of committees [45].[21] The supposed deliberations then are actually quite often just a show, with most of the work done not out in the open by the people responsible to the electorate, but by the staffers [46, 47].[22] While the staffers may consult with experts in the field [48, 49],[23] they need not do so, and

---

[18] Defines "Chairman's Mark" as a "[r]ecommendation by committee (or subcommittee) chair of the measure to be considered in a markup, usually drafted as a bill."

[19] "David Corn, who writes for the liberal Mother Jones magazine, tweeted 'Colbert is making a mockery of this hearing.' Republicans were more harsh."

[20] "The very conduct of the committee hearings undermines any serious examination of the facts; attendance is often poor, and during the testimony legislators frequently talk to one another, wander in and out to take phone calls, and engage in side conversations with their staff."

[21] Notes that Congressmen "have multiple committee assignments and, under the best of circumstances, have difficulty giving adequate time and attention to any one of them."

[22] "The Committee, however, "had not completed the final text of the bill and left the task of drafting the appropriate language to its staff." [46].

"The drafting can be done by the legislator's own staff, as Truth-in-Lending was, or by a centralized staff of one kind or another, such as committee counsel, legislative counsel, or a separate research office …." [47].

[23] Staffer "had most recently been reworking a long-pending constitutional amendment drafted in consultation with legal scholars, policy experts, and representatives of law enforcement." [48].

"Members of Congress and their staffs are most vulnerable to the problematic methods because of their reliance on reelection, the often temporary nature of their government service, and their ability to have closed door meetings with lobbyists that protect the information they receive from outside scrutiny." [49].

even when they do consult, because whatever advice is obtained is obtained through private communications, there is little chance to test these communications against criticism and opposing viewpoints [50].[24] Instead, the more likely outcome is epistemic closure where a preplanned political outcome is justified by reference to a selective presentation of information and arguments [49]. Congressional committees are then not the deliberative and fact-finding bodies portrayed in Schoolhouse Rock videos, but are rubber stamps for pre-written bills. Indeed, courts have often disregarded "Congressional findings of fact"[25] [51] precisely because quite often these "findings" are tendentious, open to much dispute, and sometimes are not even supported by actual evidence [44].

This situation would be bad enough, but that is merely the beginning of failures in the legislative process. Several additional factors ensure that the bills that come up for votes on the floor of each house are not subject to full debate, scrutiny, and relevant data. In the House of Representatives, before being reported to the floor, each bill has to be considered and reported by the Committee on Rules [52]. Whereas the various committees with subject matter jurisdiction are at least nominally specialized, with representatives assigned based on specific interest in the matters within committee's jurisdiction, and staffers being drawn from the pool of individuals with specialized knowledge in these matters, the Rules Committee is a purely political tool designed to allow the Speaker of the House to keep control of the bills brought to the floor [52]. The Rules Committee's power over all bills is nearly limitless.

> The [Rules] Committee has the authority to do virtually anything during the course of consideration of a measure, including deeming it passed. The Committee can also include a self-executed amendment which could rewrite just parts of a bill, or the entire measure. In essence, so long as a majority of the House is willing to vote for a special rule, there is little that the Rules Committee cannot do [52].

Despite this power, the Committee does not spend much time considering the bills that it reports to the floor. Nor does it often hear outsiders' testimony. Instead, the individuals testifying before the Rules Committee are usually other members of Congress who urge the committee to allow (or disallow) consideration of certain amendments on the House floor [52]. Despite the lack of deep familiarity with the bills or the factual background behind the bills, the Rules Committee can and does rewrite bills that it considers, even when such bills have been painstakingly developed in the committee of jurisdiction [52, 53]. This makes the final product even less deliberative, and even more political—in the worst sense of the word [53].

The Senate does not have a counterpart to the House Rules Committee [54].[26] Nonetheless, the Senate has its own methods of skirting committees of jurisdiction.

---

[24] Notes that the minority party is often unable "to call witnesses or otherwise define the hearing agenda."

[25] Rejecting Congress' finding of facts and noting that they "are substantially weakened by the fact that they rely so heavily on a method of reasoning that we have already rejected as unworkable if we are to maintain the Constitution's enumeration of powers."

[26] The Senate does have a Committee on Rules and Administration, but its jurisdiction is significantly narrower than that of its House counterpart. The Senate Committee deals only with the administration of the Senate itself, as well as bills on a specific, and rather limited issues.

The Senate calendar is controlled by the Majority Leader of the Senate [55].[27] The Majority Leader decides when to call up which bills, irrespective of whether they have been fully vetted (or for that matter, vetted at all) by the committee of jurisdiction [55]. In other words, a bill can be written, introduced, and then immediately called up for consideration, thus bypassing any hearings or opportunity (such as it is) for interested members of the public to offer their views and criticism [55].[28] To be fair, the Senate rules do allow Senators to force extended (and nearly limitless) debate on any bill, thus providing a bit of a safety check against bills being rushed through without due consideration [56].[29] That said, the length of the debate and speechifying (often to an otherwise empty chamber)[30] [57] does not necessarily enhance the quality of the debate or allow experts and individuals and groups most affected by the proposed legislation to offer their views or describe the likely effect the proposed legislation will have.

Related to the aforementioned problems is the fact that Congress has, over the decades, blurred the traditional line between authorizing legislation and appropriating legislation. Professor Richard Lazarus describes the distinction between the two types of bills and the consequences that flow from each:

> The decision whether to pass authorizing legislation, such as the Clean Air Act, its detailed amendments, or any other kind of substantive legislation, is almost always entirely discretionary. Because relatively few federal statutes … have sunset provisions, congressional failure to pass a new authorization statute preserves the status quo. The absence of legislative action does not create a disruptive legal vacuum. Congress need not formally reauthorize either the Clean Water Act or the Clean Air Act after a statutorily prescribed number of years for those laws to remain in effect. Hence, those seeking to pass a new authorization statute invariably face the heavy burden of demonstrating why a change is necessary.
>
> Precisely the converse is true when appropriations legislation is at stake. There is enormous political pressure to pass annual appropriations legislation because, absent its passage, the status quo is not maintained. Instead, there is a very real threat of a complete shutdown of the federal government. If the deadline for the annual appropriations bill is not met, then to avoid a shutdown Congress must at a minimum pass a continuing resolution to appropriate funds for a few more weeks or months as necessary to keep an agency in operation until passage of the annual appropriations bill [58].

As a result of the “must-pass” nature of the appropriation bills, “it is tempting to try to attach incidental provisions that otherwise might lack the political momentum (or even majority support) necessary for passage.” [58]. These riders can be quite different than stand-alone “substantive” bills, but because they are attached to appropriation bills, rather than authorization legislation, they are not considered in

---

[27] “The Senate gives its majority leader the primary responsibility for deciding the order in which bills on the calendar should come to the floor for action.”

[28] Notes that Senate Rule XIV allows any Senator to bypass referral to Committee, but because the Majority Leader controls the calendar, that power is only effective with respect to the bills that the Majority Leader wishes to have debated on the floor.

[29] Senate Rule XXII is the rule that permits the process known as filibuster as it allows the debate to be shut off only if three-fifths of the elected Senators vote to end debate.

[30] “On C-SPAN today, you can watch politicians giving speeches before what look like completely empty chambers.”

the committee of jurisdiction over the substantive matter; rather, if they are considered in the committee at all, it is in the Committee on Appropriations [58]. Quite often, these riders are not even considered in the Appropriations Committee, but are added at the last minute, during the floor debates and votes [58]. Again, in either case, the legislators are deprived of the considered views of those whom the legislation is likely to affect [58].

A final stage at which bills can be amended without much public input or debate is a conference committee formed to negotiate over different versions of a bill passed by the House and the Senate [59].[31] Much like House of Representative's Committee on Rules, conference committees have an almost unlimited authority to rewrite or modify a pending bill [60],[32] and they can do so in near-total secrecy [60, 61],[33] as meetings of conference committees are generally not open to the public, at least not for the purposes of giving testimony and illuminating the full scope of effects that the bill (or any modifications thereto) would have [62].[34]

In short, the informed, deliberative process that the public is taught to expect from Congress is quite often anything but that. Instead, the process is quite often much more haphazard, ill informed, and subject to hijacking by individuals who may not understand the full impact of the very legislation that they support and vote for.

The Dickey-Wicker Amendment

The Amendment and Its History

The above discussion is not meant to suggest that the legislative process is either irreparably broken or that the process itself is worthless. Indeed, with respect to most matters addressed by the legislature, the legislative process works the way it is intended to. Much of what Congress does centers on value judgments about the

---

[31] "A temporary, ad hoc panel composed of House and Senate conferees that is formed for the purpose of reconciling differences in legislation that has passed both chambers."

[32] Describes how a conference committee rewrote the 2003 Medicare bills, including reinserting the language previously rejected in floor votes.

[33] Reference [60] describes that the conference committee excluded not only the public but even Members of Congress with opposing viewpoints.

According to Rep. Jerry Nadler, "[t]he conference committee, [dealing with a Patriot Act reauthorization] met only once, and only so that members could deliver opening statements. The rest of the work of the conference committee consists of Republican staff working behind the scenes to draft a compromise bill .... That is to say that the Republican staff of the Senate negotiated with the Republican staff of the House." (Internal quotations omitted) [61].

[34] The bill went to the Senate Appropriations Energy-Water Subcommittee, where the second Tennessee senator, Jim Sasser, left the language intact. The full Senate voted to remove Duncan's language from the bill, but after the conference committee concluded, the bill returned to the Senate with the Tellico exemption again present. The senators, now weary of the issue, voted to allow the dam to be completed.

appropriate role of government, level of taxation, proper foreign policy, etc [63, 64].[35] In those circumstances, Congressional majorities are more concerned with building public support for their proposed public policy solutions [65].[36] In that posture, the "dog and pony" congressional hearings make perfect sense. The hearings here are not meant to illuminate the issues for debate, but rather to bolster the political support for (or to drum up opposition to) a preformulated political position [65]. It is for this reason that the "courts accord substantial deference to the predictive judgments of Congress," [66] even when such judgments prove to be wrong.

The deference, however, is due only to the *predictive* judgments of Congress, not necessarily due to its judgment as to the facts as they already exist in the real world [67]. With respect to these facts, Congress gets much less deference, as it should [67]. Nonetheless, Congress, in making its decisions, does have to rely on its understanding of the facts as they do exist in the real world. When the facts are common or undisputed knowledge (e.g., the distance between two cities, the number of days in a year, the revenues and expenditures of the government in the years past) there is not much danger that Congress will misunderstand the content, scope, or import of the factual basis (though it may choose to assign whatever weight it chooses to these facts). However, when the facts concern complicated scientific issues requiring specialized knowledge for full comprehension, Congressmen untrained in science are unlikely to fully understand either the predicate for their actions or the full effect that the actions will have [68].[37] As a result, Congress often enacts laws that have a devastating effect on the speed and scope of scientific progress. It does so not out of any malice for scientific advances, but out of misunderstanding of the issues.

The DWA [69] is a perfect example of Congress acting without understanding the full effect that the legislation would have on scientific exploration. Since 1974, the federal law had already imposed restrictions on the use of federal funds with respect to fetal research [70]. Those restrictions have been part and parcel of the abortion debate and legislative skirmishes [71].[38] In the 1990s, however, as scientific horizons began to expand, and the research began to focus on the earliest stages of human development, the ethical and political concerns over such research began to extend to not just fetal tissue but also embryonic tissue. The issue was studied by the National Institute of Health's Human Embryo Research Panel, composed of 19

[35] "[E]very statute encapsulates legislative value judgments regarding foreseeable situations at the time of enactment." [63].

"Whether legislation is generally reasonable largely depends on value judgments that vary from nation to nation." [64].

[36] "In order to enact effective securities regulation on the federal level, the Pecora Hearings sought to 'galvanize broad public support for direct federal regulation of the stock markets.'"—quoting Joel Seligman, THE TRANSFORMATION OF WALL STREET: A HISTORY OF THE SECURITIES AND EXCHANGE COMMISSION AND MODERN CORPORATE FINANCE 2 (3rd ed. 2003).

[37] Notes that scientists are "unable to translate their ideas into language that Congressmen understand."

[38] "Roe produced a rash of hastily prepared … statutes designed to prohibit the same type of fetal experimentation that had occurred prior to recent liberalized abortion laws."

leading scientists and ethicists [72]. The panel issued its report on September 27, 1994, and recommended making federal funding available for research using "spare" embryos, embryos obtained from consenting IVF patients, embryos created specifically for research, and research using "parthenotes" [72]. I will discuss the science of parthenotes below, and why the distinction is important despite being overlooked by Congress. President Clinton declined to follow the recommendation in full, and under the executive order issued in 1994, federal funding was not made available for embryos created specifically for research [73].[39] What is interesting about Clinton's executive order was that it was made after a period of study, comments, and a report by a body of experts [73]. The fact that the President did not fully endorse the recommendations of the expert panel does not diminish the importance of having had the benefit of the expert input.

Congress, however, was not satisfied with the Clinton compromise. In response, in 1996, it enacted the DWA [29],[40] which prohibited funding for any research that involved "(1) the creation of a human embryo or embryos for research purposes; or (2) research in which a human embryo or embryos are destroyed, discarded, or knowingly subjected to risk of injury or death …." [69, 74, 75]. The DWA defined "human embryo" as "any organism … that is derived by fertilization, parthenogenesis, cloning, or any other means from one or more human gametes." [69, 74, 75]. Although Congress, like the President, had access to the NIH report, there is no evidence that it ever considered either the findings of the report or the distinctions drawn therein. The reason is that the DWA, being a "rider" on a must-pass appropriations bill, was never debated in any committee or on the floor. Instead, it was attached to a bill that resolved a longest federal government shutdown in American history [29]. The entire Act was introduced, debated, and voted on in the US House of Representatives in less than two-and-a-half hours [28]. The Senate considered the entirety of the bill, including three separate amendments (none of which dealt with embryonic research), and voted on it the next day [28]. President Clinton signed it immediately upon Senate's passage [28]. This legislative rider has been reenacted every year since 1996 [76]. As with the initial enactment, there is no evidence that the amendment was ever debated in any committee or on the floor of either house.

The DWA and its restrictions became particularly salient in 1998, with the discovery of a successful method to isolate and grow human embryonic stem cells in culture [77].[41] Embryonic stem cells are a potential treasure-trove of future research and treatment [77].

[39] "On the very same day that the NIH approved the report, however, President Clinton issued an executive order forbidding the use of federal funds for embryo research in which embryos were created or destroyed."

[40] "The momentum for a more inclusive ban, however, began a month earlier, when, in the 1994 elections, Republicans regained control of both Congressional houses. For many of those elected, Clinton's prohibition was not enough."

[41] "The right-to-life versus scientific research fault-line surfaced again in debates over federal funding of embryonic stem cell research. That debate began in 1998 when researchers at Johns Hopkins University and the University of Wisconsin developed ways to culture human embryonic stem cells indefinitely in the laboratory, opening the door to directing them to produce replacement tissue to treat disease."

Three different Presidents have had to issue contradictory executive orders on NIH funding of such research [78–80]. The most recent NIH policy, one enacted pursuant to President Obama's Executive Order [80], has been challenged in courts as contravening DWA's clear statutory language [81]. The US Court of Appeals disagreed that the language was sufficiently clear to allow only one interpretation, thus permitting the challenged regulations to stand [81]. The point is that because Congress never debated the DWA, it has never made a record as to what evils it was meant to prevent, leaving each administration somewhat free to adopt broad or narrow interpretation of the law, and fund or not fund various research projects. This, of course, is highly detrimental to the scientific community which, as a result, is plagued by uncertainty over whether research will continue to be funded or whether the change in administration will result in a funding cutoff. With scientific progress dependent on long-term research projects, this state of affairs is hardly ideal.

The Science of Parthenotes

The DWA is part of the perennial fight and debate over abortion and the question of when life actually begins [82].[42] To be sure, these are not scientific issues, and are not amenable to any falsifiable experimentation [83].[43] As the Supreme Court pointed out, even "those trained in the respective disciplines of medicine, philosophy, and theology are unable to arrive at any consensus" as to when life begins [84]. In that sense, DWA's effect on science and scientific exploration is secondary to its proponents [82].[44] Nonetheless, even those who espouse the view that life begins at conception and merits protection from that point in time do not generally take the view that research on any cell that contains the full complement of human chromosomes is improper [85, 86].[45] Indeed, opponents of abortion and embryonic research often tout research on human non-embryonic cells as a viable alternative to embryonic research [85, 86]. The reason for treating embryos (even single-cell ones) differently from other cells with full chromosomal complement is the notion that embryos, given enough time and the right environment, can develop into full adult human organism, whereas other cells cannot do so. It is for this reason that the two sets of cells that would otherwise look nearly identical under the microscope are accorded a different moral status [87].[46] The moral and philosophical aspects of this

[42] Discusses the enactment of DWA as part of the effort "to uphold the sanctity and intrinsic value of life, and to prevent the dehumanization and commodification of human life."

[43] Discusses the lack of scientific consensus on the question of when life begins.

[44] "Congress voiced its response as a rider to the appropriations bill and made it clear that beneficence to the embryo rather than utility to the populace should be the governing value."

[45] Reference [85] notes that there is "little ethical debate" about the use of adult stem cells. Reference [86] discusses support of various religious groups for adult stem cell research.

[46] States that the reason for much of opposition to embryonic research stems from the fact that "some view embryos as human persons with the same moral status as adults and children."

valuation, however, are undergirded by a purely factual scientific inquiry: Can this particular cell develop into an adult human organism? If so, then, and only then, does it stand on a higher moral plane [87, 88].[47] Thus, in order to make that judgment, an individual needs to be familiar with the answers to certain basic scientific questions. Unfortunately, the Congress that enacted the DWA (and subsequent Congresses) never considered this issue when they enacted the broad funding prohibition that covered research on parthenotes [69]. Had Congress understood the nature and the science of parthenotes and parthenogenesis, the scope of the DWA may have well been narrower, and the effect on scientific exploration less dramatic.

Parthenogenesis is a portmanteau [89][48] word derived from Greek *parthenos* meaning *virgin*, and *genesis* meaning *birth*. The term is used to denote asexual reproduction [90]. Unlike sexual reproduction that involves the contribution of genetic materials from both an egg and a sperm, parthenogenesis involves contribution from the egg only [29]. This form of reproduction is naturally occurring and is common to a number of invertebrate species [29]. It is also present in all classes of vertebrates except mammals [29]. In non-mammals, this form of reproduction "can occur spontaneously (i.e., naturally) as a continuous reproductive strategy or as a response to environmental or nutritional changes." [29]. In mammals (including humans, of course), spontaneous parthenogenesis cannot result in a viable full-term offspring because this form of reproduction has been, evolutionarily speaking, abandoned [29]. Instead, when mammalian ova are spontaneously activated, they result not in an offspring, but in an ovarian tumor [29]. Thus, spontaneous "parthenogenesis" can occur in humans, but it is not a genesis or a birth of a new life, but rather of cancerous lesions [29].

Parthenotes (defined as ova activated via parthenogenesis) can also be created in vitro "through chemical stimuli that mimic fertilization, but the lack of required genetic imprinting rules out further development." [29]. These "activated" ova do begin to divide as if they were fertilized, but the division is halted at an early stage of cell differentiation, eventually resulting in the death of the parthenote [29]. Thus, human parthenotes, whether created spontaneously in vivo or during the course of an experiment in vitro, are intrinsically incapable of becoming viable human embryos [29]. Their potential for developing into an adult organism is no greater than the potential of an unfertilized egg or a tumor cell. Yet, despite this obvious difference between parthenotes and embryos, the DWA treats them as one and the same, and it does so without anyone in Congress ever explicitly considering this difference [69].

While parthenotes are not a perfect research substitute for embryos, they do have valuable uses. First, because parthenotes involve the initial activation of an ovum,

---

[47] "Proponents believe *that the embryo's potential to develop into a human person* confers upon it full moral status as a person …." (emphasis added) [87].

"Proponents of th[e] view [that embryos have the same moral status as humans], including many Roman Catholics, believe that when genetic material is joined *there is a unique potential for life*, therefore the embryo holds independent moral status and should have the same rights that all living people have."(emphasis added) [88].

[48] "You see it's like a portmanteau—there are two meanings packed up into one word."

they can be used to study the early stages of pregnancy and embryonic development [29]. For instance, it has been reported that implantation of fertilized eggs as part of assisted reproductive technology (ART) processes often fails because the egg activation process does not function properly [29]. Studying the intricacies of that process would help perfect ART processes and ultimately lead to higher rate of success with in vitro fertilization and therefore fewer abandoned or "spare" embryos [29]. Next, parthenotes are useful in studying miscarriages [29]. It has been suggested that many miscarriages are due to the "very early loss of nonviable parthenotes caused by spontaneous egg activation in the female." [29]. Identifying a biological marker that differentiates parthenotes from fertilized ova would help study the causes of miscarriage [29].

Third, parthenotes are useful in studying certain tumors [29]. As mentioned above, in mammals, spontaneous in vivo parthenogenesis leads not to an offspring, but to a gonadal tumor [29]. Despite tremendous advances in knowledge about cancer causes and treatments, ovarian cancer is still one of the most complicated diseases from the viewpoint of its etiology, diagnosis, and progression, as well as treatment [91]. Any advances in understanding cancer processes, its diagnosis, and treatment would be valuable for the preservation of both extant human life as well as potential human life, by helping to preserve fertility in the affected population.

Finally, parthenotes may serve as a source of stem cells akin to those extracted from embryos [29]. It is generally believed that stem cell research can lead to breakthrough advances in the understanding and treatment of spinal cord injuries, Alzheimer disease, Parkinson disease, and a number of other ailments [92]. Whereas extraction of embryonic stem cells generally involves destroying an embryo, thus raising the concerns about the destruction of potential viable human life [86], extraction of similar stem cells from parthenotes avoids these concerns because, as discussed above, parthenotes are never viable and will not, under any circumstances, develop into an adult human [29]. Thus, parthenotes can be a point of compromise between proponents of full federal funding for embryonic stem cell research and opponents of such funding.

Yet all of these advances are now precluded because of the broad language of the DWA—a provision that was enacted with no debate and no understanding of the crucial biological differences between embryos and parthenotes.

I do not intend to take a specific position on the propriety of embryonic or parthenote research because the ultimate outcome of legislative debate is not where I think the problem lies [86].[49] After all, on any contentious issue, after the votes are counted, one side has to win and the other has to lose. That has to happen even if there has been the most exhaustive and informative of debates. My point is not that the decision on the DWA should have been different either in whole or in part. It may very well be that, even after hearing all of the arguments and scientific data differentiating parthenotes from embryos, Congress would still have enacted the DWA in its present form. One reason they could have done so is to create a "fence of protection" around human life, much like Talmudic scholars impose requirements on

[49] For my views on the embryonic research, see [86].

observant Jews that go beyond the bare minimum commands of the Torah so as to make sure that the actual precepts are not violated [93, 94].[50] Second, it is quite possible that even given an identical set of facts, people of different political and religious persuasions will, after viewing the facts through their own lens, come to radically different conclusions as to what is the "right solution" [95], and therefore choose not to fund parthenote research. Again, whether such a decision would have been a good one from the perspective of public policy is not what concerns me at present. Rather, my concern is that the decision, whatever it is, should be made after the legislators are fully apprised of the scientific underpinnings of their proposals and the likely effect that the proposal would have on the progress of science and scientific research. In the next part of this chapter, I suggest how to ensure that this informational and deliberative part of the decision-making process actually occurs.

The Congressional Science Office and Legislative Notice and Comment Process

The Congressional Science Office

As I discussed in the Introduction, there are three distinct major problems with Congressional decision-making, especially when it affects science. First, there is a lack of an independent, nonpartisan forum for discussing and evaluating proposals. Second, there is a lack of sufficient training in the subject matter of proposals to fully understand their scope, and third, there is no meaningful ability for the public to contribute to the debate and discussion of the proposals. Thus, any system designed to fix the current flaws would necessarily have to address each of these shortcomings. Luckily, there are systems currently in place that can be used as models for addressing the shortcomings in Congressional deliberations when it comes to scientific issues. Specifically, the role and function of the CBO is a useful point of departure in creating a nonpartisan body of experts to advise Congress on specific and technical matters for which Congressmen themselves may not have full appreciation.

The CBO was created in 1974 by the Congressional Budget Act, to provide "independent analyses of budgetary and economic issues to support the Congressional budget process. The agency is strictly nonpartisan and conducts objective, impartial analysis …." [96]. The CBO "produce[s] a formal cost estimate for nearly every bill that is 'reported' (approved) by a full committee of either House of Congress …." [96]. The CBO also provides an annual report called "Budget and Economic Outlook," which "includes an economic forecast and projections of spending and revenues under current law over the next 10 years." [97]. Thus, the CBO not only evaluates likely prospective effects of proposed legislation but also yearly reevaluates the effect of current policy and estimates the effect of these policies if they are continued [96]. Finally, the CBO "prepares analytic reports at the

[50] Discuss the Talmudic principle specifically in the context of cloning debate.

request of the Congressional leadership or Chairmen or Ranking Minority Members of committees or subcommittees." [96]. These reports analyze proposals that may or may not be in a form of a formal bill or an amendment, but help Congressmen evaluate ideas that are being discussed either formally or informally [96].

In producing its reports, the CBO relies on the internal government data available from agencies like the Census Bureau, Federal Bureau of Labor Statistics, Bureau of Economic Analysis, and Bureau of Justice Statistics [96]. Government agencies, however, are not the sole source of information for the CBO. A particularly interesting aspect of the CBO's operation is that it "seeks input from outside experts, including professors, analysts at think tanks, private-sector experts, and employees at various government agencies." [96]. This input "complement[s] the knowledge and insights of … the agency's staff." [96].

CBO reports are not "binding" on Congress in a sense that an unfavorable CBO "score" (i.e., a report that projects that a given proposal would increase the deficit) does not preclude Congress from adopting the proposed bill [98].[51] Indeed, Congress often votes to enact bills that increase the deficit [99].[52] Nonetheless, the CBO reports are discussed during committee and floor debates, as well as during election campaigns [100, 101].[53] As a result, politicians, even when they ultimately decide to enact a law that is unfavorably scored by the CBO, must take that score into account and come up with coherent arguments as to why they voted the way they did [102].[54]

Though there has been some criticism of the CBO's methods [98, 103],[55] the CBO is generally viewed as a nonpartisan body, not beholden to either political party [104].[56] Indeed, despite the criticism leveled at the CBO, it is generally viewed as a neutral arbiter of budgetary disputes (even if certain political actors disagree with the underlying methodology) [98].[57] The CBO's estimates are often the

[51] "In principle, Budget Committee Chairmen could ignore the CBO score or the Congress could amend its own rules or the Budget Act to allow the legislative amendment of a CBO score or to allow a PAYGO-violating measure to proceed without a supermajority."

[52] "Despite the requirements [of the Gramm-Rudman Act], Congress took little notice of the CBO-OMB report."

[53] Reference [100] notes the political effect of a CBO report on various stimulus proposals. Reference [101] quotes then-Sen. John Kerry relying on CBO scoring to criticize President George W. Bush's Social Security reform plans.

[54] Describes different political justifications used to support tax cuts enacted during the Bush Administration, despite the unfavorable CBO score.

[55] "Capital gains proponents have argued that both the Joint Committee on Taxation and the Congressional Budget Office have historically erred in calculating capital gains revenues. Opponents of dynamic scoring, on the other hand, argue that CBO estimates of revenue gains from new tax provisions have tended to err on the high side …" [103].

"[W]ork done by the CBO is credible and subject to intense review and criticism by interested parties …." [98].

[56] Notes that the CBO "has a reputation for impartiality."

[57] "The near-constant carping by dissatisfied members of Congress, interest groups, or journalists that the CBO estimates are 'wrong' misses the point of the exercise. The CBO score is *deemed* to be correct by the agreements on how the budget process is to work, and all legislative rules and actions follow from it." (emphasis in original).

centerpiece of political and campaign debates and are relied on by members of both parties to tout their own agenda or to criticize their opponents' plans [100, 101, 105].[58] The CBO ensures that it remains a neutral arbiter (and is perceived as such) by limiting the political activities of its staff [96], requiring that the Director of the Office be appointed after consultations with the members of the committees having jurisdiction over budgetary matters [96], giving the Director a fixed 4-year term (irrespective of the political vicissitudes of the individuals originally responsible for the Director's appointment) [96], and seeking input from a variety of outside experts [96]. Additionally, and perhaps most importantly, the CBO makes no policy recommendations to Congress [96]. Instead, the CBO's role is limited to evaluating and scoring Congressional policy proposals [96].

The CBO model is a good starting point for the creation of a system that would illuminate and evaluate Congressional proposals that would have an effect on the progress of scientific research. If Congress had a Congressional Science Office (CSO), with a mission similar to that of the CBO but focused on matters of science, the debates over legislation that has an impact on scientific progress would be better informed and more substantive. Indeed, a similar congressional office used to exist. From 1972 to 1995, an Office of Technology Assessment (OTA) produced studies on a wide range of topics from acid rain to payment for physician services and to wood use [106, 107].[59] The OTA was abolished in 1995 by the new Republican majority as part of the *Contract with America* [106, 107]. The abolition of the office was criticized at the time [108],[60] and there have been calls to resurrect it [106, 109]. In my view, a resurrected OTA would indeed be a good first step; however, the "new OTA," or as I call it, the CSO, should have a somewhat different mission from the original OTA.

The OTA prepared reports on scientific issues of the day but without being tied to any specific legislation [110, 111].[61] Such reports are certainly useful as background information, and as prods for Congress to act on issues that they might not have otherwise considered. Nonetheless, for individuals lacking scientific or technical training (as most Congressmen do) [4], applying the background information to specific legislative proposals is often just as difficult as acquiring the background knowledge in the first place [112].[62] For that reason, I am of the opinion that the

[58] "Congress created the Congressional Budget Office and required the CBO to calculate the costs incurred over a 4 year period by each bill or joint resolution reported by any committee of the House or Senate [...]. The point of these disclosure requirements was to furnish Congress with detailed information concerning the budget consequences of proposed legislation so that its budget consequences form part of the legislative debate, and to provide an external measure of the budget consequences of enacted legislation." [105].

[59] Technically, Congress did not "abolish" the OTA, but it cut off all funding to the Office.

[60] Criticizes elimination of the OTA.

[61] Reference [110] states that "[t]he basic function of the Office shall be to provide early indications of the probable beneficial and adverse impacts of the applications of technology and to develop other coordinate information which may assist the Congress." Reference [111] gives the Office itself the authority to decide what issues to explore and report on.

[62] Notes that in order to be useful to Congress, information must be in a format that "Congress can readily understand and apply."

recreated CSO would be more effective if its reports were linked to specific legislative proposals, rather than general scientific issues that may be of interest to Congress and the country. On a related note, an office that chooses on its own which subject matters to report on and when is more open to the accusation of political bias [112].[63] Even when the science found in the report is sound, and the conclusions drawn true, the very act of selecting on which topics to report—and therefore highlight in the public's mind—and which to omit may create an impression that certain issues are being given more importance for political reasons [112]. That is especially true when the issues are fairly politically sensitive [112].[64] On the other hand, when the Office reports on every bill that has passed the committee of jurisdiction, as well as on any requests that are made of it by the Chairman and the Ranking Member of relevant committees, the Office itself cannot be accused of picking and choosing which issues to highlight. Instead, they would be merely a responsive body, helping Congress understand both the scientific background in the relevant area, and the likely impact of the proposed legislation. It would, however, remain entirely up to Congress whether and how much weight to give to these reports. What Congress would not be able to avoid is the debate over the actual merits of the proposed legislation, either in the halls of Congress or on the campaign trail.

Additionally, much like the CBO, the CSO would not only report on pending bills but also provide a year-end report on how previously enacted bills have actually worked in the real world. Educated predictions as to the effect that legislation will have are certainly a valuable tool for legislators deciding how to vote on a pending bill, but reporting and evaluating actual effects will help legislators decide whether to renew expiring legislation and will also serve as an annual self-check on the CSO itself. By cross-checking its predictions with actual outcomes, the CSO will be better able to fine-tune its evaluative function and insulate itself from any charges of partisanship.

The Legislative Notice and Comment Process

The creation of a CSO, charged with evaluating proposed legislation for impact on science, would solve the first problem with current Congressional decision-making in the scientific arena—the lack of an independent, nonpartisan forum for discussing and evaluating proposals. However, two additional problems would remain: lack of sufficient training in the subject matter of proposals to fully understand their scope [109], and no meaningful ability for the public to contribute to the debate and discussion of the proposals [20–22, 48–50]. Of course, the staff of the CSO would need to have scientific, technical, or engineering training, much like the staff of the

---

[63] Discusses accusations of bias lobbed at the OTA and stating that "[t]he most likely way for bias to arise is in the selection of issues to be investigated."

[64] States that much criticism was directed at the OTA following its negative review of the Strategic Defense Initiative—a top Republican priority.

CBO must have training in economics. However, with scientific knowledge proliferating and progressing at an incredible pace, it would be quite hard to hire enough people to cover all possible fields of scientific exploration, and even if such coverage were possible, it is likely that the knowledge of the Office's staff would grow stale with time. Thus, the mere existence of the CSO and quality staff, while going a long way to improving the understanding of the scope and effect of the legislative proposals, would still be insufficient to keep up with the emerging or rapidly changing science and technologies. Thus, the Office would have to look beyond its own internal expertise. I have already discussed that the CBO does just that by seeking input of independent experts of various political stripes in making its projections [96]. While that approach is laudable, I do not view it as being sufficient in the context of evaluating the impact of legislation on scientific progress. Furthermore, if the Office were able to pick its own experts, especially on highly charged issues (e.g., embryonic research, global warming, human subject research) it could again invite the accusation of bias.[65] If such an outcome were to come to pass, it would undermine the legitimacy of the CSO and its evaluations. Thus, in my view, participation in evaluating the impact of proposed legislation on matters of science should be broad. Broader engagement would also address the current lack of meaningful opportunity for the public to participate in the shaping of the legislative decisions. The question is the following: How does one achieve broad participation that results in informative and valuable input into the ultimate product—the CSO's formal evaluation of legislative proposals?

One way to involve the interested and informed public in crafting legal language has been successfully tried in the administrative arena. The Administrative Procedures Act (APA) of 1946 [113] required agencies to give notice to the public on proposed rules, to allow the public to comment on the proposal, and to consider the comments before issuing a final rule.[66] "[N]otice-and-comment rulemaking provides several interrelated benefits. It allows all stakeholders in a regulatory decision to be heard before a decision is made and ensures that the agency responds to relevant comments." [114]. As the Fourth Circuit very recently pointed out,

> The important purposes of this notice-and-comment procedure cannot be overstated. The agency benefits from the experience and input of comments by the public, which help ensure informed agency decisionmaking. The notice-and-comment procedure also is designed to encourage public participation in the administrative process. Additionally, the process helps ensure that the agency maintains a flexible and open-minded attitude towards its own rules, because the opportunity to comment must be a meaningful opportunity.[67] [115].

The agency, of course, "need not respond to every comment so long as it responds in a reasoned manner to significant comments received." [116]. In other words, the agency must simply show that it has considered the views of the public and came to a reasoned decision, even if that decision is contrary to views expressed in the

[65] In other words, the focus of bias would move from the level of congressional committees to the level of CSO.

[66] Codified as amended in scattered sections of 5 U.S.C.

[67] Internal quotations and citations omitted.

comments [117]. This process has been found to be so successful that there have been calls to export it beyond America's borders [118]. However, the successes of the notice-and-comment procedure can be applied on the home front as well, by transplanting it to the legislative arena.

Once a bill or a proposal is referred to the CSO for an evaluation and report, the CSO would identify provisions that would potentially have an impact on scientific progress. It would then invite public comments on those provisions. Those most familiar with the underlying science, as well as the likely effect that the proposed legislation will have on the research in the field, would be able to convey their understanding to the CSO via a formal comment. Furthermore, because the comments would be open to the public at large, and not just to select scientists, comments centering on ethical implications of the legislative enactments or the research itself would also be made. In that way, the CSO would be able to present a full range of views of the scientific community, including any concerns raised about the propriety of certain methods and avenues of research. The CSO would serve as an aggregator and a filter for this commentary, evaluating, compiling, and summarizing it in a language accessible to Congressmen. It is Congress, however, that will ultimately decide what weight, if any, to give to the concerns and critique of the individuals and groups that have commented on the proposed legislation.

Of course, the process would not be identical to that in the administrative agencies. Administrative agencies' rules and actions can be judicially set aside for failure to follow the proper notice-and-comment procedure or for failure to consider comments submitted [119].[68] No such sanction could be imposed on Congress if it itself or its own advisory body failed to fully consider the concerns of the public. After all, unlike administrative agencies, which have only whatever authority that was delegated to them by Congress, the Congress itself retains sovereign authority to enact whatever laws it deems fit (subject only to the constitutional constraints on its power) [120].[69] Nonetheless, though the courts would not be in a position to invalidate congressional laws as "inadequately considered or debated," the legislative notice-and-comment will still have a salutary and constraining function.

As an initial matter, the notice-and-comment process will, of necessity, slow down some legislative activity because some time will have to be allocated to actually receive and evaluate the comments. Though it is true that Congress has not been a bastion of rapid and efficient decision-making, it may be a good thing if an additional brake is placed on legislation that may have a far-reaching negative impact on science, technology, and medicine. As Professor Lazarus points out, oftentimes slowing down such laws simply preserves the legislative and legal status quo—stability that is usually beneficial for scientific progress [58].

Second, the notice-and-comment mechanism, by permitting broader public participation combined with the reasoned responses from other members of the public,

[68] States that courts shall set aside agency actions that were arrived at "without observance of procedure required by law."

[69] Holds that once Congress attests that the bill was properly passed, the judiciary will not inquire into the procedures.

the scientific community, and the CSO, will lead to a broader acceptance of the legislative outcome [106]. By giving individuals a real voice in the legislative process, Congress will help grow confidence that at least with respect to issues that turn on objective understanding of scientific realities and definitions, it has considered and properly weighed the objective evidence, even if a particular individual disagrees with the weight assigned to his or her own comments and arguments [121]. Additionally, under an open notice-and-comment regime, the CSO is less likely to be lobbied or captured by special interest groups. If the CSO, like an administrative agency, by its rules is required to "respond in a reasoned manner to significant comments received" [116], it will be less likely that a few influential individuals or groups would be able to sway the Office's views. Indeed, to the extent necessary, the Office can anonymize the comments (beyond the educational and experience qualifications) so as not to be swayed by any personal connections or partisan leanings of the commenter. The fact that the CSO would not offer any policy prescriptions, but will limit itself only to analyzing legislation, will further insulate it from the danger of capture.

Next, and related to the second point, ignoring clear and specific criticisms and warnings issued by a neutral, nonpartisan body would serve as good fodder for intra-Congressional criticism, as well as campaign commercials. Much like how candidates are consistently criticized in campaign ads for disregarding the opinion of the CBO and voting for additional spending or tax cuts that have been scored as adding to the deficit [100–102], so too will candidates be criticized for adopting legislation that the CSO warned would lead to slowing of scientific progress. This will be an especially potent tool if in its "progress reports" the CSO reconfirms its initial predictions.

Finally, to the extent the courts consider the "legislative history" of any particular enactment, especially when applying the *Chevron* analysis [122] to the administrative interpretations of the law (as was the case with *Sherley v. Sebelius* [81]), or when attempting to figure out whether a particular interpretation would be an "absurd result," subject to the rule of the *Church of the Holy Trinity* [123], CSO reports would be of tremendous help. Courts will actually be able to see whether Congress was warned of the "absurd results," and whether it enacted legislation despite such warnings [124, 125].[70] Similarly, the courts (and administrative agencies) will be able to better evaluate whether the language and intent of the statute are indeed ambiguous, or whether the particular problem, in all its details, was considered by Congress, and a definitive decision was reached.

Anticipated Criticisms and the Responses

Had the proposed notice-and-comment followed by a full CSO report procedure been in place in 1996, the DWA may have encountered a different fate. On one

[70] Reference [124] is arguing that despite majority's view that a different outcome would lead to "absurd results," "[t]he legislative branch fully considered the possibility of [such results] and took that risk advisedly." Judge Cardamone's view was vindicated by the Supreme Court [125].

hand, it is true that the legislative vehicle to which the DWA was attached was considered, voted, enacted by Congress, and signed by the President in less than 48 h, thus leaving very little time for any, much less exhaustive, debate on the riders attached to the bill [28]. Furthermore, given the "must-pass" nature of the bill and the background of the government shutdown that the bill was attempting to resolve, there was likely no appetite to debate the particulars. Thus, it is unlikely that the process I am proposing would have had much impact at that initial stage. Indeed, this criticism can be generalized to argue that the process I am proposing is unlikely to solve many problems, and will accomplish little more than creating another government bureaucracy that will succeed only in the proliferation of reports that no one reads. While certainly my proposal is not a panacea to legislation gratuitously injurious to the progress of science and scientific research, it is an improvement over the current process. In the case of the DWA, though Congress attached the rider to an emergency, must-pass bill, it does not mean that (a) the proposed system would have had no impact at all on the likelihood of DWA being enacted, or (b) that the DWA would have continued to survive, essentially unchanged, to the present day.

It is certainly the case that when operating under exceedingly narrow time constraints, the proposed CSO would not be able to engage in a full-blown notice-and-comment period, analysis of comments received, and creation of a comprehensive report for Congressmen to debate and consider. But such situations arise presently both in Congress and in the administrative agencies. The CBO often has to work under very tight time constraints to produce cost estimates for last-minute budgetary compromises [126–128].[71] Perhaps such reports are not as comprehensive as the reports that allow for more detailed study, broader consultations, and deeper reflection. But such reports are still given significant weight by Congressmen and eventually the electorate. There is no reason to believe that the CSO would be unable to produce its own reports and estimates on an expedited basis, even if in those cases they would have to forgo the notice-and-comment mechanism. Similarly, administrative agencies also occasionally issue rules and regulations without engaging in the notice-and-comment process. The APA permits agencies to forego the process in "emergency situations" [129, 130].[72] This exception recognizes that though notice-and-comment is important, agencies do have their own expertise and can, in exceptional circumstances, be allowed to rely on that expertise alone [131].[73]

[71] The estimate was prepared on January 1st, the very same day the Senate passed the bill [126]. The actual text of the bill was only agreed upon the previous day [127].

Reference [128] is the amendment by Sen. Reid to strike all previously considered text and substitute the text of the amendment.

[72] Reference [129] permits agency to forego the notice-and-comment process "when the agency for good cause finds … that notice and public procedure thereon are impracticable, unnecessary, or contrary to the public interest." Reference [130] states that "[P]romulgation of order without notice-and-comment procedures under 5 U.S.C. § 553(b)(B) is proper only if the agency concludes there is an 'emergency situation … [where] delay would do real harm'."

[73] Notes that in a situation where emergency environmental regulations are called for, the relevant agency would "exercise its own expertise in environmental matters."

These exceptions are generally permitted only when the promulgated rule is temporary, with the permanent rule subject to the full scope of the APA procedures [132].[74]

Likewise, legislative riders on annual appropriation bills remain in effect only for so long as the underlying bill does, and because annual appropriation bills never last more than 1 year, neither do restrictions contained therein. Thus, though the initial restriction may have been enacted under emergency circumstances leaving no time for full public participation in the CSO process, nothing would prevent the CSO from conducting a full notice-and-comment procedure in anticipation of the rider potentially being renewed in a subsequent year. Thus, though in emergency circumstances similar to the ones that attended the passage of the DWA, the initial report would potentially be truncated and somewhat superficial, in the long term, the process would still provide the benefits that I have previously identified. Relatedly, the CSO would be charged with not just making reports on pending bills but also producing year-end estimates on the effect of all statutes presently in force (as they relate to science and technology) have. Thus, even if there were no opportunity to provide notice-and-comment at the time of a bill's initial consideration, there would still be an opportunity to comment on how the enacted bill has *actually* affected the progress of science, thus permitting Congress to reconsider the bill's scope when it comes up for reauthorization. Had this process been in place, the public would have had over a dozen annual opportunities to comment on the scope and effect of the DWA and explain the difference between parthenotes and embryos. Congress, presented with formal report from the CSO, would then have had an opportunity to debate and rethink the renewal of the Amendment as originally written. (Of course, Congress may well have remained unpersuaded, but at least Congressmen would have to justify their approach to each other and/or their constituents.)

The second objection to the proposed system—and one that also casts doubt on the proposition that, had the system been in place, the DWA would have likely encountered a different fate—is that there are already ways for Congress to obtain detailed reports on matters of science, and that an additional report-producing body would do little to change the legislative dynamic. After all, the National Institute of Health's Human Embryo Research Panel did issue a two-volume report on embryonic research, and that report did discuss the difference between parthenotes and embryos, yet Congress enacted the DWA anyway [72]. I readily concede that Congress could ignore the reports of the CSO just like it ignored the report of the Human Embryo Research Panel. I do not, however, agree that the adoption of my proposed system would be simply duplicative of existing resources and advisory bodies.

---

[74] "[A]ny administrative action taken in a rare 'emergency' situation … need only be temporary, pending public notice-and-comment procedures …. [O]nce an emergency situation has been eased by the promulgation of interim rules, it is crucial that the comprehensive permanent regulations which follow emerge as a result of the congressionally-mandated policy of affording public participation …."

I again begin by referring to the CBO. By the time the Congressional Budget Act created the CBO, the Office of Management and Budget (OMB) had been in existence for over half a century [133]. Yet, Congress saw fit to establish its own independent nonpartisan office. Though the OMB is well respected, it is viewed as more partisan than the CBO [134, 135].[75] It is now the CBO, not its older sibling, the OMB, which has grown to be an authoritative arbiter on budgetary matters [134, 135]. Perhaps this stems from the fact that Congress is by its very nature bipartisan (even when a single party has a majority in both chambers) and therefore each party has to try to accommodate the other to a certain extent, whereas the Presidency is, of necessity, uni-partisan, and the President need not accommodate anyone in selecting those of his advisors that are not subject to Senate confirmation. The same dynamic is likely to play out with the CSO. Though Presidents have had various bodies advising them on scientific and bioethical issues since 1974, each President has changed the scope and the focus of these commissions, thus giving the commissions a flavor of partisanship and allegiance to the appointing Administration's priorities [136]. In contrast, the proposed CSO would be charged with reporting on every bill having potential impact on science and technology, thus avoiding the perception that it is focusing on issues favored by a particular party or individual. Furthermore, the various Presidential commissions were designed to recommend a specific course of action. Indeed, the present Presidential Commission for the Study of Bioethical Issues was created explicitly to "offer practical policy options," to the administration [136]. Commissions with such a charge can be perceived as having a stake in the political outcome rather than serving as a neutral evaluator of Congressional proposals. That posture necessarily makes these bodies partisan, even if not in the traditional Republican-Democratic sense. In my view, such a perception would undermine the value of such a body to Congress, and therefore to the legislative process.

There is another reason that a Congress-based body for evaluating scientific issues is preferable to that based in the Executive Branch. As Congressman Rush Holt pointed out,

> *Congress needs access to unbiased technical and scientific assessments finished in a time frame appropriate for Congress,* written in a language that is understood by members of Congress, and crafted by those who are familiar with the functions of Congress .... *[M] embers of Congress do not suffer from a lack of information, [but they] lack time and resources to assess the validity, credibility, and usefulness of the large amount of scientific information and advice we receive as it affects actual policy decisions. The purpose of the [former Office of Technology Assessment] was to assist members of Congress in this task. It both provided an important long-term perspective and alerted Congress to scientific and technological components of policy that might not be obvious.*[76] [109].

[75] Reference [134] states that members of both parties view OMB as more partisan and more "likely to distort its projections of the budget deficit in accordance with the chief executive's wishes."

[76] Emphasis added.

Simply put, scientific advisors based in the Executive Branch (or independent of political branches altogether) are not ideal because they are insufficiently familiar with Congressional procedures, schedules, and language to serve Congressional needs. Furthermore, unless Congress has some level of control over the advisors, it cannot demand timely reports on matters that are of importance to Congress, rather than those that are of importance to the Executive.

Finally, though the various Presidential commissions have done an admirable job in soliciting views of a broad range of scientists, ethicists, patients, and others, they still lack the formal notice-and-comment format that I am proposing. The formal notice-and-comment mechanism with an invitation to participate extended to every interested individual, rather than just to those that the commission finds to be worthy of attention, will improve both the legislative process itself and the public perception of and confidence in the process.

Conclusions

Mark Twain once quipped, "Suppose you were an idiot. And suppose you were a member of Congress. But I repeat myself." [137]. I am somewhat less cynical about Congress than Mark Twain, and I tend to think that the real problem with Congress is not idiocy, but lack of digestible, objective, and timely information on complex scientific and technical issues. In today's environment, where even scientific issues are politicized and the public trust in legislators is at an all-time low, we sorely need a mechanism that provides unbiased assessment of legislative proposals while increasing public participation in the legislative process, diminishing the influence of special interests, and educating legislators on the complex scientific and technical issues. An independent, nonpartisan, CSO modeled on the CBO, which would provide an opportunity for the experts and public at large to weigh in with comments on the likely effect of the proposed bills on scientific issues, and which would evaluate these comments and produce reports "written in a language that is understood by members of Congress, and crafted by those who are familiar with the functions of Congress," would go a long way towards improving the legislative process and reducing damage that haphazardly considered legislation can inflict on scientific progress. Creating a legislative notice-and-comment process would therefore improve legislation and public confidence and have beneficial effects on science. While Congress may not always defer to the concerns raised by the commenters or the staff at the CSO, the improved quality of Congressional debates, and the increased accountability that will come with forcing Congress to confront explicit warnings from the scientific community, will be a marked improvement over the current process of legislating in matters of science and technology.

Acknowledgements This work was supported by the Oncofertility Consortium NIH 5UL1DE019587. A version of this chapter appears in Utah Law Review, v. 2014.

References

1. Block CD. Pathologies at the intersection of the Budget and Tax legislative processes. B.C. L. Rev. 2002;43(28):863, 870.
2. Sanders AM Jr. Newgarth revisited: Mrs. Robinson's case. S.C. L Rev. 1998;49(18):407, 412.
3. Bowen J. Behind closed doors: re-examining the Tennessee open meetings act and its inapplicability to the Tennessee General Assembly. Colum J L Soc Probs. 2002;35:133.
4. Dean C. Groups call for scientists to engage the body politic. N.Y. *Times*. 9 Aug 2011 at D1.
5. Randsell Act. Pub. L. No. 71-251. Stat. 1930;46:379.
6. An act to incorporate The National Academy of Sciences (NAS) 1863.
7. National Aeronautics and Space Act, Pub. L. No. 85-568. Stat. 72:429 (codified as amended at 42 U.S.C. § 429).
8. Consolidated Appropriations Act. 2004, 108 P.L. 199. Stat. 2004;118:3; Consolidated Appropriations Act, 2012, Pub. L. No. 112-74. Stat. 2011;125:786.
9. Goldberg S. The Reluctant Embrace: Law and Science in America. Geo L J. 1987;75:1341, 1366.
10. Treaty Banning Nuclear Weapon Tests in the Atmosphere, in Outer Space and Under Water, 5 Aug 1963, 14 U.S.T. 1313, T.I.A.S. 5433, 480 U.N.T.S. 43 (effective 10 Oct 1963).
11. Schmitt E. Experts Say Test Ban Could Impair Nuclear-Arms Safety. N.Y. *Times*. 8 Oct 1999, at A11.
12. Nagan WP, Slemmens EK. Developing U.S. Nuclear Weapons Policy and International Law: The Approach of the Obama Administration. Tul J Int'l Comp L. 2010;19:41, 76.
13. 145 Cong Rec 1999;25:143 (rejecting the Treaty by a vote of 48–51).
14. Fogleman VM. Regulating science: an evaluation of the regulation of biotechnology research. Envtl L. 1987;17:183, 192
15. Roberts CL. Discretion and deference in senate consideration of judicial nominations. U. Louisville L Rev. 2012;51:1, 6.
16. Lund N. Capitalism, Markets, and The Constitution: The Thirtieth Annual Federalist Society National Student Symposium on Law and Public Policy—2011: ii. Economic Theory, Civic Virtue, and the Meaning of the Constitution: Judicial Independence, Judicial Virtue, and the Political Economy of the Constitution. Harv J L Pub Pol'y. 2012;35:47.
17. Editorial. How conservative is judge Roberts? N.Y. *Times*. 15 Sept 2005, at A30.
18. McCann MA. Antitrust, Governance, and Postseason College Football. B.C. L. Rev. 2011;52(147):517, 541.
19. Indiana State Bar Association Conference on Relations Between Congress and the Federal Courts: Conference on Relations Between Congress and the Federal Courts: A Stenographic Record. Ind L Rev. 2008;41:305, 327.
20. Monaco LO. Give the People What They Want: The Failure of "Responsive" Lawmaking. 3 U. Chi L Sch Roundtable. 1996;735, 761–762.
21. DiCola P, Sag M. An Information-Gathering Approach to Copyright Policy. Cardozo L Rev. 2012;34:173, 189.
22. Calvert C. The First Amendment, the media and the culture wars: eight important lessons from 2004 about speech, censorship, science and public policy. Cal W. L. Rev. 2005;41:325, 341–347.
23. Feinberg LE. Open government and freedom of information: fishbowl accountability? In: Cooper PJ, Newland CA, editors. Handbook of public law and administration. NJ, USA: Jossey-Bass Hoboken; 1997.
24. Alonzo JS. Restoring The Ideal Marketplace: How Recognizing Bloggers As Journalists Can Save The Press, 9 N.Y.U. J Legis Pub Pol'y. 2005/2006;751, 752.
25. Balanced Budget Downpayment Act. Pub. L. No. 104-99, § 128. Stat. 1996;110:26, 34.
26. Omnibus FY 96 Bill Ties Loose Ends. Congressional Quarterly Almanac. 1996;LII: 10-5–10-19.
27. Sneed OC. Science, Public bioethics, and the problem of integration. U.C. Davis L Rev. 2010;43:1529, 1546.

28. H.R. 2880 (104th Cong. 1996). Bill summary and status. The Library of Congress. http://thomas.loc.gov/cgi-bin/bdquery/D?d104:1:./temp/~bd4W4C:@@@X|/home/LegislativeData.php?n=BSS;c=104. Accessed 12 Jan 2012.
29. Rodriguez S, et al. An obscure rider obstructing science: the conflation of parthenotes with embryos in the Dickey-Wicker amendment. Am J Bioethics. 2011;11:20.
30. An Introduction to the Congressional Budget Office (2012). http://www.cbo.gov/sites/default/files/cbofiles/attachments/2012-IntroToCBO.pdf. Accessed 12 Jan 2012.
31. Administrative Procedures Act. 5 U.S.C. § 553.
32. Schoolhouse Rock: I'm Just a Bill (ABC television broadcast 1975). http://vimeo.com/24334724. Accessed 12 Jan 2012.
33. Mr. Smith Goes to Washington (Columbia Pictures Corp. 1939).
34. Keohane NO, Revesz RL, Stavins RN. The choice of regulatory instruments in environmental policy. Harv Envtl L Rev. 1998;22(99):313, 344.
35. Pildes RH, Anderson ES. Slinging arrows at democracy: social choice theory, value pluralism, and democratic politics. Colum L Rev. 1990;90:2121, 2137.
36. Berke RL, Myers SL. In Washington, Few Trifle With Jesse Helms, *N.Y. Times*. 2 Aug 1997, at A1.
37. Newshour: Helms v. Weld (PBS television broadcast 12 Sept 1997). Transcript. http://www.pbs.org/newshour/bb/latin_america/july-dec97/helms_9-12.html.
38. Katharine Q. Seelye. With Iron Gavel, Helms Rejects Vote on Weld. 13 Sept 1997 at A1.
39. Neikirk W. Weld Whiffs on Helms Hardball. *Chicago Tribune*. 16 Sept 1997, at 1.
40. TheCapitol.Net. Glossary of congressional terms. http://www.thecapitol.net/glossary/c.htm#Chairman's Mark/Staff Draft. Accessed 12 Jan 2013.
41. *C-SPAN:* Stephen Colbert's opening statement. http://www.youtube.com/watch?v=k1T75jBYeCs. Accessed 12 Jan 2013.
42. Allen J. Colbert Knocks Dems Off Message. Politico.com. 2010. http://www.politico.com/news/stories/0910/42692.html. Accessed 12 Jan 2013.
43. Parker A. A Comic Twist on Political Chatter. *NY Times*. 25 Sept 2012, at A11.
44. Borgmann CE. Rethinking Judicial Deference to Legislative Fact-Finding. Ind L J. 2009; 84:1, 41.
45. Marvin C. Ott. Partisanship and the Decline of Intelligence Oversight. 16 Int'l J Intelligence Counterintelligence 2003;69, 87.
46. Andreen WL. Beyond Words of Exhortation: The Congressional Prescription for Vigorous Federal Enforcement of the Clean Water Act. Geo Wash L Rev. 1987;55:202, 237.
47. Rubin EL. Legislative Methodology: Some Lessons from the Truth-in-Lending Act. Geo L J. 1991;80:233, 285.
48. Nourse VF. The politics of legislative drafting: a congressional case. N.Y.U.L. Rev. 2002;77:575, 584.
49. Mayer LH. What Is This "Lobbying" That We Are So Worried About? Yale L. Pol'y Rev. 2008;26:485, 552.
50. Devins N. Why Congress Did Not Think About the Constitution when Enacting the Affordable Care Act. NY U. L. Rev Colloquy. 2012;106:261, 267.
51. U.S. v. Morrison. U.S. 2000;529:598, 615.
52. U.S. House of Representatives. Committee on Rules, About the Committee, http://www.rules.house.gov/singlepages.aspx?NewsID=1&RSBD=4. Accessed 12 Jan 2012.
53. Solomon GBH, Wolfensberger DR. The Decline of Deliberative Democracy in the House and Proposals for Reform. Harv J Legis. 1993;31:321, 358–359.
54. U.S. Senate, Committee on Rules and Administration, About the Committee. Purpose and jurisdiction. http://www.rules.senate.gov/public/index.cfm?p=PurposeJurisdiction. Accessed 12 Jan 2013.
55. Congressional Research Service. Valerie Heitshusen, The Legislative Process on the Senate Floor at 5, 28 Nov 2012, at 2. http://www.senate.gov/CRSReports/crs-publish.cfm?pid=%26*2D4Q%5CK3%0A. Accessed 12 Jan 2013.
56. Senate Rule XXII.

57. Banner S. Childress lecture: trials and other entertainment. St. Louis L J. 2011;55:1285, 1289.
58. Lazarus RE. Congressional Descent: The Demise of Deliberative Democracy in Environmental Law. Geo L J 2006;94:619, 634–635.
59. TheCapitol.Net. Glossary of congressional terms. http://www.thecapitol.net/glossary/c.htm#Conference Committee. Accessed 12 Jan 2013.
60. Houck OA. Things fall apart: a constitutional analysis of legislative exclusion. Emory L J. 2006;55:1, 12.
61. Jaffer J. Secret Evidence and the Courts in the Age of National Security: Panel Report: Secret Evidence in the Investigative Stage: FISA, Administrative Subpoenas, and Privacy. Cardozo Pub L Pol'y Ethics J. 2006;5:7, 15.
62. Sher V. Carol Hunting. Eroding the Landscape: Congressional Exemptions from Judicial Review of Environmental Laws. Harv Envtl L Rev. 1991;15:435, 443–444.
63. Jiang G. Rain or shine: fair and other non-infringing uses in the context of cloud computing. J Legis. 2010;36:395, 395.
64. Seibert-Fohr A. The Rise of Equality in International Law and its Pitfalls: Learning from Comparative Constitutional Law. Brooklyn J Int'l L. 2010;35:1, 38.
65. Castelluccio JA III. Sarbanes-Oxley and Small Business: Section 404 and the Case for a Small Business Exemption. Brooklyn L Rev. 2005;71:429, 435–436.
66. Turner Broad. Sys. v. FCC, U.S. 1994;512:622, 665.
67. Carhart v. Ashcroft, 331 F. Supp. 2d 805, 1006 (D. Neb. 2004), *rev'd on other grounds by* Gonzales v. Carhart. U.S. 2007;550:124.
68. Cote AJ Jr. Who Tells Congress About Technology? *Indus Res* Sept 1967, at 80.
69. Pub. L. No. 104-99, § 128. Stat. 1996;110:26, 34.
70. Public Health Service Act. Pub. L. No. 93-348, 213. Stat. 1974;88:342, 353 (codified at 42 U.S.C. 289l-1 (1978)).
71. Note. Fetal experimentation: moral, legal, and medical implications. Stan L Rev. 1974;26:1191, 1207.
72. Nat'l Inst. of Health. Report of the Human Embryo Research Panel at vii-viii. 1994. http://bioethics.georgetown.edu/pcbe/reports/past_commissions/human_embryo_vol_1.pdf. Accessed 20 Jan 2013.
73. Spar D, Harrington A. Selling stem cell science: how markets drive law along the technological frontier. Am J L Med. 2007;33:541, 556.
74. Department of Labor, Health and Human Services, and Education, and Related Agencies Appropriations Act 2006. Pub. L. 109-149, § 509. Stat. 2005;119:2833, 2880.
75. Omnibus Appropriations Act 2009. Pub. L. No. 111-8, § 509. Stat. 2009;123:524, 803.
76. Bigloo K. Aggregation of powers: stem cell research and the scope of presidential power examined through the lens of executive order jurisprudence. Psych Pub Pol L. 2012;18: 519, 523.
77. Robertson JA. Procreative liberty in the era of genomics. Am J L Med. 2003;29:439, 483.
78. 30 Weekly Comp Pres Doc. 1994;2459 (President Clinton's Executive Order).
79. 37 Weekly Comp Pres Doc. 2001;1149, 1151 (9 Aug 2001) (President Bush's Executive Order).
80. Exec. Order No. 13,505, 74 Fed. Reg. 10,667. 2009; (President Obama's Executive Order).
81. Sherley v. Sebelius, 644 F.3d 388. D.C. Cir. 2011.
82. Makdisi JMZ. The slide from human embryonic stem cell research to reproductive cloning: ethical decision-making and the ban on federal funding. Rutgers L J. 2003;34:463, 475–478.
83. Robbins LR. Open Your Mouth and Say "Ideology": Physicians and the First Amendment. U. Pa. J Const L 2009;12:155, 183–186.
84. Roe v. Wade. U.S. 1973;410:113, 159.
85. James J. McCartney Ph.D. Embryonic stem cell research and respect for human life: philosophical and legal reflections. 65 Alb L Rev. 2002;597, 624.
86. Dolin G. A defense of embryonic stem cell research. Ind L J. 2006;84(56):1203, 1257.

87. Kukla HJ. Embryonic stem cell research: an ethical justification. Geo L J. 2002;90:503, 517–518.
88. Ayer AC. Stem cell research: the laws of nations and a proposal for international guidelines. Conn J Int'l L. 2002;17:393, 399.
89. Carroll L. Through the Looking Glass, and What Alice Found There. University of California Press; 1983. p. 67.
90. Aloni E. Symposium: from page to practice: broadening the lens for reproductive and sexual rights: cloning and the LGBTI family: cautious optimism, N.Y.U. Rev L Soc Change 1. 2011;35(268):80.
91. Kolata G. In long drive to cure cancer, advances have been elusive. N.Y. *Times*. 24 Apr 2009, at A1.
92. Silfen M. How Will California's Funding of Stem Cell Research Impact Innovation? Recommendations for an Intellectual Property Policy. Harv J Law Tech. 2005;18:459, 468.
93. The Babylonian Talmud. Pirkei Avot ("Ethics of the Fathers"). 1:1.
94. Werber SJ. Cloning: a Jewish law perspective with a comparative study of other Abrahamic traditions. Seton Hall L Rev. 2000;30(1):1114.
95. Kahan DM, Braman D. Cultural cognition and public policy. Yale L Pol'y Rev. 2006;24:149.
96. Congressional Budget Office. An Introduction to the Congressional Budget Office at 1. http://www.cbo.gov/sites/default/files/cbofiles/attachments/2012-IntroToCBO.pdf. Accessed 19 Jan 2013 (hereinafter "CBO, *Introduction*").
97. Congressional Budget Office. Budget and Economic Outlook. https://cbo.gov/topics/budget/budget-and-economic-outlook. Accessed 20 Jan 2013.
98. Westmoreland T. Standard errors: how budget rules distort lawmaking. Geo L J. 2007; 95:1555, 1578.
99. Gramm-Rudman-Hollings: Forgotten. But Not Yet Gone. *Cong Q Weekly Rep*. 1986:2526.
100. Herszenhorn DM. Wrangling over stimulus is one-sided so far. *N.Y. Times*. 16 Jan 2008, at A15.
101. Transcript of Debate Between Bush and Kerry, With Domestic Policy the Topic. *N.Y. Times*. 14 Oct 2004, at A15.
102. Bartlett B. The Fiscal Legacy of George W. Bush. *N.Y. Times*, Economix. 12 June 2012. http://economix.blogs.nytimes.com/2012/06/12/the-fiscal-legacy-of-george-w-bush/. Accessed 20 Jan 2013.
103. Lee JW. Critique of current congressional capital gains contentions, 15 VA. Tax Rev. 1 at 72–73.
104. Hahn RW. Achieving real regulatory reform. 1997 U. Chi Legal F 1997;143, 153.
105. Stack KM, Vandenbergh MP. The one percent problem. Colum L Rev. 2011;111:1385.
106. Lin AC. Technology assessment 2.0 revamping our approach to emerging technologies. Brooklyn L Rev. 2011;76:1309, 1332.
107. Legislative Branch Appropriations Act 1996. Pub. L. No. 104-53, 112. Stat. 1995;109:468, 525–526.
108. Glicksman RL, Chapman SB. Regulatory reform and (breach of) the Contract with America: improving environmental policy or destroying environmental protection? Kan J L Pub Pol'y. 1996;5:9, 16, 19.
109. Holt R. Reversing the congressional science lobotomy. Wired.com. 2009. http://www.wired.com/wiredscience/2009/04/fromthefields-holt/. Accessed 20 Jan 2013.
110. 2 U.S.C. § 472(c).
111. 2 U.S.C. § 472(d)(2-3).
112. Peha JM. Science and technology advice for congress: past, present, and future. 24 Renewable Resources J. 2006;19:20. http://repository.cmu.edu/cgi/viewcontent.cgi?article=1054&context=epp. Accessed 23 Jan 2013.
113. Pub. L. No. 79-404. Stat. 1946;60:237 (codified as amended in scattered sections of 5 U.S.C.).
114. Kolber M. Rulemaking without rules: an empirical study of direct final rulemaking. Alb L Rev 2009;72:79, 86.

115. N.C. Growers' Ass'n, Inc. v. United Farm Workers, No. 11-2235, ___ F.3d ___, 2012 WL 6634773 at *5 (4th Cir. 21 Dec 2012).
116. U.S. Satellite Broad'ing Co., Inc. v. F.C.C., 740 F.2d 1177, 1188 D.C. Cir. 1984.
117. Rodway v. U.S. Dept. of Agric., 514 F.2d 809, 817 D.C. Cir. 1975.
118. Bignami FE. The democratic deficit in European Community rulemaking: a call for notice-and-comment in comitology. Harv Int'l L J. 1999;40:451.
119. 5 U.S.C. § 706(2)(D).
120. Cf. Marshall Field & Co. v. Clark, U.S. 1892;143:649, 671.
121. Rawls J. The domain of the political and overlapping consensus. N.Y.U. L. Rev. 1989;64:233, 250.
122. Chevron U.S.A. Inc. v. NRDC, U.S. 1984;467:837.
123. Church of the Holy Trinity v. United States, U.S. 1892;143:457.
124. Sedima, S.P.R.L. v. Imrex Co., 741 F.2d 482, 510 2d Cir. 1984.
125. Sedima v. Imrex Co., U.S. 1985;473:479, 486–488.
126. Cost Estimate of H.R. 8, American Taxpayer Relief Act of 2012. http://www.cbo.gov/sites/default/files/cbofiles/attachments/American%20Taxpayer%20Relief%20Act.pdf. Accessed 20 Jan 2013.
127. H.R. 8 (112th Cong. 2013). Bill Summary and Status. The Library of Congress. http://thomas.loc.gov/cgi-bin/bdquery/z?d112:HR00008:@@@X. Accessed 12 Jan 2012.
128. 158 Cong. Rec. S8592 (31 Dec 2012).
129. 5 U.S.C. § 553(b)(3)(B).
130. Action on Smoking and Health v. Civil Aeronautics Board. 713 F.2d 795, 800 D.C. Cir. 1983.
131. Orsi R. Emergency exceptions from NEPA: who should decide? B.C. Envtl Aff L Rev. 1987;14:481, 517.
132. American Federation of Government Employees. AFL-CIO v. Block, 655 F.2d D.C. Cir. 1981;1153, 1157–1158.
133. Wieser MJ. Beyond Bowsher: a separation of powers approach to the delegation of budgetary authority. Brooklyn L Rev 1990;55:1405, 1408.
134. Entin JL. The removal power and the federal deficit: form, substance, and administrative independence. Ky L J. 1986;75(267):699, 792.
135. Fram A. Despite GOP Laughter, Congress' Budget Office Gets High Marks With PM-CBO vs. OMB Numbers, AP News Archive. 1993. http://www.apnewsarchive.com/1993/Despite-GOP-Laughter-Congress-Budget-Office-Gets-High-Marks-With-PM-CBO-vs-OMB-Numbers/id-0cdd51362adc82226be3ecd79e86c657. Accessed 23 Jan 2013.
136. Wade N. Obama Plans to Replace Bush's Bioethics Panel. *N.Y. Times*. 18 June 2009, at A24.
137. 2 Albert Bigelow Paine. Mark Twain, A Biography 724. Harper & Brothers;1912.

Chapter 17
The Role of Popular Media in Oncofertility Communication

Donna Rosene Leff

Introduction

In this chapter, we will take a look at popular media stories about fertility preservation in young cancer patients, reviewing a variety of stories in national newspapers, such as *The New York Times*, *The Washington Post*, and *USA Today*; National Public Radio; national and local network news broadcasts; and news media affiliated Web sites, such as Time.com. A small review of three examples of entertainment (as opposed to news) media follows, including two television shows and a popular movie that introduce the concept of oncofertility. The chapter concludes with some observations and analysis on how popular media coverage might more effectively encourage communication about oncofertility and fertility preservation in general.

Use of the Term Oncofertility Versus "Fertility Preservation" in the Popular Media[1]

Popular media cover oncofertility, but the stories rarely use the term. A Google search of the term "oncofertility" yielded 39,500 hits, but after screening the first 100, we found that only one was an actual media story about oncofertility

[1] In this chapter, we describe our findings of popular media coverage of oncofertility; I limited my review to articles after 2007 when the multicenter Oncofertility Consortium was launched with funding from the National Institutes of Health and the term "oncofertility," coined by Teresa Woodruff the year before, began appearing in the popular media.

D.R. Leff, Ph.D. (✉)
Medill School of Journalism, Media, Integrated Marketing Communications,
Northwestern University, 105 West Adams Street, Suite 200, Chicago, IL 60603, USA
e-mail: d-leff@northwestern.edu

T.K. Woodruff et al. (eds.), *Oncofertility Communication: Sharing Information and Building Relationships across Disciplines*, DOI 10.1007/978-1-4614-8235-2_17,

(The Time.com Mother's Day feature that will be discussed in detail below) [1–4].[2,3] The references were dominated by Northwestern University's Oncofertility Consortium, with other hits linking to health and medical Web sites, published by academic institutions or advocacy groups.[4]

Entering the term "oncofertility" in major media Web site search engines yielded similar results, with no stories returned in searches of *The Wall Street Journal*, *The Boston Globe*, and the *Los Angeles Times*. The *San Francisco Chronicle* yielded two mentions [5],[5] and *The New York Times* (described below) [6] and *The Washington Post* had one mention each [7]. The *Chicago Tribune* Web site search yielded more mentions [8–10],[6] but because of the way it is archived (with a firewall and free abstracts), many of the articles were referenced multiple times and the actual number was fewer than five, beginning with the announcement in September 2007 of a $21 million federal grant that established the Oncofertility Consortium at Northwestern University [9],[7] and including a feature on the Consortium's Saturday Academy [10].

Entering the term "infertility treatment after cancer not experimental" yielded 3.97 million Google hits, but again, the bulk of the articles weren't from the popular

---

[2] This early story on fertility and cancer was a harbinger of the future, describing the then experimental procedure performed by Kutluk Oktay of New York Methodist Hospital in Brooklyn (He is now at New York Medical College) in which the ovaries from a cervical cancer patient were removed and then strips of ovarian tissue were implanted in her arms before radiation treatment in an attempt to prevent premature menopause. The story begins:

"In an experimental operation last Thursday that one doctor called 'great work' but another called 'preposterous,' surgeons in Brooklyn removed a woman's ovaries, sliced them into thin strips and implanted them into her arm. The patient, in her 30's, has cervical cancer, and the reason for the seemingly outlandish procedure was to protect her ovaries from the radiation treatment she will be getting."

Oktay is quoted in the story speculating that although this patient simply wanted to protect herself from osteoporosis and other effects of early menopause, perhaps in the future the treatment could lead to successful fertility treatments. The article also said that unlike sperm, eggs could not be frozen, which turned out to be incorrect but was accurate in 1999 when the article was published.

[3] In her 2004 piece, Grady reported that a woman in Belgium had become the first to give birth after having ovarian tissue removed, frozen, and then implanted in her body (as Oktay had speculated in her 1999 piece).

[4] See: Fertile Hope Foundation, www.fertilehope.org; Oncofertility Consortium at Northwestern University, http://oncofertility.northwestern.edu; and the related patient-directed Web site, www.myoncofertility.org.

[5] This story reports on a 9-year-old boy from Florida who has Ewing sarcoma. Partway through chemotherapy, his mother realizes the fertility threat of his cancer treatment and goes to Pittsburgh to harvest stem cells that may be able to later produce sperm.

[6] Story about a 17-month-old girl with cancer in Rhode Island who underwent fertility preservation.

[7] Announcement of Oncofertility Consortium funding at Northwestern University.

media. Searching the first 250 hits, we found five mentions (all discussed in greater detail below):

NBC News.com story featuring Dr. Nancy Snyderman reporting on freezing ovarian tissue [11].

The Huffington Post: Young cancer patients rarely get help, information on fertility issues [12].

Chicago Tribune Lifestyles, Reuters story about women getting less information than men about post-cancer fertility [13].

King5.com (Seattle), local television news report on preserving fertility after a cancer diagnosis [14].

The Washington Post AP story on a new surgery to help some men regain fertility after cancer treatment [7].

We then entered the term "infertility treatment after cancer," which yielded between nine and ten million hits (varied on different search dates), but of these, only three stories on two topics hadn't come up in the previous search. One, on the ABC News medical blog, was headlined "Fertility After Cancer Treatment Aim of New Free Program," and gave an account of the Sher Institutes for Reproductive Medicine's program to treat cancer patients for infertility free of charge. The story did not give a location for the patient featured and the center is a large commercial fertility group with seven locations nationally [15].

The other two stories were about a Monash University (Melbourne, Australia) study—published in the journal *Molecular Cell*—one that appeared in Mail Online, the Web site of the UK's *Daily Mail*, under the headline: "Women undergoing cancer therapy could still have children thanks to protein breakthrough" [16] and another in *The New Scientist* [17]. The September 2012 article from *The New Scientist* reported research that involved the removal of two proteins from the eggs of women exposed to radiation and chemotherapy [17]. Of all the popular media reports examined, this one was the most technical and was based on a press release from the university [posted on EurekAlert! (www.eurekalert.org), the American Association for the Advancement of Science news Web site, which is restricted to credentialed science writers but has a public version for older news].

The 2009 *New York Times* story [6] was exceptional in that it specifically mentioned oncofertility, after Teresa Woodruff coauthored a February 2009 paper in the *New England Journal of Medicine* that reported an estimated 16,000 women younger than 45 each year learn they have breast cancer [18]. "Many of these young women were planning to have children or contemplating the possibility. In some, but not all patients, options for the preservation of fertility can be explored before the initiation of therapy," quoting the study's coauthors, Brody writes in her personal health column [6]. Brody goes on to report the launch of myoncofertility.org, led by the Northwestern researchers of the Oncofertility Consortium and supported by funding from the National Institutes of Health [6].

The Power of Personal Anecdote: Melissa Brown's Mother's Day Story

Brody's 2009 column was one of several stories she published over the next 3 years, and each followed a similar pattern: an anecdote at the beginning to interest the reader, followed by scientific information, often based on new studies or guidelines from the medical community. In the 2009 story, the anecdote was about Dan Shapiro, a 20-year-old college junior whose mother happened to have a waiting room conversation with another cancer patient's mother [6]. That conversation led the young Shapiro to bank sperm prior to treatment for stage 2 Hodgkin's disease, making possible the birth of his two children 9 years after his initial diagnosis, writes Brody.

At its most robust, popular media can alert young cancer patients and their families to the possibilities for preserving fertility despite facing treatments that might otherwise make childbearing impossible. When the storytelling is rich, journalists can reach this audience in an impactful way. A Mother's Day feature in May, 2012, published in Time Magazine's online health section, reported the story, "My Sister, My Surrogate: After Battling Cancer, One Woman Receives the Ultimate Mother's Day Gift" [4]. The story focuses on one sister serving as a surrogate for another, Melissa Brown, 26, who was newly diagnosed with breast cancer. Before it gets to their story, writer Bonnie Rochman discusses oncofertility in the context of Melissa's experiences [4]:

> But before the first toxic chemical dripped into her bloodstream, Melissa's oncologist—the same doctor who'd cared for her mother for more than 20 years—recommended a sort of insurance policy for the future. If you want children, he told her, preserve your fertility now. Along with killing the bad cells, cancer treatment can wreak havoc on a woman's ability to bear children. It can catapult you into early menopause. You may stop ovulating—or you may not—but if you know you want children, rolling the dice on whether you'll be able to conceive post-treatment is probably not a risk you want to take.
>
> Melissa was lucky. Not all oncologists advise their patients to freeze their embryos or eggs before treatment. Increasingly, though, doctors are addressing the issue. Men, and more notably women, with their incredibly complex reproductive systems, are being routinely advised to consider their future fertility before rushing ahead with cancer therapy. Melissa immediately started taking fertility drugs designed to spur the release of multiple eggs (Fig. 17.1).

The piece continues with excerpts from Melissa's journal, including this entry [4]: "They were able to remove ten eggs but only four fertilized. They froze the four. I am devastated. There is nothing more I can do." As readers can discern from the headline, the story has a happy ending, with Melissa's sister delivering healthy twins from the two embryos that were implanted.

While the *Time* online story might be viewed as a feel-good Mother's Day story, and the headline is about surrogacy, the article focuses on information that accurately describes oncofertility, though the term itself is not used. The story of a successful surrogacy, using embryos created just prior to the mother's chemotherapy,

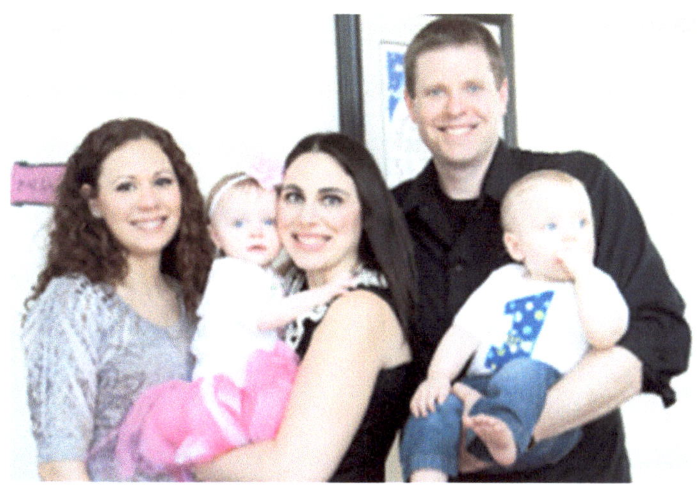

Fig. 17.1 Melissa Brown, at center of photo, chose to harvest eggs before undergoing chemotherapy for breast cancer. Her sister, Jessica, at *left*, was the surrogate who carried Melissa's twins with Melissa's husband, Steve Mohler, at right in the family photo published with the "My Sister, My Surrogate," story in *Time* (Brown/Mohler family photo, courtesy of Melissa Brown)

offers hope to readers. More importantly, the article alerts readers, including medical professionals and future patients, to the importance of fully informing cancer patients about preserving fertility.

Prior to the online article, Rochman had written about fertility preservation for cancer patients when she put a face on Northwestern's Oncofertility Consortium in *Time Magazine* in 2010, with a long print feature on a woman who froze five embryos after receiving counseling from the Consortium's patient navigator [19]. The story recounts the Consortium's founding, Dr. Woodruff's coining of the term "oncofertility," and the effort to make more young cancer patients aware of their fertility preservation options. Rochman also blogged on the issue under the headline, "First Comes Cancer, Then Come Children: The New World of Oncofertility," and with a graphic of the ubiquitous breast cancer awareness pink ribbon pierced by a diaper pin [20, 21][8] (Fig. 17.2).

After the flurry of initial stories, however, and a couple of popular television stories we'll cover later in this chapter, journalists only occasionally write about fertility preservation and even less frequently use the term oncofertility.

[8] This article follows the format of starting with an anecdote and then giving information about oncofertility.

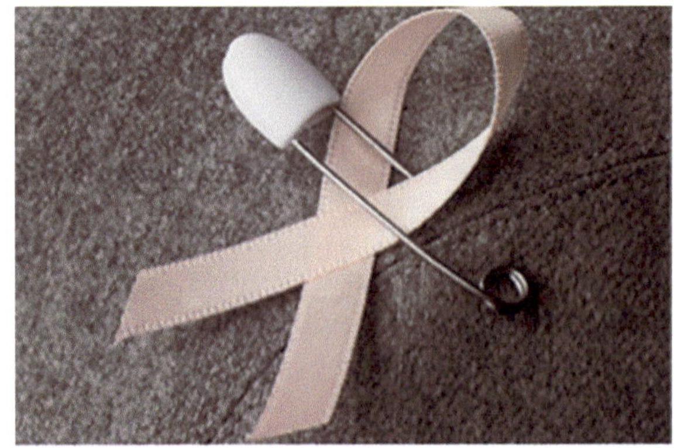

Fig. 17.2 Graphic artists Tamara Shopsin and Jason Fulford looped the iconic breast cancer awareness pink ribbon through a diaper pin for this image in Time (Courtesy of the artists)

Framing Issues in the Popular Media: Freezing Eggs No Longer "Experimental"

When the American Society for Reproductive Medicine (ASRM) declared in October 2012 that egg freezing was no longer experimental, it triggered widespread popular media coverage. The Associated Press (AP) wrote a story that was picked up by major media outlets across the country. *USA Today* carried a 900-word version of the AP story, reporting accurately on the society's recommendations, including references to studies showing that frozen eggs were as likely to be viable as fresh eggs [22]. The story's "angle," however, was really about what one might call elective fertility preservation, as opposed to oncofertility—a medical practice entirely devoted to preserving fertility in people with cancer. Thus, the AP story notes [22],

> Here's the controversy: Should otherwise healthy women freeze their eggs as sort of an insurance policy against infertility in case they do not meet Mr. Right—or just are not ready for motherhood—until their late 30s or beyond, when the childbearing window is closing fast?

The AP story quotes Dr. Samantha Pfeifer of the University of Pennsylvania, who chaired the ASRM guideline committee, as noting that egg freezing wouldn't necessarily be successful in older women and that women in their 30s and 40s "may have the worst success of anybody." The reporter also quotes a fertility specialist at New York University whose center has frozen more than 1,100 batches of eggs "mostly for elective fertility preservation," and a single woman from San Francisco who paid $15,000 at age 39 to freeze 11 eggs, hoping for a future baby; this woman started a Web site, eggsurance.com, targeted to women like her [22].

Only two sentences in the story speak to oncofertility. In the third paragraph, the story notes, "The move is expected to help cancer patients preserve their fertility, by pushing more insurers to pay for their procedure," but then quickly changes the subject to women who electively delay childbearing [22]. Finally, the story notes that "For a number of years, egg-freezing has been offered experimentally for young women or girls who are diagnosed with cancer or other serious illnesses that would destroy their ovaries."

The focus on elective preservation over medical necessity was nearly universal in the coverage following the release of the ASRM guidelines. For example, in a nearly 9-min report on the PBS NewsHour that aired on the same day the society issued its guidelines, less than a minute was spent on the topic of cancer and fertility preservation [23]. Margaret Warner opens her report by noting that the practice of freezing and thawing eggs has been used for years, but only 1,000 births had been reported using the technique, as opposed to approximately five million born through traditional (fresh egg) in vitro fertilization (IVF). She interviews two experts: Dr. Eric Widra, a coauthor of the society's new standards, and an ethicist from Berkeley. As in the AP stories, Warner almost immediately pivots the discussion from the topic of fertility preservation in patients with cancer to a lengthy discussion of whether infertility treatment for women who delay childbearing is ethical.

Dr. Widra, speaking for the ASRM, says the society has three points [23]: "One is, that we do think we should be recommending this procedure for women who may become infertile from medical treatment, such as cancer and chemotherapy." He then moves quickly to add that though the technology is "reasonable," it is "premature" to recommend that patients store eggs for later fertility; yet he also acknowledges that many will choose to do so. As the reporter, Warner, puts it: "Something that is elective. You're not really afraid of losing your fertility, other than from age." The ethicist then raises questions about the marketing of egg freezing, an obvious source of revenue for fertility clinics, and the issue of preserving fertility in cancer patients is never mentioned again during the segment.

The society's recommendations also caught the attention of local broadcasters, who kept the focus on preserving fertility in people with cancer. King5.com, the Web site of Seattle's NBC affiliate, and owned by Belo Corp., featured video and a post by Jean Enersen under the headline "Preserving Fertility After Cancer Diagnosis" [14]. News organizations try to find "local angles" to important national stories and King5's handling of the Society for Reproductive Medicine's new standards was a textbook example. Enersen's report spotlights Nina Garkavi, 24, who was diagnosed with brain cancer soon after graduating from college. The tone of the piece is intimate and upbeat, opening with Garkavi playing with her dog and closing with her ebulliently jumping from a skydiving plane, clinging to an unidentified man, presumably her instructor [14] (Fig. 17.3).

In the segment, Garkavi describes her feelings on being told she has cancer [14], "What I remember is a blur. But what I took from it is, it will affect your fertility." Her comment essentially serves to focus the piece, which in 2.2 min manages to capture the important facts about preserving fertility in patients with cancer, including a description of the new guidelines designating egg freezing as non-experimental and an interview with a clinical nurse specialist at Seattle Children's Hospital. The nurse notes that staff at the hospital always raise the topic of posttreatment fertility with patients and their families. The video plays loud, optimistic music over the

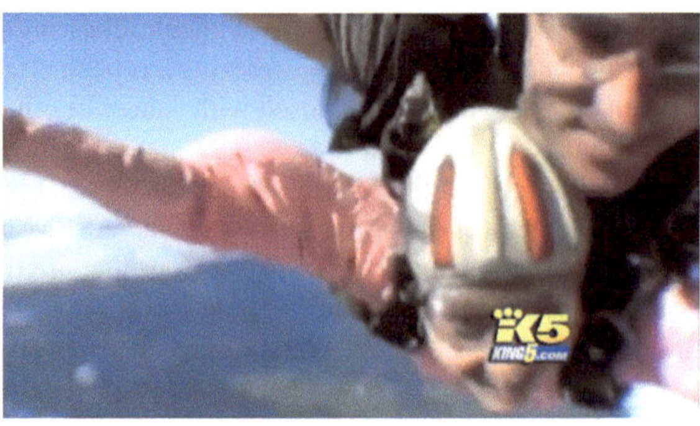

Fig. 17.3 Cancer survivor Nina Garkavi shared this image of her leap from a skydiving plane with King5 television news in Seattle (Courtesy of Nina Garkavi)

skydiving scene but it is entirely responsible journalism, concluding with the nurse's caution that [14], "…no patients from Seattle Children's cancer program have gone on to become parents. But adult cancer survivors have." She notes that, in general, *…children born to cancer survivors don't have any greater risk than other children of getting cancer.*

Presumably, the new recommendations also led Dr. Nancy Snyderman—reporting on NBC's Nightly News with Brian Williams, as well as on the Today Show—to go more deeply into the subject of oncofertility [11]. She explains that egg freezing isn't always a good option for women who have aggressive or hormone-sensitive cancers and therefore can neither delay treatment nor take the hormones necessary to harvest eggs. She interviews surgeons who have removed ovarian tissue for preservation, noting this procedure still is experimental, although 20 babies have been born to women who have had tissue reimplanted after cancer treatment [11].

Another Angle: Studies Show Women Get Less Information than Men on Post-cancer Fertility

The bread-and-butter of science writing is reporting on studies published in peer-reviewed medical journals, and in this respect, research on oncofertility, while not necessarily referred to by that term, does get covered in the popular media. These reports are generally shorter (typically 300–400 words) and expositive, without anecdotal narrative. For example, Swedish researchers reported in the *Journal of Clinical Oncology* in May 2012 that among almost 500 cancer survivors 18–45 years of age, 80 % of men and only 48 % of women were informed by their doctors that cancer treatment could lead to infertility [24]. Moreover, only 14 % of women, but 68 % of men, reported getting information about options for preserving fertility. The Reuters story on this research ran in newspapers world wide, including the *Chicago Tribune*, and included information about the American Society of Clinical Oncology (ASCO) recommendation that doctors discuss and offer fertility options to all patients of reproductive age [13]. The reporter highlights cost differences between sperm banking and storage (maximum cost $1,500) and embryo and egg banking (as much as $20,000), the latter being technically more difficult [13]. The story also mentions the findings of a University of California, San Francisco (UCSF) School of Medicine survey, published in the *Journal of Cancer Survivorship*, of 1,000 cancer patients under the age of 40 at the time of diagnosis; more than half of the respondents said they would still like to have children despite their cancer [24].

The same California study also generated several print and broadcast stories, frequently tied to an individual woman's specific—and poignant—struggle with cancer and fertility. Sarah Lisle, featured in a Tribune Company newspapers story, began her cancer journey with a diagnosis of breast cancer at the age of 25 in Austin, Texas [25]. She took a 5-year course of tamoxifen, hoping to prevent a recurrence of the cancer, and went on to marry and finish a graduate degree. At age 31, she found a new lump, which turned out to be estrogen-sensitive cancer requiring treatment that would have obvious implications for fertility. This time, however, her oncologist recommended she freeze eggs before further treatment. The story then cites both the Swedish study and the California survey described above, noting that fewer than half of the young female cancer survivors surveyed recalled receiving reproductive counseling, and 88 % failed to recall receiving any information about preserving fertility [25]. The story quotes Emily Eargle, navigation manager for national services for the Lance Armstrong Foundation's Fertile Hope Initiative [25], "The biggest error that we're seeing is that people are not having the conversation based on assumptions—that they're too old, or too young, or that it's not safe or they don't think it's affordable." The Fertile Hope Initiative helps underwrite fertility treatment costs by getting providers to reduce their costs. With a 50 % discount, Lisle was able to undergo IVF and have a daughter through a surrogate.

Gina Danford's story was featured in *The Huffington Post* in November 2012, following the same pattern [12]. It opens with Danford being diagnosed with an 8-lb ovarian tumor at age 19, then tells of Danford's 10-year remission, followed by two recurrences, each benign. Finally, 12 years after her first tumor, an oncologist encourages her to see a reproductive endocrinologist; according to Danford, this is the first time a doctor had spoken to her about her fertility options [12]. At the time of the report, Danford was 37 years of age and observes [12], "It was hard to think beyond the next doctor's appointment and what that meant, and what we would find out at the next test. It was extremely difficult for me to plan for a future when I knew I may not be there to see it." The post goes on to cite several studies on fertility after cancer treatment, including one published in 2011 in the journal *Cancer*, coauthored by Danford's reproductive endocrinologist at UCSF, Dr. Mitchell Rosen [26], as well as the UCSF survey study lead by Dr. Rosen and published in the *Journal of Cancer Survivorship*, described above [24]. The post also cites the Oncofertility Consortium as the source for estimating the cost of women's treatment options, starting at $10,000 and going up to $20,000, but also notes that lack of counseling is probably a bigger barrier to oncofertility procedures than cost, along with the factors noted by the UCSF survey respondents (and echoed by the Fertile Hope Initiative source) [12]:

> When asked why they felt their doctors hadn't brought it up, women's reasons were consistent—among them, an uncertain prognosis, the fact that they already had children, and age—being seen as too young or too old to worry about having kids.

The post ends with the happy outcome that is common in these popular press stories [12]:

> In Danford's case, being urged by her oncologist to speak with a fertility specialist led to her having a baby. Though she said she underestimated how grueling fertility treatment would be, both physically and emotionally, she is thrilled to be mom to Samantha Grace, now 2.
>
> She's incredible," Danford said. "She's a little person now—she's talking. She was frozen for almost 4 years, but she's healthy as can be.

ABC news covers the same ground, airing after the publication of the Rosen UCSF survey, but including information that the 1,000 women studied were between the ages of 18 and 40 years and were diagnosed with leukemia, Hodgkin lymphoma, non-Hodgkin lymphoma, breast cancer, and gastrointestinal cancer [27]. The story notes that only 4 % of women overall pursued fertility preservation but, as in the other popular media stories about the survey, focuses on one woman who did pursue fertility treatment. Unlike the other stories, however, the ABC report leaves open the question whether the woman, who has the BRCA-2 gene mutation for breast cancer, would eventually have a baby. The reporter notes that the women harvested and froze seven eggs when she was 32 years old. Three years earlier, she had been diagnosed with breast cancer during a routine preoperative examination for elective mastectomy, which she chose because of her high genetic risk of breast cancer. The reporter omits any explanation of genetic factors in breast cancer, only saying the woman's sister died of the disease after 7 years [27].

Entertainment Media and Oncofertility

The term "oncofertility" made its entertainment television debut on an episode of ABC's *Private Practice* called *Contamination*, which aired on January 8, 2009 [28]. One minute into the hour-long show, a doctor says, "Oncofertility is new and it's interesting." In the episode, the doctors try an operation to reimplant ovarian tissue that had been removed from "Claudia," a cancer patient who learns she doesn't have enough blood supply for the ovary to implant (she nearly dies during the failed surgery). But the surgeons offer her hope—they still have some of her ovarian tissue frozen and perhaps a specialist might implant it deeper, closer to a vigorous blood supply. Viewers never learn whether Claudia goes on to have a child, but the depiction of oncofertility is dramatic and scientifically accurate, although not terribly complete. Further, the focus in this case is not on egg freezing but on ovarian tissue preservation, which has gotten little popular media attention since a 1999 story in the *New York Times* introduced the subject [1].

Viewers of CBS's *The Young and The Restless* daytime serial were privy to the latest in cancer fertility preservation in a pair of episodes that aired in July 2009 [29, 30],

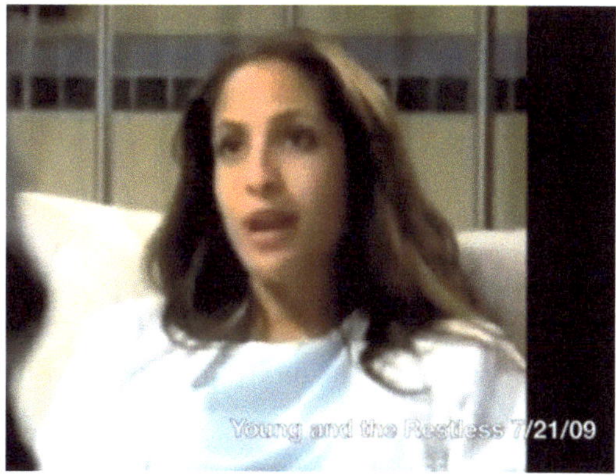

Fig. 17.4 In this July 9, 2009 episode of CBS's "The Young and the Restless," Lily Winters says, "Take me to Chicago," where she'll seek to preserve her fertility before undergoing cancer treatment (The Young and the Restless" © 2013 CPT Holdings, Inc. courtesy Sony Pictures Television)

when the character Lily Winters (played by Christel Khalil) is diagnosed with cancer and refuses immediate treatment:

> But I have been on the internet and I have read that there's a good chance the surgery means that I'll never be able to have children…But first I want to harvest and freeze my eggs… And then I will have the surgery. My mind is made up. I'm going to harvest my eggs.

In the next day's episode, the argument with her father, husband, and doctor continues, "You want to support me? Then you understand why I have to freeze my eggs first. Listen, you want to support me? Then take me to Chicago, okay, and I will find a doctor that will help me keep my eggs…". The performance led to a daytime Emmy nomination for Khalil in 2010, for Outstanding Actress in a Drama Series. Although Khalil didn't win the Emmy, Lily, her character, did become the mother of twins—a boy and a girl—carried by a surrogate using Lily's harvested eggs (Fig. 17.4).

While these television dramas offered at least a few lines of dialogue devoted to explaining fertility preservation in cancer patients, the 2011 movie *50/50,* which tells the story of Adam, a 27-year-old with rare spinal cancer, has exactly one phrase about fertility, quoted below in its entirety, in a scene where he has just been told of the diagnosis [31][9]:

> *Dr. Ross*: I think that given the placement and size of your particular tumor, the wisest course of action is to see if we can possibly reduce this thing down to a more manageable size before we consider surgery. *Now chemotherapy can often result in fertility issues* (emphasis added).
>
> [Adam unable to cope with the news, gets up and walks over to the office window and looks out].
>
> *Adam*: But I'm gonna be okay?
>
> *Dr. Ross:* If you need someone to talk to uh… we have an excellent staff here at the hospital of social workers and psychologists. They specialize in these matters and they would be able to help you.
>
> [Adam stares out the window as the doctor carries on talking]

[9] Riser was diagnosed with spinal cancer at 25.

While the physician offers Adam psychosocial help, he glosses over the issue of fertility and never circles back to the subject. Thought the movie is fiction, it is based on the true story of its screenwriter Will Reiser, who was diagnosed at age 25 with cancer.

Conclusions

A review of popular media coverage of infertility shows some common threads.

- Personal stories of patients, especially success stories, capture media attention. Failed fertility treatments seem almost entirely absent from the popular media.
- Studies in peer-reviewed journals are likely to be covered, especially if they lend themselves to narrative journalism. Not unexpectedly, we find only rare instances of reports on the technical aspects of oncofertility, but widespread coverage of the reproductive medicine society's guidelines and the results of patient surveys.
- The term "oncofertility" is used less frequently in the popular media than more generic descriptors, such as "fertility preservation in cancer patients" or just "fertility preservation."
- Popular media stories are scattered and hard to locate or catalogue through search-engine research, in part because the term "oncofertility" is absent from the majority of relevant stories.

These findings suggest that if providers want to use popular media to communicate information about oncofertility to young cancer patients and their families, they should tell stories as often as they can. At medical meetings and conferences, through press releases and Web sites, providers should gather information about patient successes and new developments as they occur. They should also seek out bloggers as well as newspaper and television reporters and national as well as local reporters. It helps to be aware of the reporters who specialize in health stories: most of the stories we identified were written by a network's health or science team, a newspaper's health beat reporter, or a news magazine's women's health specialist. Increasingly, popular media are establishing blogs in conjunction with their regular print or broadcast coverage, in an effort to broaden their publication's reach.

We conclude with an example of one such blog that underscores the power of narrative to educate. *The New York Times* blog called *Well, Tara Parker-Pope on Health* has been featuring *Life, Interrupted*, a column by Suleika Jaquad, age 23 [32]:

> Last spring, I found out I had leukemia. Before the horror of the news even had time to sink in, I had to absorb a second shock: The chemotherapy treatments that could save my life would also make me infertile….It was only after I asked about fertility that the doctors told me about the available options. While my oncologists are intent on saving my life—and I am forever indebted to them for this—preserving my chance to be a mother someday just didn't seem to be on their radar.

References

1. Denise Grady. Experiment seeks to protect ovaries from cancer treatment. The New York Times. 26 Oct 1999. http://www.nytimes.com/1999/10/26/health/experiment-seeks-to-protect-ovaries-from-cancer-treatment.html?pagewanted=all&src=pm. Accessed 27 Nov 2012.
2. Jane E. Brody. Cancer and childbirth: mutually exclusive no longer. The New York Times. 28 May 2002. http://www.nytimes.com/2002/05/28/health/cancer-and-childbirth-mutually-exclusive-no-longer.html?pagewanted=all&src=pm. Accessed 19 Dec 2012.
3. Denise Grady. Report of first birth for cancer survivor in a tissue implant. The New York Times. 24 Sept 2004. http://www.nytimes.com/2004/09/24/health/24baby.html. Accessed 21 Feb 2013.
4. Bonnie Rochman. Family matters. My sister, my surrogate: after battling cancer, one woman receives the ultimate mother's day gift. Time. 9 May 2012. http://healthland.time.com/2012/05/09/my-sister-my-surrogate-after-cancer-one-sister-gives-another. Accessed 19 Dec 2012.
5. Lauran Neergaard, AP. Doctors aim to save fertility of kids with cancer. San Francisco Chronicle. 11 March 2011. http://www.sfgate.com/default/article/Doctors-aim-to-save-fertility-of-kids-with-cancer-1139123.php. Accessed 19 Dec 2012.
6. Jane E. Brody. Personal health, family planning when cancer intrudes. The New York Times. 21 April 2009. http://www.nytimes.com/2009/04/21/health/21brod.html?_r=0. Accessed 19 Dec 2012.
7. Associated Press. Surgery helps men regain fertility after cancer. The Washington Post. 14 March 2011. http://www.washingtonpost.com/wp-dyn/content/article/2011/03/14/AR201103 1403626_pf.html. Accessed 19 Dec 2012.
8. Heidi Stevens. Fertility on hold for child cancer patients. Chicago Tribune. 30 May 2012. http://articles.chicagotribune.com/2012-05-30/health/sc-health-0530-freezing-kids-eggs-20120530_1_ovarian-tissue-fertility-preservation-reproductive-tissue. Accessed 19 Dec 2012.
9. Bonnie Miller Rubin. Fight cancer, save moms. Chicago Tribune. 6 Sept 2007. http://articles.chicagotribune.com/2007-09-06/news/0709050795_1_cancer-treatment-breast-cancer-reproductive-health.
10. Kathy Peyton. Program opens girls' eyes to science. Chicago Tribune. 17 March 2010. http://articles.chicagotribune.com/2010-03-17/news/ct-x-c-science-academy-20100317_1_cancer-patients-program-science. Accessed 19 Dec 2012.
11. Linda Carroll. Cancer survivors keep fertility with new treatment. Vitals on NBCnews.com. http://vitals.nbcnews.com/_news/2012/10/23/14651535-cancer-survivors-keep-fertility-with-new-treatment?lite. Accessed 20 Feb 2013.
12. Catherine Pearson. Huff post generation why young cancer patients rarely get help, information on fertility issues. The Huffington Post. 29 Nov 2012. http://www.huffingtonpost.com/2012/11/20/cancer-fertility-young-adult_n_2123477.html. Accessed 23 Dec 2012.
13. Amy Norton, Reuters. Women get less information on post-cancer fertility. Chicago Tribune. 25 May 2012. http://articles.chicagotribune.com/2012-05-25/lifestyle/sns-rt-us-women-post-cancerbre84o13i-20120525_1_fertility-preservation-cancer-treatment-cancer-patients. Accessed 18 Dec 2012.
14. Jean Enersen. Preserving fertility after cancer diagnosis. King5.com website. 30 Oct 2012. http://www.king5.com/health/childrens-healthlink/Preserving-fertility-after-cancer-diagnosis-176331251.html#. Accessed 18 Dec 2012.
15. Cara Lemieux. Fertility after cancer treatment aim of new free program. ABC News Medical Unit website. 9 Nov 2011. http://abcnews.go.com/blogs/health/2011/11/09/fertility-after-cancer-treatment-aim-of-new-free-program/. Accessed 21 Feb 2013.
16. Claire Bates. Women undergoing cancer therapy could still have children thanks to protein breakthrough. Mail Online. 24 Sept 2012. http://www.dailymail.co.uk/health/article-2207760/Cancer-treatment-fertility-Women-undergoing-cancer-therapy-children-thanks-protein-breakthrough.html. Accessed 21 Dec 2012.

17. Jessica Hamzelou. Block egg suicide to guard fertility after cancer therapy. New Scientist. 22 Sept 2012. http://www.newscientist.com/article/dn22296-block-egg-suicide-to-guard-fertility-after-cancer-therapy.html. Accessed 21 Feb 2013.
18. Jeruss JS, Woodruff TK. Preservation of fertility in patients with cancer. N Engl J Med. 2009;360:902–11.
19. Bonnie Rochman. Fertility and cancer: surviving and having kids too." Time Magazine. 11 Oct 2010. http://www.time.com/time/magazine/article/0,9171,2022642,00.html?xid=rss-topstories. Accessed 21 Feb 2013.
20. Bonnie Rochman. First comes cancer, then come children: the new world of oncofertility. Time Magazine. 15 Oct, 2010. http://healthland.time.com/2010/10/15/first-comes-cancer-then-come-children-the-new-world-of-oncofertility/. Accessed 14 Nov 2012.
21. Anna Kuchment. Survive cancer, have baby. Newsweek. 25 July 2008. http://www.thedailybeast.com/newsweek/2008/07/25/survive-cancer-have-baby.html. Accessed 15 Oct 2012.
22. Associated Press. Freezing eggs for fertility works. USA Today. 19 Oct 2012. http://www.usatoday.com/story/news/nation/2012/10/19/egg-freezing-fertility/1643937/. Accessed 18 Dec 2012.
23. Margaret Warner. Freezing human eggs for in vitro fertilization no longer experimental procedure. PBS NewsHour. PBS television. 19 Oct 2012. http://www.pbs.org/newshour/bb/health/july-dec12/eggs_10-19.html, Accessed 20 Oct 2012.
24. Niemasik EE, Letourneau J, Dohan D, Katz A, Melisko M, Rugo H, et al. Patient perceptions of reproductive health counseling at the time of cancer diagnosis: a qualitative study of female California cancer survivors. J Cancer Surviv. 2012;6:324–32.
25. Alexia Elejalde-Ruiz. Planning for children: only half of women facing breast cancer treatment are given reproductive counseling. The stakes are high and there are options. Chicago Tribune. 26 Sept 2012. http://articles.chicagotribune.com/2012-09-26/health/sc-health-0926-bc-infertility-20120926_1_tamoxifen-fertility-preservation-breast-cancer. Accessed 21 Feb 2013.
26. Letourneau JM, Ebbel EE, Katz PP, Katz A, Ai WZ, Chien AJ, et al. Pretreatment fertility counseling and fertility preservation improve quality of life in reproductive age women with cancer. Cancer. 2012;118(6):1710–7.
27. Mikaela Conley. Few young women with cancer freeze eggs to preserve fertility. ABC News Web site. 26 March 2012. http://abcnews.go.com/Health/women-cancer-freeze-eggs/story?id=15988472#.UOo4jbZGHu0. Accessed 21 Dec 2012.
28. Contamination. Season 2, episode 11. Private practice. ABC Television. 8 Jan 2009.
29. The young and the restless. CBS Television. 21 July 2009.
30. The young and the restless. CBS Television. 22 July 2009.
31. Will Reiser. 50/50 [transcript]. http://www.moviequotesandmore.com/50-50-movie-quotes.html#.UNFJq4VGG9Y. Accessed 21 Feb 2013.
32. Suleika Jaquad. Life, interrupted: a young cancer patient faces infertility. Well—Tara Parker-pope on health blog. The New York Times. http://well.blogs.nytimes.com/2012/04/19/life-interrupted-a-young-cancer-patient-faces-infertility/. Accessed 21 Feb 2013.

Index

T.K. Woodruff et al. (eds.), *Oncofertility Communication: Sharing Information and Building Relationships across Disciplines*, DOI 10.1007/978-1-4614-8235-2,

MIX
Papier aus verantwortungsvollen Quellen
Paper from responsible sources
FSC® C105338

If you have any concerns about our products,
you can contact us on
ProductSafety@springernature.com

In case Publisher is established outside the EU,
the EU authorized representative is:
Springer Nature Customer Service Center GmbH
Europaplatz 3, 69115 Heidelberg, Germany

Printed by Libri Plureos GmbH
in Hamburg, Germany